Books are to be returned on or before
the last date below.

Immunotherapy for Infectious Diseases

Infectious Disease

SERIES EDITOR: *Vassil St. Georgiev*
National Institute of Allergy and Infectious Diseases
National Institutes of Health

Immunotherapy for Infectious Diseases

Edited by

Jeffrey M. Jacobson, MD

Mount Sinai School of Medicine, New York, NY

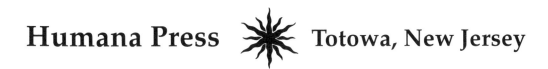

Humana Press ✳ Totowa, New Jersey

Production Editor: Diana Mezzina

Cover design: Patricia Cleary

For additional copies, pricing for bulk purchases, and/or information about other Humana titles, contact Humana at the above address or at any of the following numbers: Tel.: 973-256-1699; Fax: 973-256-8341; E-mail: humana@humanapr.com; or visit our Website: www.humanapress.com

Printed in the United States of America. 10 9 8 7 6 5 4 3 2 1

Library of Congress Cataloging in Publication Data

Immunotherapy for infectious diseases / edited by Jeffrey M. Jacobson.
        p. ; cm. -- (Infectious disease)
   Includes bibliographical references and index.
   ISBN 0-89603-669-3 (alk. paper)
   1. Immunotherapy. 2. AIDS (Disease)--Immunotherapy. I. Jacobson, Jeffrey M. II.
Infectious disease (Totowa, N.J.)
   [DNLM: 1. Communicable Diseases--therapy. 2. Immunotherapy--methods. 3. HIV
Infections--immunology. 4. HIV Infections--therapy. 5. Immunity. 6. Viral Vaccines.
WC 100 I33373 2002]
RM275 .I484 2002
616.9'046--dc21

2002017246

Preface

The HIV epidemic has brought renewed attention to the immune system and an enhanced understanding of its mechanisms for defending against infection. Despite the development of potent chemotherapeutic agents against HIV, chronic HIV infection cannot be cured over the long term with this approach. Chronic exposure to these medications is limited by debilitating toxicities and the development of drug resistance. Hence, there is a need to understand how the immune system can be manipulated to effect better control of viral replication and disease progression. This effort is proceeding in tandem with progress toward development of an effective vaccine.

Other infections, particularly those for which the development of safe, effective chemotherapy has proved difficult, have been targeted with specific immunotherapeutic approaches, from monoclonal antibodies to vaccines to interferons and cytokines.

Immunotherapy for Infectious Diseases is intended to review the state-of-the-art developments of this rapidly emerging and evolving field. Much of the work in this area is only beginning to be appreciated by clinicians and medical scientists. We hope *Immunotherapy for Infectious Diseases* will not only serve as a useful guide to current knowledge of the field, but will also stimulate readers to contribute to its further development. As such, the book should be of interest to basic scientists and clinicians active in the fields of immunology and infectious diseases, particularly HIV infection.

Immunotherapy for Infectious Diseases is divided into four sections. The first section provides an overview of the basic principles of immune defense, as seen in the context of developing strategies of immunotherapy. Humoral and cellular immunity are reviewed. Because many infectious agents enter and exit through mucosal surfaces, there has been growing appreciation of the role of mucosal immunity in protection against infection and immunopathogenesis. Therefore, a chapter on mucosal immunity is included.

The second section discusses the principles of immunotherapy on a molecular level. There are discussions of monoclonal antibodies, types of vaccines, methods of antigen presentation, cytokines, and cytokine antagonists.

The third section reviews the current state of anti-HIV immunotherapy. The current knowledge of HIV immunopathogenesis is reviewed, as is the degree of immune reconstitution that occurs as a result of anti-HIV chemotherapy. Chapters dealing with HIV-specific passive and active immunization strategies, gene therapy, and host cell-targeted approaches for treating HIV infection and restoring immune function are presented.

The fourth section reviews immunotherapy for additional infections and virus-associated malignancies.

I am grateful to all of our experts who contributed chapters to the book. They represent some of the finest minds working in this area, and did superb jobs in reviewing the latest information in their areas of expertise. I am deeply appreciative of Dr. Vassil St. Georgiev, the series editor, for inviting me to edit this book, and Thomas Lanigan, Sr., Elyse O'Grady, Craig Adams and Diana Mezzina, at Humana Press for their support in compiling it. Thanks also to the secretaries and copy editors who diligently worked to put together the elements of the book. Finally, I wish to thank the readers, who I hope will use the knowledge gained from this book to advance our ability to treat infectious diseases.

Jeffrey M. Jacobson, MD

Contents

Contributors

CONSTANTIN A. BONA, MD, PhD • *Department of Microbiology, Mount Sinai School of Medicine, New York, NY*

PROSPER N. BOYAKA, PhD • *Immunobiology Vaccine Center, University of Alabama at Birmingham, Birmingham, AL*

R. PAT BUCY, MD, PhD • *Department of Pathology, University of Alabama at Birmingham, Birmingham, AL*

ARTURO CASADEVALL, MD, PhD • *Department of Microbiology and Immunology, Albert Einstein College of Medicine, Bronx, NY*

ELIZABETH CONNICK, MD • *Division of Infectious Diseases, University of Colorado Health Sciences Center, Denver, CO*

SAM T. DONTA, MD • *Department of Medicine, Divisions of Infectious Diseases and Biomolecular Medicine, Boston University School of Medicine, Boston, MA*

RALPH DORNBURG, PhD • *Division of Infectious Diseases, Jefferson Medical College, Philadelphia, PA*

EDGAR G. ENGLEMAN, MD • *Stanford Blood Center, Palo Alto, CA*

LAWRENCE M. FOX, MD, PhD • *HIV Research Branch, Division of AIDS NIAID, NIH, Bethesda, MD*

PAUL GOEPFERT, MD • *Department of Pathology, University of Alabama at Birmingham, Birmingham, AL*

HELEN HESLOP, MD • *Departments of Medicine, Pediatrics, and Center for Cell and Gene Therapy, Baylor College of Medicine, Houston, TX*

JEFFREY M. JACOBSON, MD • *AIDS Center, Mount Sinai School of Medicine, New York, NY*

JOHN L. JOHNSON, MD • *Case Western Reserve University School of Medicine, Division of Infectious Diseases, Cleveland, OH*

SPYROS A. KALAMS, MD • *Partners AIDS Research Center, Massachusetts General Hospital, Charlestown, MA*

HERMANN KATINGER, PhD • *Institute of Applied Microbiology, University for Agricultural Sciences, Vienna, Austria*

J. MICHAEL KILBY, MD • *Department of Pathology, University of Alabama at Birmingham, Birmingham, AL*

SMRITI K. KUNDU-RAYCHAUDHURI, MD • *Division of Infectious Diseases, Department of Medicine, Stanford University, Stanford, CA*

RENATE KUNERT, PhD • *Institute of Applied Microbiology, University for Agricultural Sciences, Vienna, Austria*

BARBARA G. MATTHEWS, MD, MPH • *FDA/CBER/OTRR, Rockville, MD*

JERRY R. MCGHEE, PhD• *Department of Microbiology, University of Alabama at Birmingham, Birmingham, AL*

PETER L. NARA, DVM, MSc, PhD • *Biological Mimetics Inc., Frederick, MD*

MICHELLE ONORATO, MD • *Division of Infectious Diseases, University of Texas Medical Branch, Galveston, TX*

RICHARD B. POLLARD, MD • *Division of Infectious Diseases, University of California, Davis Medical Center, Sacramento, CA*

ROGER J. POMERANTZ, MD • *Division of Infectious Diseases, Center for Human Virology, Jefferson Medical College, Philadelphia, PA*

CLIONA M. ROONEY, PhD • *Departments of Molecular Virology and Microbiology, Pediatrics, and Center for Cell and Gene Therapy, Baylor College of Medicine, Houston, TX*

ULUHAN SILI, MD • *Departments of Molecular Virology and Microbiology, Pediatrics, and Center for Cell and Gene Therapy, Baylor College of Medicine, Houston, TX*

ROBERT S. WALLIS, MD • *UMDNJ New Jersey Medical School, Division of Infectious Diseases, Newark, NJ*

I
Basic Principles of Immunity

1
Humoral Immunity

Peter L. Nara

INTRODUCTION

It has been almost 100 years since Emil von Behring and Shibasaburo Kitasato received the first Nobel Prize for the discovery of passive immunotherapy. In 1888 Emile Roux and Alexandre Yersin isolated a soluble toxin from cultures of diphtheria. The bacterium itself is only found in the throat, but its destructive effects are found throughout the body. Clearly, the bacteria must be sending out an invisible factor, most likely chemical in nature, to cause the body-wide destruction. This idea was the hypothesis of Roux and Yersin. They filtered diphtheria cultures to remove the bacteria and then injected the remaining fluid filtrate (which we call the supernatant) into healthy animals. As expected, the animals showed diphtheria lesions but without any obvious presence of bacteria.

They then took serum from animals infected with diphtheria and injected it into healthy animals. When these animals were later inoculated with diphtheria, they were found to be resistant to infection. We now know this method of conferring infection resistance as *passive immunity*. This first demonstration of defense against infection was described as mediated by *antitoxin. (1)*. It was clear to von Behring and Kitasato *(2)* that the antitoxin was specific only for diphtheria; it did not confer any defense against other forms of infection. We now know that this antitoxin is composed of antibodies produced specifically against the diphtheria microbe. In 1897, Rudolf Kraus first visualized the reaction of antitoxins to bacteria by simply adding serum from infected animals to a culture of the bacteria and seeing a cloudy precipitate develop as the antibodies bound the bacteria together.

Other scientists took different approaches and revealed serum-based responses toward bacteria and their products. Initially these serum properties were given a range of different names, such as precipitins, bacteriolysins, and agglutinins. Immunologic research would have to wait until 1930 before these subtly different properties were unified and recognized as a single entity. Long before antibodies were actually isolated and identified in serum, Paul Erlich had put forward his hypothesis for the formation of antibodies. The words *antigen* and *antibody* (intentionally loose umbrella terms) were first used in 1900. It was clear to Erlich and others that a specific antigen elicited production of a specific antibody that apparently did not react to other antigens.

From: *Immunotherapy for Infectious Diseases*
Edited by: J. M. Jacobson © Humana Press Inc., Totowa, NJ

Erlich introduced a number of ideas that were later to be proved correct. He hypothesized that antibodies were distinct molecular structures with specialized receptor areas. He believed that specialized cells encountered antigens and bound to them via receptors on the cell surface. This binding of antigen then triggered a response and production of antibodies to be released from the cell to attack the antigen. He understood that antigen and antibody would fit together like a "lock and key." A different key would not fit the same lock and vice versa. However, he did get two important points wrong. First, he suggested that the cells that produced antibody could make any type of antibody. He saw the cell as capable of reading the structure of the antigen bound to its surface and then making an antibody receptor to it in whatever shape was required to bind the antigen. He also suggested that the antigen-antibody interaction took place by chemical bonding rather than physically, like pieces of a jigsaw puzzle.

Thus, by 1900, the medical world was aware that the body had a comprehensive defense system against infection based on the production of antibodies. They did not know what these antibodies looked like, and they knew little about their molecular interaction with antigens; however, another major step on the road had been made. We can see that the antibody system of defense was ultimately a development of the ancient Greek system of medicine that believed in imbalances in the body humors. The antibody response later became known as the *humoral* arm of the immune system. The term humoral (from the Latin word *humors*) refers to the fluids that pass through the body like the blood plasma and lymph. The blood plasma is the noncellular portion of the blood, and the lymph is the clear fluid that drains via lymph ducts to the lymph glands and finally into the venous circulation. These fluids carry the antibodies, which mediate the humoral immune response (Fig. 1).

BASIC STRUCTURE OF ANTIBODIES

Antibodies (immunoglobulins, abbreviated Ig) are proteins of molecular weight 150,000–900,000 kD. They are made up of a series of domains of related amino acid sequence, which possess a common secondary and tertiary structure. This conserved structure is frequently found in proteins involved in cell-cell interactions and is especially important in immunology. Some examples of other members of the immunoglobulin supergene family are the T-cell receptor; the adhesion molecules intercellular cell adhesion molecule (ICAM)-1, -2, and -3 and vascular cell adhesion molecule (VCAM); the coreceptors CD4 and CD8; the costimulatory pairs CD28, CTLA4, B7.1, and B7.2; and all or parts of many other proteins. The proteins utilizing this structure are members of the immunoglobulin supergene family. All antibodies have a similar overall structure, with two light and two heavy chains. These are linked by both covalent (disulphide bridges) and noncovalent forces.

One end of the Ig binds to antigens (the Fab portion, so called because it is the fragment of the molecule that is antigen binding); the other end which is crystallizable, and therefore called Fc, is responsible for effector functions (Fig. 2).

There are five classes (isotypes) of Ig: IgM, IgG, IgA, IgD, and IgE, plus four subtypes of IgG (IgG1–4) and two subtypes of IgA (IgA1 and IgA2). Light chains exist in two classes, λ and κ. Each antibody molecule has either λ or κ light chains, not both. Igs are found in serum and in secretions from mucosal surfaces. They are produced and

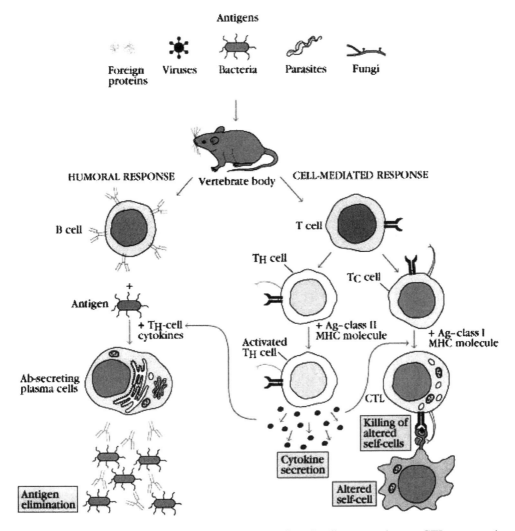

Fig. 1. Humoral and cell-mediated responses of antibodies to antigens. CTL, cytotoxic T-lymphocyte.

secreted by plasma cells, which are found mainly within lymph nodes and which do not circulate. Plasma cells are derived from B-lymphocytes (Fig. 3).

As seen in Fig. 2, the immunoglobulin molecule consists of two light chains, each of approximate molecular weight 25,000, and two heavy chains, each of approximate molecular weight 50,000. IgA exists in monomeric and dimeric forms and IgM in a pentameric form of 900,000 kD. The links between monomers are made by a J chain.

Additionally, IgA molecules receive a secretory component from the epithelial cells into which they pass. This is used to transport them through the cell and remains attached to the IgA molecule within secretions at the mucosal surface. The heavy and light chains consist of amino acid sequences. In the regions concerned with

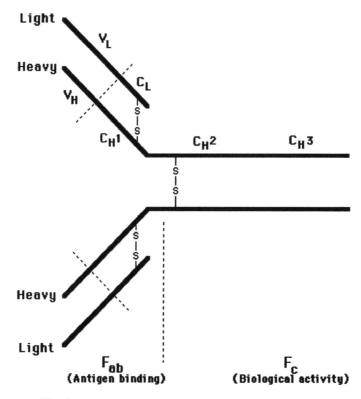

Fig. 2. Immunoglobulin structure. s-s, disulfide links.

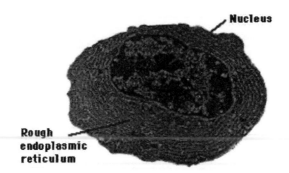

Fig. 3. The immunoglobulin molecule.

antigen binding, these regions are extremely variable, whereas in other regions of the molecule, they are relatively constant. Thus each heavy and each light chain possesses a variable and a constant region. The isotype of an Ig is determined by the constant region. L chains are separated from H chains by disulphide (S-S) links. Intrachain S-S links divide H and L chains into domains, which are separately folded. Thus, an IgG molecule contains three H chain domains, C_H1, C_H2, and C_H3 (Fig. 2). Between C_H1 and C_H2, there are many cysteine and proline residues. This is known as the hinge region and confers flexibility to the Fab arms of the Ig molecule. It is used when

Table 1
Properties of Human Immunoglobins (Igs)

Property	Ig class				
	IgG	IgM	IgA	IgE	IgD
Heavy chains	γ	μ	α	ε	δ
Light chains	κ or λ	κ or λ	κ or λ	κ or λ	κ or λ
Four-chain units	1	5	1 or 2	1	1
Serum conc. (mg/mL)	8–16	0.5–2	1.4–4	<0.5	0–1
% Total serum Ig	75	10	15	<1	<1
Activates C′ (classic pathway)	+	+ +	−	−	−
C′ activation (alternative)	−	−	+/−	−	−
Crosses placenta	+	−	−	−	−
Binds to macrophages and PMNs	+	−	−	−	−
Binds to mast cells and basophils	−	−	−	+	−

Abbreviations: PMNs, polymorphonuclear neutrophils.

antibody interacts with antigen. The properties of immunoglobulins are summarized in Table 1.

ANTIBODY RECEPTORS

There are various Fc receptors (R) with different properties. Monocytes and neutrophils express receptors (FcγR) for the Fc region of IgG. They constitutively express FcγRIIa and FcγRIIIa (monocytes) and FcγRIIIb (neutrophils). Mature tissue macrophages additionally express FcγRI, as do activated neutrophils. The principal difference between these receptors is that FcγRI is a high-affinity receptor ($K_d \sim 10^{-9}$) and therefore can bind monovalent antibody/complexes, whereas FcγRII and -III are low-affinity receptors ($K_d \sim 10^{-6}$) and thus only bind multivalent antibody-antigen complexes. The receptors are described in Table 2.

SOURCES OF ANTIBODIES

Antibodies are synthesized by lymphocytes. Lymphocytes may be T (= thymus)-processed or B (= bone marrow)-processed. Antibodies are made by B-lymphocytes and exist in two forms, either membrane bound or secreted. B-lymphocytes use membrane-bound antibody to interact with antigens. A B-cell makes antibodies all of the same specificity, i.e., able to react with the same antigenic determinants; its progeny (as a consequence of mitotic division) are referred to as a clone. The clone will continue making antibody of the same specificity. Simultaneously, there will be many other clones of different specificity. This is known as a polyclonal response. Antigens have determinants called epitopes. Epitopes are molecular shapes recognized by antibodies, which recognize one epitope rather than whole antigen. Antigens may be proteins, lipids, or carbohydrates, and an antigen may consist of many different epitopes and/or may have many repeated epitopes.

B-lymphocytes evolve into plasma cells under the influence of T-cell released cytokines. Plasma cells secrete antibodies in greater amounts but do not divide. They exist in lymphoid tissues, not blood. Other B-cells circulate as memory cells.

Table 2
Receptors for the Constant (Fc) Region of IgG

Family	CD	Affinity for IgG	Cell distribution/function
FcγRI	CD64	High	Mφ activated PMNs, phagocytosis
FcγRIIa	CD32	Low	Phagocytes, phagocytosis
FcγRIIb	CD32	Low	B-cells, antibody feedback
FcγRIIIa	CD16	Low	PMNs, phagocytosis
FcγRIIIb	CD16	Low	Mφ, phagocytosis
FcγRIIIb	CD16	Low	NK cells, ADCC

Abbreviations: ADCC, antibody-dependent cell-mediated cytotoxicity; NK, natural killer; PMNs, polymorphonuclear neutrophils.

The Life of the B-Cell

B-lymphocytes are formed within the bone marrow and undergo their development there. They have the following functions:

1. to interact with antigenic epitopes, using their immunoglobulin receptors
2. to subsequently develop into plasma cells, secreting large amounts of specific antibody, or
3. to circulate as memory cells
4. to present antigenic peptides to T-cells, consequent upon interiorization and processing of the original antigen.

FUNCTIONS OF ANTIBODIES

Antibodies exist free in body fluids, e.g., serum, and membrane-bound to B-lymphocytes. Their function when membrane-bound is to capture antigen for which they have specificity, after which the B-lymphocytes will take the antigen into its cytoplasm for further processing. Free antibodies have the functions given below.

Agglutination. Antibodies can agglutinate particulate matter, including bacteria and viruses. IgM is particularly suitable for this, as it is able to change its shape from a star form to a form resembling a crab.

Opsonization. Opsonization involves the coating of bacteria for which the antibody's Fab region has specificity (especially IgG). This facilitates subsequent phagocytosis by cells possessing an Fc receptor, e.g., neutrophil polymorphonuclear leukocytes (polymorphs). Thus it can be seen that in opsonization and phagocytosis both the Fab and the Fc portions of the immunoglobulin molecule are involved.

Neutralization. Toxins released by bacteria, e.g., tetanus toxin, are neutralized when specific IgG antibody binds, thus preventing the toxin binding to motor end plates and causing persistent stimulation, manifest as sustained muscular contraction, which is the hallmark of tetanic spasms. This applies particularly to IgG. In the case of viruses, antibodies can hinder their ability to attach to receptors on host cells. Here, only Fab is involved.

Immobilization of bacteria. Antibodies against bacterial ciliae or flagellae will hinder their movement and ability to escape the attention of phagocytic cells. Again, only Fab is involved.

Complement Activation. Complement activation (by the classical pathway), especially the Fc region of IgM and IgG, eventually leads to death of bacteria by the terminal complement components, which punch holes in the cell wall, leading to an osmotic death. Complement components also facilitate phagocytosis by cells possessing a receptor for C3b, e.g., polymorphs.

Mucosal protection. This is provided mainly by IgA and, to a lesser degree, IgG. IgA acts chiefly by inhibiting pathogens from gaining attachment to mucosal surfaces. This is a Fab function.

Expulsion as a consequence of Mast cell degranulation. As a consequence of antigen, e.g., parasitic worms, binding to specific IgE attached to mast cells by their receptor for IgE Fc, there is release of mediators from the mast cell. This leads to contraction of smooth muscle, which can result in diarrhea, and expulsion of parasites. Here we see involvement of both Fab versus parasite antigen, with Fc anchoring the reacting participants.

Precipitation of soluble antigens by immune complex formation. These consist of antigen linked to antibody. Depending on the ratio of antigen to antibody, they can be of varying size. When fixed at one site, they can be removed by phagocytic cells. They may also circulate prior to localization and removal and can fix complement. Here Fab and Fc are involved.

Antibody-dependent cell-mediated cytotoxicity (ADCC). Antibodies bind to organisms via their Fab region. Large granular lymphocytes (natural killer [NK] cells)—attach via Fc receptors and kill these organisms not by phagocytosis but by release of toxic substances called perforins.

Conferring immunity to the fetus by the transplantal passage of IgG. IgG is the only class (isotope) of immunoglobulin that can cross the placenta and enter the fetal circulation, where it confers immune protection. This is of great importance to the fetus in the first 3 months. The precise function of IgD is not known. It may serve as a maturation marker of B-lymphocytes.

Primary and Secondary Responses

When we are exposed to an antigen for the first time, there is a lag of several days before specific antibody becomes detectable. This antibody is IgM. After a short time, the antibody level declines. These are the main characteristics of the primary response. If at a later date we are reexposed to the same antigen, there is a far more rapid appearance of antibody, and in greater amounts. It is of the IgG class and remains detectable for months or years. These are the features of the secondary response. If at the same time we are reexposed to an antigen, we are exposed to a different antigen for the first time, the properties of the specific response to this antigen are those of the primary response, as shown in Fig. 4.

The characteristics of the two responses may be outlined as follows:

Primary response
   Slow in onset
   Low in magnitude
   Short lived
   IgM
Secondary response
   Rapid in onset
   High in magnitude
   Long lived
   IgG (or IgA, or IgE)

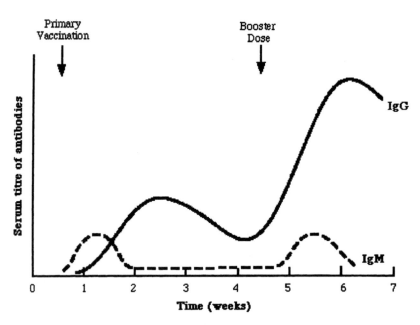

Fig. 4. Primary (dotted line, vaccination; IgM) and secondary (solid line, booster; IgG) antibody responses.

Thus the secondary response requires the phenomenon known as class switching. This requires cooperation with T-cells of various types, which release cocktails of substances called cytokines. These cytokines induce gene rearrangements culminating in class switching (described below).

This phenomenon is possible because the immune system possesses specific memory for antigens. It occurs because during the primary response, some B-lymphocytes, in addition to those differentiating into antibody-secreting plasma cells, become memory cells, which are long lived.

GENERATION OF ANTIBODY DIVERSITY

A major question is how antibodies recognize so many different epitopes. The antigen-combining site of the antibody molecule is in the variable region of Fab. Actually, this site is even more variable than the immediately adjacent sites and is known as the hypervariable region. The bond with antigen is of a physical, non-covalent nature.

As mentioned before, variable (V), and constant (C) regions are genetically encoded. If we bear in mind that we need to be capable of responding to something on the order of 1018 antigens, we can appreciate the need for the enormous number of genes necessary to provide this. In fact, the amount of DNA that this would involve would be quite profligate, and nature has solved this problem very ingeniously by a neat little trick.

In the germline DNA, the V genes encoding the antigen-combining sites need to combine with the C genes. Additional interposed genes bring about diversity of specificity. In light chains, these are the J genes, which link V to C, i.e., we have V-J-C. Joining is imprecise, causing further variation, or *combinatorial diversity.* In the case of H chains, there is yet another region interposed between V and J, the D (for diversity) gene segment. Thus, in H chains, we have V-D-J-C, again with combinatorial diversity. So, if there are 25 λ light chain V genes, and 5 J genes, constituting light chain variable regions, there are already 125 possible combinations, disregarding imprecision of joining. For κ light chains, there are 5 V genes and 70 J genes, yielding 350 combinations. For H chains, there are 100 V genes, 50 D genes, and 6 J genes, giving 30,000 combinations. Overall, disregarding combinatorial diversity, this yields more than 109 combinations. When we multiply this by joining imprecision, plus a heightened mutation rate of genes in the hypervariable region, we can see that from 261 genes, we can easily exceed 1018 variations.

The C regions are also genetically encoded, there being four genes for λ light chains, one for κ light chains, and nine H chain C genes (IgM, IgD, IgG1–4, IgA1, IgA2, and IgE).

IgG is the only class of immunoglobulin capable of crossing the placenta (an Fc-mediated event) (Table 1).

The mechanisms for generating antibody diversity may be summarized as follows:

1. Multiple germline V genes
2. V-J and V-D-J recombinations
3. Combinatorial diversity (= recombinational inaccuracies)
4. Somatic point mutation
5. Pairing of heavy and light chains.

Millions of antibody genes come from diverse combinations of gene parts. (Fig. 5). Antibodies have a variable region (binding site) and a constant region (holds binding sites together, interacts with cells). B-cell maturation joins V (variable), D (diversity), and J (segments) to form a variable gene region, connected to a constant region. Post-transcriptional processing removes introns (and extra J regions) to form mRNA.

Class switching changes the constant region type (Fig. 6). Each stem cell produces an antibody with a different specificity, because it combines a different combination of V, D, and J exons for both light and heavy chains (Fig. 7).

ANTIBODY ENGINEERING YESTERDAY AND TODAY

The discovery of monoclonal antibody (MAb) technology in the late 1970s and early 1980s opened a new era in human therapeutics *(3).* The economic promise of MAbs was said to be limitless. In fact, MAbs, could be selected with exquisite specificity. They were found to orchestrate various components of the immune system such as ADCC and complement, and they showed a high biologic half-life in blood and tissues, rendering them effective for prophylactic use. The toxicity of infused MAbs was expected to be low because of their biologic nature. This concept was further supported by the successful clinical results of mouse antiidiotypic MAbs in the treatment of lymphoma and leukemias and by U.S. Food and Drug Administration (FDA) approval in 1986 of the OKT3 and anti-CD3 mouse MAb for acute renal transplant rejection.

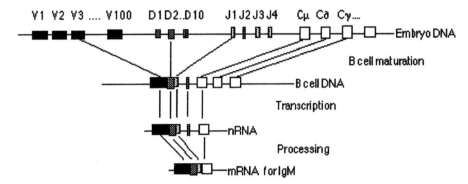

Fig. 5. Diagram showing how antibody genes are combined (see text).

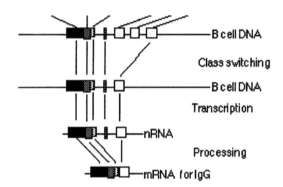

Fig. 6. Diagram of class switching.

This excess of optimism was soon followed by a period of skepticism after adverse clinical and laboratory findings with rodent MAbs when they were used clinically in humans: up to 50% of treated patients developed antimurine antibody responses. In addition, the effector functions and biologic half-life were much less efficient. Adding to the skepticism were the additional failures of the clinical trials of the anti-lipopolysaccharide (LPS) mouse IgME5 MAb from Zoma, which was completed between 1992 and 1993, and the human IgM HA-1A (for septic shock) from Stanford/Centocor. However, in 1994, the FDA approved the antiplatelet mouse MAb ReoPro to treat the complications of angioplasty. This modest success was followed by FDA approval of six other engineered antibodies between 1997 and 1999.

The resurgence of interest in antibody-based therapeutics was the direct consequence of the introduction of genetically engineered immunoglobulins and the refinement of targets for antibody therapy. MAbs or their recombinant derivatives now account for the single largest group of biotechnology-derived molecules in clinical trials and have a prospective market of several billion dollars. Their applications include the prophylaxis, therapy, or control of allergic and autoimmune diseases; complications of angioplasty; sepsis; a variety of inflammatory diseases; many viral and bacterial infections; organ transplantation rejections; and solid and hematologic tumors *(4–10)*.

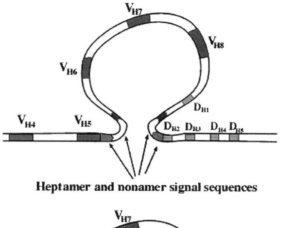

Heptamer and nonamer signal sequences

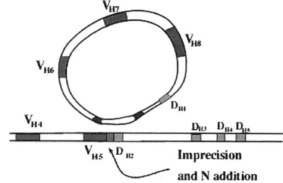

Fig. 7. VDJ joining occurs through DNA recombination.

ANTIGEN-PRESENTING CELLS AND T-CELLS

MHC and Antigen Presentation

Class II major histocompatibility complex (MHC) is an antibody-like protein representing an extension of the principles by which antibodies are made: MHCs in different clones have different specificities (like antibodies) but otherwise different structures and functions. MHCs have α and β chains with binding sites (rather than small and large chains) and a constant region that anchors the molecule to the plasma membrane (with a binding site outside the cell) (Fig. 8).

Cytokines

This is a generic term for messenger molecules (polypeptides) secreted by lymphoid and nonlymphoid cells that form a mediator network regulating the growth, differentiation, and function of cells involved in immunity, hematopoiesis, and inflammation. Cytokines secreted by lymphocytes are also called lymphokines, and those secreted by monocytes/macrophages are known as monokines. An interleukin (IL) is a cytokine that carries a message between leukocytes. Cytokines involved in the regulation of T-cells, B-cells, and macrophages were mentioned previously and are summarized in Table 3. CD 4+ helper T-cells are now divided into two subsets based on cytokine profile and predominant function:

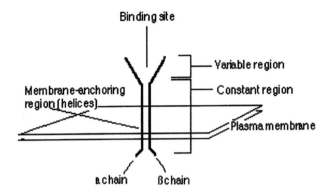

Fig. 8. Macrophages with class II MHC take up antigen and break it into pieces; the pieces of the MHC are displayed on the surface.

Table 3
Cytokines in Immunity

Cytokine	Source	Action and target
IL-1	Macrophages	Growth of activated T- and B-cells
IL-2	Activated T-cells	Growth of activated T-, B-, and NK cells
IL-3	Activated T-cells	Growth and differentiation of hematopoietic precursors
IL-4	Activated T-cells	Growth of activated B- and T-cells
IL-5	Activated T-cells	Growth of activated B-cells
IL-6	Activated T-cells and macrophages	Growth and maturation of activated B- and T-cells
IL-10	Activated T-cells	Inhibits IFN-γ secretion
IFN-γ	Activated T-cells	Activates macrophages and increases their expression of MHC I and II
TNF	Macrophages, activated T- and NK cells	Helps activate cytolytic T-cells; cytotoxic to tumor; activates phagocytic cells

Abbreviations: IL, interleukin; IFN, interferon; TNF, tumor necrosis factor; NK, natural killer.

1. Type 1 (Th1) cells produce interferon (IFN)-γ, tumor necrosis factor (TNF)-α and -γ, and IL-2 (but not IL-4, IL-5, or IL-10) and regulate classical delayed (type IV) hypersensitivity reactions centered around macrophage activation and T-cell-mediated immunity.
2. Type 2 (Th2) cells elaborate IL-4, IL-5, IL-6, and IL-10 and participate in immediate (type 1) hypersensitivity reactions and B-cell antibody-mediated immunity *(11)*.

Proinflammatory cytokines, such as TNF (α and β) and IL-1, which are produced by activated macrophages, mediate local and systemic effects, including the induction of the acute-phase reactions of inflammation.

Chemokines (chemotactic cytokines) belong to a family of low-molecular-weight proteins (with complex names/eponyms) that are secreted by monocytes (e.g., monocyte chemotactic protein [MCP]), macrophages (e.g., macrophage inflammatory protein [MIP]), and T-cells (e.g., regulated upon activation normal T-cell expressed and secreted [RANTES]) that influence leukocyte motion and that attract leukocytes to

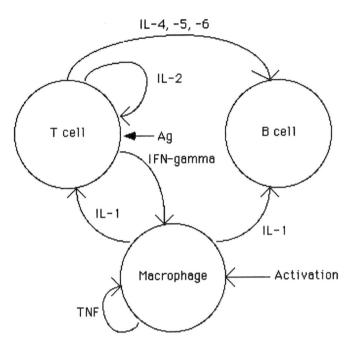

Fig. 9. Messenger molecule (cytokine) mediator circuits involved in immunity. Ag, antigen; IFN, interferon; IL, interleukin; TNF, tumor necrosis factor. (Modified from ref. *56.*)

sites of tissue inflammation or infection (Fig. 9). Surprisingly, in HIV infection, specific chemokine receptors on CD4+ target cells are now known to function as coreceptors required for viral entry.

B-CELLS

Early Development of the Repertoire

The evolutionary selection pressure guiding T-cell and B-cell repertoire development is the same in each case: to generate a range of specificities that will protect against various and unpredictable infectious disease challenges while limiting the potential for reactivity against self. This selection pressure acts on the level of the individual animal, such that the individual with the most effective repertoire in a particular time and place is most likely to survive and reproduce. The selection pressure also acts on the level of the population, such that repertoire diversity maintained within a population makes it more likely that some individuals will survive to reproduce after an infectious outbreak.

The downside of clonal deletion as a mechanism for tolerance is that it creates holes in the repertoire. A pathogen could take advantage of these holes by mimicking self to evade immune recognition. For T-cells, this problem is dealt with by balanced polymorphism of MHC within a species. T-cell recognition of peptide in the context of polymorphic MHC molecules provides each individual with a different T-cell repertoire complete with different holes *(12–14)*. Thus MHC polymorphism provides protection against disease at the level of the population. Because B-cells recognize native antigen, and most of us express the same set of native proteins, any holes in the B-cell repertoire created by clonal deletion would be the same across the population, putting the entire population at great risk from infectious agents that mimic "self" proteins. Whereas the recognition of polymorphic MHC by T-cells protects populations from this sort of threat, B-cell recognition of native antigen precludes a similar strategy.

Antigen Recognition and Lymphocyte Development

B-cell development differs significantly from T-cell development in that negative selection of autoreactive B-cells can occur in the same microenvironment in which productive immune responses begin, the outer T-cell zone of the spleen. The maturation of B-cells in this more public environment has important implications for the mechanisms that maintain self-tolerance and contribute to the development of autoimmunity. This type of development allows for the shaping of the B-cell repertoire with multiple specificities, including weakly autoreactive and crossreactive specificities, into the functional repertoire. The evolution of the humoral immune system was challenged by having on hand as diverse an array of antibody-producing cells as possible to address the multiple types of invaders discussed earlier.

Much of T-cell development occurs in the thymus, geographically sequestered from the sites of active immune responses. This cloistered environment ensures that many self-reactive T-cells are eliminated before joining the mature T-cell repertoire. B-cells also undergo several forms of negative selection of self-reactive specificities. Recent experiments suggest that, in contrast to T-cell development, much B-cell negative selection occurs in the same location in which immune responses to foreign antigens are initiated—the outer T-cell zone of the spleen (reviewed in ref. 15). This maturation of B-cells in a public environment has important implications for the mechanisms that maintain self-tolerance and that might contribute to the development of autoimmune disease. Here, we suggest that the public shaping of the B-cell repertoire allows the recruitment of multiple specificities, including weakly self-reactive specificities, into the functional immune repertoire and that this mechanism for increasing repertoire diversity offsets the risk of autoimmunity.

B-cell selection, like T-cell selection, functions to balance the need for repertoire diversity with the need to protect against autoimmunity. T-cells and B-cells recognize antigen in fundamentally different ways, and these differences in recognition are reflected in differences in the mechanisms of repertoire generation. T-cell recognition is inexorably associated with recognition of self. T-cells recognize peptide antigen complexed with MHC molecules, constraining recognition to antigen processed and presented by cells *(16–18)*. T-cell selection reflects this recognition by allowing only those T-cells with receptors that bind MHC to mature, while eliminating those T-cells that strongly bind self-peptide—MHC complexes during development in the thymus *(19–24)*. Signals to the T-cell that stimulate activation of T-cell immune responses in the periphery induce deletion of maturing, self-reactive cells in the thymus *(25)*. Thymic T-cells that have yet to complete development and selection are prevented from joining the functional immune repertoire; the cloistered environment of the thymus thus protects against autoimmunity.

In contrast to T-cell recognition, B-cells recognize native antigen that is not necessarily associated with cells. B-cell development also begins in an isolated environment in the bone marrow, where high avidity self-reactive B-cells are deleted *(26,27)*. Although it was generally thought that most B-cell-negative selection occurred in the bone marrow *(28)*, several lines of evidence point to a key distinction from T-cell development. First, the bone marrow appears to export a larger proportion of the B-cells that it produces than the thymus *(29,30)*. These newly exported B-cells are relatively immature cells that migrate from the bone marrow to the outer T-cell zones of the white pulp of the spleen *(31)*. These newly emigrated splenic B-cells express high levels of the heat-stable antigen (HSA), a maturation marker common to developing B- and T-cells *(32)*. By contrast, HSA^{hi} T-cells are found only in the thymus, as maturing T-cells lose HSA expression before migrating to the periphery *(33–36)*. Second, when the recirculating B-cell repertoire has attained an adult size and steady state, only a small fraction of these recent bone marrow emigrants persists after reaching the splenic T-cell zone *(31,37,38)*. The cells that do persist have a skewed V-region repertoire *(39,40)*. This splenic restriction point in B-cell production eliminates unwanted B-cells by the same order of magnitude as occurs for T-cells exclusively in the thymus. A key question is whether immature B-cells are selected against within the splenic T-cell zone because they fail a positive selection step for particular specificities or because they trigger a negative selection step against particular specificities.

The first evidence that immature B-cells are negatively selected in the spleen came from Cyster et al. *(41)*, who showed that self-reactive B-cells recognizing circulating lysozyme antigen accumulate in the T-cell zone of the spleen and are excluded from migration into the B-cell follicles, with an efficiency that is directly proportional to the level of self-ligand present, the affinity of the receptor, its signaling properties, and the presence of competing B-cells *(41–44)*. Self-reactive cells that are excluded from the follicular recirculating repertoire are short lived (1–3 days), whereas, cells that enter the B-cell follicles are long lived and recirculate for 1–4 weeks *(42)*.

The significance of this follicular exclusion checkpoint in negative selection of self-reactive B-cells has recently been extended by studies tracking the development of B-cells specific for double-stranded DNA (anti-dsDNA), a clinically important specificity, in the context of a polyclonal B-cell repertoire. Mandik-Nayak et al. *(45)* have shown that prototypic anti-dsDNA B cells are not deleted in the bone marrow but are exported to the spleen as relatively immature cells with a short half-life relative to the bulk of the repertoire. They also show that these autoreactive cells localize to the interface between the B-cell and T-cell zones of the spleen. Together with the lysozyme model antigen data, and the evidence that many immature cells are competitively selected against at this site, it seems likely that B-cells bearing many different autoreactive specificities will join the peripheral B-cell population and be subject to selection at this stage and site within the spleen.

The exclusion of newly produced autoreactive B-cells from the B-cell follicles places these potentially pathogenic cells in a site known to be important for the initiation of antibody responses to foreign antigens—the outer T-cell zone *(46, 47)*. Indeed, autoantibody-producing cells in autoimmune mice appear and accumulate in the outer T-cell zone *(48)*, and it has been proposed that the pathogenic autoantibody production results from a failure of B-cell tolerance in this site *(49)*. Self-reactive cells that are excluded from follicles are also functionally anergic—that is, signaling by their B-cell receptors (BCRs) is reversibly altered so that they make weak mitogenic responses to antigen *(45,50)*. Nevertheless, antigens with high avidity binding can deliver strong signals to the B-cells that partially override anergy and induce modest proliferation and antibody production by maturing self-reactive B-cells *(50)*. Thus self-reactive B-cells that have yet to complete development and negative selection might be recruited into the functional immune repertoire if they crossreact avidly with a foreign antigen; the public environment of the spleen seems to encourage this recruitment at the risk of autoimmunity. Why risk autoimmunity by requiring so much of B-cell-negative selection to occur where immune responses begin?

The Autoimmune Solution

The export of self-reactive short-lived cells into a splenic B-cell pool, in which lifespan is inversely proportional to the degree of self-reactivity, might solve the problem of holes in the B-cell repertoire, much as MHC polymorphism serves to solve the hole problem in the generation of the T-cell repertoire. In any one individual in a population, at a particular time, a proportion of the B-cell repertoire is contained in the short-lived B-cell pool, being excluded from entry into the B-cell follicles. In the absence of infection, self-reactive cells within this population will die within a few days and so pose little risk of causing a pathogenic autoimmune response. Autoimmunity is also avoided by requiring stronger signals to recruit autoreactive B-cells into an immune response than are required to recruit naive B-cells and by producing smaller bursts of progeny when autoreactive cells clear the higher activation hurdle *(50)*. Because of the huge potential B-cell repertoire encoded in the genome, the actual B-cell repertoire available at any one time is likely to differ between individuals based on the probable recombination and expression of BCRs. Accordingly, each individual within a population will express a different B-cell repertoire, with varying propensity toward autoimmunity when an infectious agent appears.

The repertoire diversity provided by the short-lived pool of B-cells might work in concert with the probable differences in B-cell pool composition between individuals to ensure that some individuals will mount effective B-cell responses against an infection. This solution to plugging the holes in the repertoire might be buttressed by the unique ability to fine-tune B-cell specificity further, by hypermutation and additional rounds of negative selection in germinal centers. The independent processes of anergy and negative selection in germinal centers might account for why these modest autoantibody responses do not achieve high concentrations and do not normally exhibit sustained or recall characteristics.

The effectiveness of this system depends on the availability of a diverse pool of B-cells within each individual at any one time, as well as differences in pools between individuals. Whereas T-cell deletion in the thymus helps to protect against self-reactivity within the T-cell repertoire, the inherent short lifespan and more rigorous signaling requirements of self-reactive B-cells helps to protect against self-reactivity within the B-cell repertoire. Whereas MHC polymorphism provides diversity in T-cell repertoires within populations, the probable generation of BCR specificities and the short-term inclusion of weakly self-reactive specificities might provide diversity among the B-cell repertoires within populations. Seen in this light, there might be a clear advantage to transiently maintaining weakly self-reactive B-cells in the periphery, where they can potentially contribute to an acute immune response to infection.

CONCLUSIONS

The presence of nonpathogenic anti-self antibodies and antibodies derived against the normal bacterial flora colonizing the vertebrate host in the serum of normal individuals and their non-anamnestic rise and fall during immunization provides evidence that self-reactive B-cells that secreting IgM and in some cases IgG autoantibodies exist and are activated in the peripheral B-cell pool *(51–55)*. One source of these relatively low-avidity autoantibodies is likely to be activation of short-lived B-cells in the outer T-cell zone by high-avidity foreign antigens. The relative contribution of these preexisting reactive B-cells to total repertoire diversity is not known; however, their influence on disease resistance and susceptibility are profoundly observed during the parasitic infection known as leishmania in mice.

Experimental leishmaniasis offers a well-characterized model of Th1-mediated control of infection by an intracellular organism. Susceptible BALB/c mice aberrantly develop Th2 cells in response to infection and are unable to control parasite dissemination. A previously identified antigen, *Leishmania* homolog of receptors for activated C kinase (LACK), was found to be the focus of this initial response. The early CD4+ T-cell response in these mice is oligoclonal and reflects the expansion of memory, Vβ4/Vα8-bearing T-cells in response to the LACK antigen. It appears the T-cells were initially derived to a specific and crossreactive antigen found on a bacterial species colonizing the mouse gastrointestinal tract during its early lifetime. IL-4 generated by these cells is believed to direct the subsequent Th2 response. Mice made tolerant to LACK by the transgenic expression of the antigen in the thymus exhibited both a diminished Th2 response and a healing phenotype. Thus, T-cells that are activated early and are reactive to a single antigen play a pivotal role in directing the immune response to the entire parasite.

Thus, breakthroughs in our knowledge of humoral immunity may be coming with our understanding of its development during differentiation and initial repertoire development as the host establishes itself in the environment. It seems that successful pathogens may have explored these subtle overlaps between self and the normal colonizing flora, which in a distant way is part of self in that they permit the survival of the host through numerous important symbiotic mechanisms *(57–59)*.

REFERENCES

1. Casadevall A, Schaarff MD. Return to the past: the case for antibody based therapies in infectious diseases. Clin Infect Dis 1995; 2:200–208.
2. von Behering E, Kitasato S. Ueber Zusttandekommen der Diptheria-Immunitat und der Tetanus-Immuniat bei Thiern. S Dtsch Med Wochenschr 1890; 16:1113–1116.
3. Kohler G, Milstein. Continuous cultures of fused cells secreting antibody of predefined specificity. Nature 1975; 256:52–53.
4. Gavilondo JV, Larrick JW. Antibody engineering at the Millennium. Biotechniques 2000; 29:128–145.
5. Casadevall A. Antibody-based therapies for emerging infectious diseases. Emerging Infect Dis 1996; 2:200–208.

6. Seledtsov VI, Seledtsova GV. A possible role of pre-existing IgM/IgG antibodies in determining immune response type. Immunol Cell Biol 1997; 2:176–180.

7. Day ED. Advanced Immunochemistry, 2nd ed. New York: Wiley-Liss, 1990.

8. Lutz HU. How pre-existing, germline-derived antibodies and complement may induce a primary immune to nonself. Scand. J Immunol 1999; 49:224–228.

9. Townsend SE, Weintraub BC, Goodnow CC. Growing up on the streets: why B-cell development differs from T-cell development. Immunol Today 1999; 20:217–220.

10. Krause RM, Dimmock NJ, Morens DM. Summary of antibody workshop: the role of humoral immunity in the treatment and prevention of emerging and extant infectious diseases. J Infect Dis 1997; 176:549–59.

11. Kay AB. Origin of type 2 helper T cells. N Engl J Med 1994; 8:567–569.

12. Schwartz R. Immune response (Ir) genes of the murine major histocompatibility complex. Adv Immunol 1986; 38:31–201.

13. Vidovic D, Matzinger P. Unresponsiveness to a foreign antigen can be caused by self-tolerance. Nature 1998; 336:222–225.

14. Lawlor DA, Zemmour J, Ennis PD, Parham P. Evolution of class-I MHC genes and proteins: from natural selection to thymic selection. Annu Rev Immunol 1990; 8:23–63.

15. Liu Y-J. J Exp Med 1997; 186:625–629.

16. Zinkernagel RM, Doherty PC. H-2 compatability requirement for T-cell-mediated lysis of target cells infected with lymphocytic choriomeningitis virus. Different cytotoxic T-cell specificities are associated with structures coded for in H-2K or H-2D. J Exp Med 1975; 141:1427–1436.

17. Kappler JW, Skidmore B, White J, Marrack P. Antigen-inducible, H-2-restricted, interleukin-2-producing T cell hybridomas. Lack of independent antigen and H-2 recognition. J Exp Med 1981; 153:1198.

18. Bjorkman PJ, Saper MA, Samraoui B, et al. The foreign antigen binding site and T cell recognition regions of class I histocompatibility antigens. Nature 1987; 329:512–518.

19. Blackman MA, Marrack P, Kappler J. Influence of the major histocompatibility complex on positive thymic selection of V beta 17a$^+$ T cells. Science 1998; 244:214–217.

20. Kisielow P, Teh HS, Blüthmann H, von Boehmer H. Positive selection of antigen-specific T cells in thymus by restricting MHC molecules. Nature 1988; 335:730–733.

21. von Boehmer H. Thymic selection: a matter of life and death. Immunol Today 1992; 13:454–458.

22. Sha WC, Nelson CA, Newberry RD, et al. Positive and negative selection of an antigen receptor on T cells in transgenic mice. Nature 1988; 336:73–76.

23. Kappler JW, Roehm N, Marrack P. T cell tolerance by clonal elimination in the thymus. Cell 1987; 49:273–280.

24. Robey E, Fowlkes BJ. Selective events in T cell development. Annu Rev Immunol 1994; 12:675–705.

25. Murphy KM, Heimberger AB, Loh DY. Induction by antigen of intrathymic apoptosis of CD4+ CD8+TCRlo thymocytes in vivo. Science 1990; 250:1720–1722.

26. Hartley SB, Crosbie J, Brink R, et al. Elimination from peripheral lymphoid tissues of self-reactive B lymphocytes recognizing membrane-bound antigens. Nature 1991; 353:765–769.

27. Nemazee DA, Börki K. Clonal deletion of β lymphocytes in a transgenic mouse bearing anti-MHC class I antibody genes. Nature 1989; 337:562–566.

28. Nossal NG. Prokaryotic DNA replication systems. Annu Rev Immunol 1983; 52:581–615.

29. Osmond DG, Nossal NG. Differentiation of lymphocytes in mouse bone marrow. II. Kinetics of maturation and renewal of antiglobulin-binding cells studied by double labeling. Cell Immunol 1974; 13:132–145.

30. Osmond DG. The turnover of B-cell populations. Immunol Today 1993; 14:34–37.

31. Lortan JE, Roobottom CA, Oldfield S, MacLennan IC. Newly produced virgin B cells migrate to secondary lymphoid organs but their capacity to enter follicles is restricted. Eur J Immunol 1987; 17:1311–1316.

32. Allman DM, Ferguson SE, Cancro MP. Peripheral B cell maturation. I. Immature peripheral B cells in adults are heat-stable antigen and exhibit unique signaling characteristics. J Immunol 1992; 149:2533–2540.

33. Crispe IN, Moore MW, Husmann LA, et al. Differentiation potential of subsets of CD4-8-thymocytes. Nature 1987; 329:336–339.

34. Crispe IN, Bevan MJ. Expression and functional significance of the Jlld marker on mouse thymocytes. J Immunol 1987; 138:2013–2018.

35. Alterman LA, Crispe IN, Kinnon C. Characterization of the murine heat-stable antigen: an hematolymphoid differentiation antigen defined by the Jlld, MI169 and B2A2 antibodies. Eur J Immunol 1990; 20:1597–1602.

36. Niklolic-Zugic J, Bevan MJ. Functional and phenotypic delineation of two subsets of CD4 single positive cells in the thymus. Int Immunol 1990; 2:135–141.

37. Ho F, Lortan JE, MacLennan IC, Khan M. Distinct short-lived and long-lived antibody-producing cell populations. Eur J Immunol 1986; 16:1297–1301.

38. MacLennan I, Chan E. The dynamic relationship between B-cell populations in adults. Immunol Today 1993; 14:29–34.

39. Malynn BA, Yancopoulos GD, Barth JE, Bona CA, Alt FW. Biased expression of JH-proximal VH genes occurs in the newly generated repertoire of neonatal and adult mice. J Exp Med 1990; 171:843–859.

40. Gu H, Tarlington D, Muller W, Rajewsky K, Forster I. Most peripheral B cells in mice are ligand selected. J Exp Med 1991; 173:1357–1371.

41. Cyster JG, Hartley SB, Goodnow CC. Competition for follicular niches excludes self-reactive cells from the recirculating B-cell repertoire. Nature 1994; 371:389–395.

42. Cyster JG, Goodnow CC. Antigen-induced exclusion from follicles and anergy are separate and complementary processes that influence peripheral B cell fate. Immunity 1995; 3:691–701.

43. Cook MC, Basten A, Fazekas de St Groth B. Outer periarteriolar lymphoid sheath arrest and subsequent differentiation of both naive and tolerant immunoglobulin transgenic B cells is determined by B cell receptor occupancy. J Exp Med 1997; 186:631–643.

44. Schmidt KN, Hsu CW, Griffen CT, Goodnow CC, Cyster JG. Spontaneous follicular exclusion of SHPI-deficient B cells is conditional on the presence of competitor wild-type B cells. J Exp Med 1998; 187:929–937.

45. Mandik-Nayak L, Bui A, Noorchashm H, Eaton A, Erikson J. Regulation of anti-double-stranded DNA B cells in nonautoimmune mice: localization to the T-B interface of the splenic follicle. J Exp Med 1997; 186:1257–1267.

46. Liu YJ, Zhang J, Lane PJL, Chan EYT, MacLennan ICM. Sites of specific B cell activation in primary and secondary responses to T cell-dependent and T cell-independent antigens. J Eur Immunol 1991; 21:2951–2962.

47. Van den Eertwegh AJM, Noelle RJ, Roy M, et al. In vivo CD40-gp39 interactions are essential for thymus-dependent humoral immunity. I. In vivo expression of CD40 ligand, cytokines, and antibody production delineates sites of cognate T-B cell interactions. J Exp Med 1993; 178:1555–1565.

48. Jacobson BA, Panka DJ, Nguyen K-A, et al. Anatomy of autoantibody production: dominant localization of antibody-producing cells to T cell zones in Fas-deficient mice. Immunity 1995; 3:509–519.

49. Jacobson BA, Rothstein TL, Marshak-Rothstein A. Unique site of IgG2a and rheumatoid factor production in MRL/lpr mice. Immunol Rev 1997; 156:103–110.

50. Cooke MP, Heath AW, Shokat KM, et al. Immunoglobulin signal transduction guides the specificity of B cell-T cell interactions and is blocked in tolerant self-reactive B cells. J Exp Med 1994; 179:425–438.

51. Guilbert B, Dighiero G, Avrameas S. Naturally occurring antibodies against nine common antigens in human sera. I. Detection, isolation and characterization. J Immunol 1982; 128:2779–2787.

52. Chen ZJ, Wheeler CJ, Shi W, et al. Polyreactive antigen-binding B cells are the predominant cell type in the newborn B cell repertoire. J Eur Immunol 1998; 28:989–994.
53. Nemazee DA, Sato VL. Induction of rheumatoid antibodies in the mouse. Regulated production of autoantibody in the secondary humoral response. J Exp Med 1983; 158:529–545.
54. Tarkowski A, Czerkinsky C, Nilsson LA. Simultaneous induction of rheumatoid factor- and antigen-specific antibody-secreting cells during the secondary immune response in man. Clin Exp Immunol, 1985; 61:379–387.
55. Logtenberg T, Melissen PMB, Kroon A, Gmelig-Meyling FHJ, Ballieux RE. Autoreactive B cells in normal humans. Autoantibody production upon lymphocyte stimulation with autoantigen-xenoantigen conjugates. J Immunol 1988; 140:446–450.
56. Old LL. Nature 1987; 326:330–331.
57. Nara PL, Goudsmit J. Clonal dominance of the neutralizing response to the HIV-1 V3 epitope: evidence for originial antigenic sin during vaccination and infection in animals, including humans. In: Lerner RA, Ginsheng H, Chanock RH, Brown F (eds.) Vaccines 91. Cold Spring Harbor Laboratory Press, Cold Spring Harbor, NY. pp. 51–58.
58. Kohler H, Muller S, Nara P. Descriptive imprinting in the immune response against HIV-1. Immunol Today. 1994; 13:475–478.
59. Nara PL, Garrity R. Deceptive imprinting: a cosmopolitan strategy for complicating vaccination. Vaccine 1998; 16:1780–1787.

2

Some Basic Cellular Immunology Principles Applied to the Pathogenesis of Infectious Diseases

R. Pat Bucy and Paul Goepfert

INTRODUCTION

In this chapter some of the functional implications of our current understanding of the basic physiology of T-cell mediated immune function for problems in infectious disease are discussed. The subtleties of the process of T-cell antigen "recognition" and the heterogeneity of kinds of functional responses within the T-cell system are a major focus. Finally, some features of the anatomic compartmentalization of the immune system and how limited access to tissue compartments skews our thinking about in vivo immunity in humans are explored. In view of our recently enhanced understanding of HIV disease, the chapter uses this viral infection as an example to illustrate relevant immune mechanisms and concepts.

MECHANISMS OF IMMUNE RECOGNITION

As outlined above, T-cells utilize a complex process to discriminate particular antigenic epitopes. Unlike antibodies that can bind with high affinity to multiple kinds of biomolecules, T-cells only recognize peptide epitopes that are embedded into one of two classes of specialized antigen-presenting structures (Fig. 1). The molecules were originally defined as strong transplantation antigens, coded for by a complex of genes termed the major histocompatibility complex (MHC). The class I MHC molecule exists on the surface of most nucleated cells, albeit at varying densities, in a complex with a small, constant component known as β_2-microglobulin. These molecules bind a selected set of peptides that are primarily derived from cytosolic proteins via degradation and transport into specialized membrane compartments by the proteosome transporter protein (TAP) complex. The peptide/class I molecules are expressed on the cell surface and serve as the antigenic stimulus for CD8+ T-cells. The CD8 molecule on the T-cell binds directly to framework portions of the class I MHC molecule, distinct from the peptide binding site and stabilizes the interaction of the T-cell receptor (TCR)/peptide/MHC complex. The class II MHC molecules serve a similar function of peptide binding and presentation, but they differ in several important ways. First, only selected cell types express class II molecules constitutively, although some cytokines (particularly interferon-γ [IFN-γ] and tumor necrosis factor-α [TNF-α]) can stimulate

From: *Immunotherapy for Infectious Diseases*
Edited by: J. M. Jacobson © Humana Press Inc., Totowa, NJ

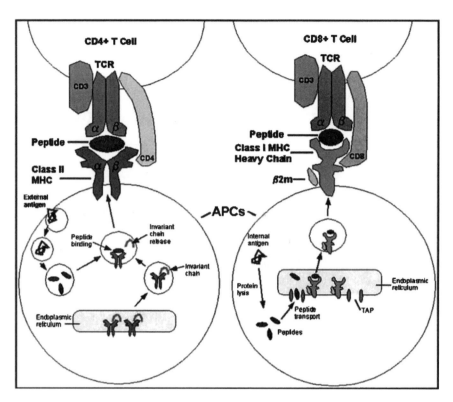

Fig. 1. Two pathways of antigen presentation correlating with two subsets of responding T cells. APCs, antigen-presenting cells; β2m, β₂-microglobulin; TCR, T-cell receptor.

other cells to express these molecules. Second, the class II molecule is a heterodimer of two different MHC-derived proteins with the peptide binding pocket having open ends allowing somewhat more flexibility in the selected peptides. Third, peptides derived from extracellular materials engulfed by the antigen-presenting cells (APCs) are loaded into class II molecules in distinct membrane-bound compartments, compared with the loading of class I molecules. Finally, CD4 binds to the framework portions of the class II MHC molecule to stabilize antigen recognition of CD4+ T-cells.

Thus, the two major sublineages of T-cells (CD4 and CD8) recognize antigens in two distinct kinds of presenting molecules that bind largely distinct universes of peptide determinants (intracellular vs extracellular), usually on distinct kinds of APCs. The binding affinity of the TCR with the MHC/peptide complex (K_d of 10^{-4}–10^{-7}M) is significantly less than typical antibody binding affinities. Several accessory membrane molecules are therefore required to increase this binding affinity. Some of the most notable of the accessory molecules include CD4 and CD8, which function by binding to specific domains of the MHC class II and class I molecules, respectively. Both the CD4 and CD8 molecules also act as signal tranducers, playing a role in intracellular signaling events. Other accessory proteins also play important roles in the TCR/MHC complex interaction, such as CD28, CD2, leukocyte function-associated antigen-(LFA-1), and CD45R *(1–8)*.

This intimate role of the MHC antigens in the process of T-cell recognition not only controls the induction of specific immune effector mechanisms, but is also critical for selection and maintenance of the repertoire of TCR specificities in the T-cell pool. During thymic development, randomly arranged TCR structures are tested out for low avidity to the available peptide/MHC molecules, presumably using peptides derived from ubiquitous self-components. Most TCR structures fail the twin selective processes of thymic repertoire selection: they either bind too strongly to available peptide/MHC molecules (functionally defined as self-antigen), or they fail to bind well enough to receive a positive survival signal *(9–11)*. In both of these situations, the T-cell is deleted, and the surviving T-cells have a low to intermediate binding affinity to a self-peptide/MHC molecular complex. The same type of low-avidity interactions with available peptide/MHC molecules also appears to be necessary for long-term survival of peripheral T-cells. Individual T-cells in the peripheral pool can undergo mitosis without developing the changes associated with specific memory function *(12,13)*, probably with one daughter cell undergoing apoptosis and the other surviving. Data from experiments using mice have shown that maintenance of the population depends on low-level TCR-mediated signals *(14–20)*.

Although most of the specific recognition characteristics inherent in the trimolecular complex mode of antigen recognition is mediated by the TCR repertoire generated during fetal development, each individual MHC molecule can only bind a fairly limited set of peptides with constrained structural features. Although this strategy apparently offers a degree of fine physiologic control (to prevent autoimmunity?), this mechanism results in alterations in the intensity of the immune response in different individuals with structurally different MHC molecules. Especially in immune responses to antigens of limited structural heterogeneity, the intensity of the response is often controlled by a genetic element linked to the MHC known as an immune response (Ir) gene. It is now clear that the structural gene that maps to the MHC is either the class I or class II antigen-presenting molecule; however, the "Ir gene phenotype" is a complex mixture of the structure of the TCR repertoire and the determinant selection activity of particular MHC molecules *(21,22)*. In some cases, there is a hole in the TCR repertoire such that a particular peptide MHC complex fails to stimulate any available T-cells; in other cases, antigenic peptides simply fail to bind with any of the available MHC restriction elements. In either case, the immune response to such an antigen is unproductive and this phenotype is a heritable genetic trait, an Ir gene.

This variability of immune response intensity due to structural constraints on permissive peptide binding by individual MHC molecules is thought to be related to the extreme polymorphism of these molecules maintained among individuals within the population. Not only are there several distinct loci for both class I and class II antigens (three for each class in humans), but there are multiple polymorphic alleles present at each locus. Since any one MHC molecule can present only a fairly limited repertoire of peptides, it is widely accepted that there is a significant selective advantage for a population to maintain great diversity of immune recognition structures. Such a diverse set of restriction elements serves to mitigate the likelihood of a single epidemic pathogen escaping detection by most individuals in a localized population.

The complex patterns of disease associations with particular alleles of the MHC, many of which involve the predisposition to autoimmune mechanisms, undoubtedly arise out of this central role of the trimolecular complex in the life, functional activity, and death of T-cells. Variation in response intensity with different MHC haplotypes can also lead to significant mechanistic insights. For example, the strong associations of rates of HIV-1 disease progression in particular MHC class I alleles *(23–25)* suggest several strong implications about the role of cellular immunity in HIV disease. First, the statistical association of MHC molecules with disease progression rates correlates with the primary effect of a relationship of MHC molecules to the initial viral load set point *(24)*, which, in turn, determines the rate of disease progression. Second, the association of particular class I alleles and the advantageous effect of heterozygosity are the molecular signature of the critical role of CD8 T-cell antigen recognition in control of the viral load set point. Furthermore, the concept that CD8 T-cells play a central role in control of HIV infection is supported by a number of other independent lines of evidence *(26–31)*. Interestingly, HIV disease progression does not correlate tightly with specific MHC class II alleles that would be indicative of a role for CD4 T-cells in the immune response to this virus. One possibility is that chronic HIV infection with persistent viremia results in the anergy of all HIV antigen-specific CD4 T-cell clones, erasing the fingerprints of the subtleties of CD4 T-cell antigen recognition via the TCR/ peptide/class II MHC interactions during chronic infection.

The complex mechanism by which T-cells recognize antigen, in comparison with B-cell/antibody antigen recognition, has several important implications for responses to infectious agents and especially the development of vaccines. First, since antibodies recognize a broad range of conformationally dependent epitopes, whereas T-cells focus on only a limited set of peptide epitopes, the degree of crossreactive immunity to different quasi-species of the same infectious agent is often greater for T-cell immunity than for antibody responses. Second, owing to the special processing mechanisms required for T-cell recognition, especially the endogenous peptides loaded into class I MHC molecules for presentation to CD8 T-cells, live viruses may stimulate significantly different T-cell specificities than purified viral proteins administered in an adjuvant fashion. The use of live attenuated viruses as vaccines or the use of pseudotyped viruses or DNA vaccines have all been suggested as a practical means to circumvent this problem, in addition to other potential advantages. Finally, for antigens of limited structural heterogeneity there may be substantial variability between individuals based on MHC haplotype in responses to particular vaccines or infectious agents. To generate strong T-cell immunity, correlation of vaccine responses to particular MHC haplotypes may be just as important as inclusion of antigens derived from diverse clades of virus in vaccine development.

FUNCTIONAL HETEROGENEITY OF T-CELL SUBSETS

The T-cell repertoire can be defined by two distinct properties: the recognition specificity of the TCR heterodimer and the functional response of the cell after TCR stimulation. It is now clear that once a particular TCR heterodimer is expressed on the T-cell surface, the antigen specificity is frozen for all the clonal progeny of that cell. The functional responses available, however, are quite extensive and range from programmed cell death to initiation of distinct modalities of immune response. The complex mechanism by which the antigen specificity is determined (random rearrangement of two distinct polypeptides with both multiple germ-line gene segments and junctional diversity followed by selection for a relatively narrow band of avidity for self-MHC peptides) imposes special characteristics on the specificity repertoire.

The mechanisms by which the functional repertoire of T-cells is developed are less well understood, but they probably involve a similar strategy to that used during thymic selection. The key element again is signaling generated from the TCR complex when it interacts with particular peptide/MHC epitopes. The TCR complex is not merely an on/off switch, but the avidity of interactions of the TCR with the myriad available peptide-loaded MHC molecules initiates biochemical cascades within the T-cell that are highly dynamic *(32)*. If the avidity of these interactions is sufficient, cooperation among other adhesion molecules, including the major coreceptors CD4 or CD8, the adhesion molecule LFA-1 (CD11a), and the CD28 molecule, stabilizes this molecular binding in a process termed the immunologic synapse *(33)*. This complex structure can deliver multiple levels of signal depending on the relative intensity and stability of the interaction. These multiple signals are most likely integrated at the level of multiple different promoter complexes, in which biochemical signals initiated at the cell surface are translated into the production of transcription complex components. In turn, these cellular signals can interact with multiple promoter motifs *(34)*, resulting in coordinated patterns of expression of multiple unlinked genes (Fig. 2).

The proteins produced by such activated genes are of several classes, including those that initiate entry into the cell cycle; expression of unique cytokine receptors; expression of various effector cytokines; expression of new surface adhesion molecules; and new transcription factors. The products of this ensemble of gene activation interact in complex ways to determine not only the fate of that particular T-cell, but also the tempo of immune activation in the immediate microenvironment in which T-cell activation occurs. Expression of new cytokine receptors (e.g., interleukin-2Rβ [IL-2Rβ]) or inactivation of existing receptors (e.g., IL-12Rβ) can alter the subsequent response pattern of the responding T-cell. Many cytokines (i.e., IL-2, IFN-γ, TNF-α, IL-4, IL-10, IL-13, granulocyte/macrophage colony-stimulating factor [GM-CSF], and transforming growth factor-β [TGF-β]) serve as growth and differentiation factors for most other cells in the local microenvironment. These include other T-cells, dendritic cells and macrophages, endothelial cells, and B-cells, in addition to the responding cell via autocrine feedback. With a longer kinetic delay, activated T-cells change the pattern of cell surface adhesion molecules that alter the subsequent recirculation and tissue distribution properties of the cell. Investigators recognize some of these adhesion molecules as memory markers (such as CD44, CD62L, and CD45 isoforms), since their differential expression on previously activated T-cells allows detection by cell surface staining with available monoclonal antibodies.

Finally, and potentially most critical, initial T-cell activation can result in the production of new transcription factors, which may differentially affect the vigor of transcriptional activation on subsequent rounds of TCR-initiated signals. It is highly likely that such factors account for the significantly lowered antigen dose threshold required for full stimulation found in previously activated (memory) T-cells *(35,36)*, compared with cells that have not been stimulated recently. Although many genes are activated in a coordinate manner, in individual cells some of the cytokine genes show distinct thresholds for activation based on different intensities of TCR/peptide/MHC stimulation. These distinct thresholds probably generate the significant clonal heterogeneity characteristic of antigen-specific T-cell activation *(37–41)*.

This hypothetical scheme of T-cell activation (incorporating the functional subtleties of T-cell antigen recognition) contrasts with the more conventional views of classes of T-cells, based on static conceptions of antigen specificity, T-cell response, and

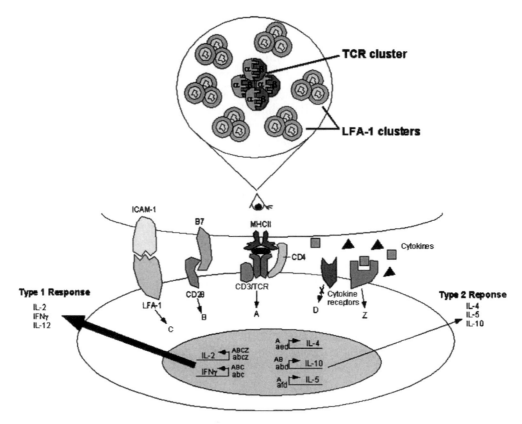

Fig. 2. Multiple distinct signal pathways converge to produce functional transcription complexes to allow coordinate activation of multiple genes. Alterations of the dominant pathway of signaling from successive cycles of antigen stimulation result in alternate pathways of functional differentiation. ICAM-1, intercellular adhesion molecule-1; IFN-γ, interferon-γ; IL, interleukin; LFA-1, leukocyte function-associated antigen; TCR, T-cell receptor.

memory versus naíve T-cells. First, antigen specificity is not a clean positive/negative phenomenon, even in response to a particular index peptide structure. All TCRs in the repertoire bind with modest avidity to ubiquitous self-antigen, and there is potential for antagonist peptides that bind to the MHC restriction element well, but fail to stimulate the particular TCRs with high avidity for the index peptide. T-cells that interact with intermediate avidity to a particular index peptide/MHC complex may show some of the features of T-cell activation, particularly entry into the cell cycle if sufficient IL-2 is available, but they do not participate in the more stringent activation pathways.

Finally, the activation signals from engagement of the TCR reflect the product of the amount of peptide/MHC complex and the inherent TCR affinity. Thus, in the presence of high doses of a particular peptide, more T-cells (including those with slightly lower avidity) can become fully activated. In the presence of lower doses of the *same* peptide, (or in the presence of peptide antagonists), these same T-cells receive suboptimal signaling that not only results in failure to reach the threshold stimulus for full activation, but probably results in a different *kind* of activation. The phenotypic characteristics among the daughter cells of such qualitatively different kinds of antigen activation are probably distinctive. Therefore, the sensitivity to TCR-initiated signal and the cytokine expression phenotype, as well as the pattern of adhesion molecule expression and tissue recirculation may all be different in these daughter cells. Thus, a static view of antigen specificity, which is implicitly defined by response to antigen, is not completely tenable, even though the actual structure of the TCR is not altered by antigen stimulation. Since the pattern of response is quite heterogeneous and dependent on the subtleties of formation and signal generation at the immunologic synapse, the range of peptides that a T-cell is specific for also depends on the circumstances of presentation and the life history of the particular T-cell. Finally, the simple dichotomy between memory and naïve T-cells is much too simple to classify different subsets of T-cells adequately. Not only is memory likely to be as heterogeneous as the response that is remembered, but many adhesion molecules used as markers of memory revert to a naïve status at different tempos.

The role of antigen dose in stimulation of responses may also be quite important in situations of persistent low-level antigen exposure, such as in chronic asymptomatic HIV infection. Persistent stimulation of high-avidity TCRs by a low concentration of HIV-derived peptides may result in exhaustion or anergy of relevant T-cells during chronic infection such that little CD4 helper activity is available for the CD8 T-cell response. A quick burst of a higher concentration of HIV peptides, such as might be experienced in a subject effectively treated with highly active antiretroviral therapy (HAART) who undergoes a scheduled treatment interruption, may allow the functional activation of these same cells to help mediate effective viral clearance. Thus, both the dynamics of antigen dose in vivo and the cytokine milieu in the histologic microenvironment may play critical roles in the ability to induce a functional immune response, beyond the mere presence of antigen-specific T-cells.

In addition to the heterogeneity that exists in concepts such as antigen specific/ nonspecific and memory/naïve, considerable heterogeneity has long been recognized in the kinds of functional effector activity mediated by different classes of T-cells. There are multiple distinct cytokines that can be expressed after TCR activation in addition to the induction of two distinct pathways of direct lytic activity for target cells (the secretory pathway and the FasL/Fas interaction). There is significant heterogeneity in the pattern of individual cytokine gene expression, even within stable in vitro passaged T-cell clones *(37,38,41)*. Although there are patterns of cytokines that tend to be coexpressed, each individual promoter is under a unique pattern of control, with a distinct threshold for activation. Furthermore, there are multiple potential phenotypes, but any one T-cell usually has a very limited subset of these alternatives actually expressed. Not only are the subtleties of TCR/peptide/MHC interaction as discussed above critical for determining the assortment of particular functional activities with different TCR structures, but the cytokine milieu in which initial T-cell activation occurs plays a dominant role in segregation of the cytokine expression phenotype *(42–45)*. The role of the innate immune system in providing the bootstrap cytokines expressed in the local environment where particular antigen-specific cells become activated is probably critical in this process *(46–48)*. Thus, one can conceptualize the T-cell repertoire as a two-dimensional classification scheme, in which each particular specificity element sorts out into distinct functional categories dependent on antigenic stimulation experience.

The determination of how many distinct functional classes of T-cells exist in the repertoire is not clear. The history of cellular immunology has been characterized by the continual subdivision of classes of cells initially thought to be homogenous (given a single name) into distinct categories based on newly discovered features. Lymphocytes have been separated into three distinct lineages and T-cells into sublineages based on both major coreceptor usage (CD4 vs CD8, which correlates with MHC restriction specificity) and distinct lineages that utilize distinct antigen receptors ($\alpha\beta$ vs $\gamma\delta$ TCR). To the first approximation, the CD4 and CD8 sublineages of T-cells are biased in the pattern of their functional differentiation to express particular patterns of cytokines (CD4 helper cells) or the induction of direct lytic activity (CD8 cytotoxic T-cells). However, exceptions to this dichotomy exist in both directions. There are CD4 T-cells that mediate direct lysis and CD8 T-cells that secrete cytokines mediating immunoregulatory activities.

There is also a further subdivision of T-cell subsets into functional classes based on the pattern of cytokine expression, the Th1/Th2 paradigm. Originally panels of murine CD4 T-cell clones were characterized that had distinctive cytokine expression phenotypes *(49)*. Clones classified as Th1 express primarily IL-2, IFN-γ, and TNF-β (LT), whereas the Th2 cells express IL-4, IL-5, and IL-10. Further work has demonstrated that these sets of cytokines are associated with functionally distinct types of immune responses, establishing a link between T-cell phenotype development and cellular versus humoral immunity *(50–52)*. In particular, IFN-γ is a potent macrophage-activating factor *(53,54)* and plays a critical role in delayed-type hypersensitivity (DTH) responses *(55,56)*, whereas IL-4 and IL-5 are potent in B-cell growth and differentiation *(57,58)*. Not only do these cytokines have distinctive biologic activities, but several lines of evidence also indicate that a reciprocal competitive relationship exists between cells with Th1 versus Th2 characteristics *(42,43,45,52,59)*. Several infectious disease models have demonstrated the critical role of Th1 and Th2 cytokines in regulating the balance in favor of the host or the pathogen *(60–64)*. Particularly clear-cut is the genetic susceptibility to *Leishmania* in mice. The disease course between inbred mouse strains is correlated with inherited tendencies to generate either a Th1 or Th2 response *(65–68)*.

The original dichotomy of cytokine expression patterns has begun to blur into many individual distinct phenotypes based on differential quantities of expression within the classical phenotypes (variation in IL-2/IFN-γ ratio in Th1, and IL-4/IL-10/IL-5 and perhaps TGF-β in Th2 cells) *(69)*. The multiplicity of functional phenotypes that have been characterized in different circumstances *(70–72)* suggests that the Th1 and Th2 designations do not represent true lineages (irreversible differentiation), but rather a useful initial distinction among a complex set of functional differentiation patterns. The general idea is that different patterns of cytokine gene transcription represent a primary functional distinction of different T-cell subsets.

Consideration of the significant heterogeneity of antigen-specific T-cell activation has several potentially important implications for the pattern of cellular immune responses to infectious agents and in particular to HIV-1 infection. First, the conventional method of measuring T-cell response to particular antigens used in most human disease clinical trials, the lymphocyte proliferation assay (LPA), is both more complicated than is usually thought and in some circumstances an unreliable guide to the potential for effective in vivo immune response. There are at least three kinds of cells required for a vigorous LPA response: 1) the availability of adequate APCs; 2) the existence of a few individual T-cells in each well that produce potent T-cell growth factors (TCGFs); and 3) the low-threshold stimulation of other T-cells to grow in the presence of TCGF. In most circumstances, IL-2 produced by CD4 T-cells is the dominant TCGF, but other cytokines may play an important role in some situations. Although a strong LPA response correlates well with effective in vivo immunity to particular pathogens, weak or negative LPA responses can result from several different circumstances. These include deficient functional APCs in the population of blood mononuclear cells, clonal anergy (deficient IL-2 production) of relevant T-cell clones, production of alternative cytokines that inhibit T-cell growth, or a low frequency of functional IL-2-producing clones. Direct measurement of the frequency of individual T-cells that produce different effector cytokines shortly after antigen stimulation may yield more insight into the status of in vivo immunity than sole reliance on the conventional LPA response.

A second practical consequence of the complexity of T-cell immunity is understanding the mechanism of insufficient immune responses to certain pathogens, especially those that maintain persistent antigen loads during chronic infection. The conventional view is that such circumstances represent deletion of the small subset of antigen-specific cells, via clonal exhaustion or pathogen-specific infection (in HIV disease for the CD4 T-cell response). An alternative possibility is that persistent antigen load results in various alternative patterns of differentiation that fail to activate effective clearance mechanisms for the infection. T-cells with sufficient TCR affinity for peptides derived from the pathogen exist, but continual low-level stimulation anergizes these cells. In this context, the term anergy simply indicates that absence of the particular function is used as the index of response, not physical absence (clonal deletion) of the relevant cells. In some circumstances, immune deviation to produce Th2-like cytokines in contrast to the Th1 pattern somewhat accounts for such unresponsiveness. Examples include lepromatous leprosy *(60,73,74)* and the well-studied *Leishmania major* infection in mice *(65–75)*.

In the case of HIV-1 infection, although such classical immune deviation has been suggested *(76)*, an alternative possibility is that direct interaction of viral particles with the CD4 molecule together with persistent low concentrations of antigens yields T-cells with low-level TCR stimulation that fail to respond with high IL-2 production. The potential role of selection of viral variants that not only escape detection by particular T-cells but also produce peptide antagonists that block the responses to other epitopes and perhaps alter the cytokine expression pattern of reactive T-cells may also play an important role in some cases. As a consequence of functional anergy of T-cells with TCRs with high affinity for HIV-derived peptides, the infection may be controlled by helper-independent CD8 T-cells that are inherently inefficient. Since persistent low-level TCR stimulation may be required to sustain this pattern of differentiation, it may be possible to reverse this pattern by first eliminating most of the persistent viral antigen (by treatment with available potent antiretroviral drugs) followed by therapeutic immunization. If clonal deletion of HIV-specific T-cells during primary infection is responsible for the deficient CD4 T-cell responses in chronic HIV infection, the prospects for successful therapeutic immunization are fairly dim, given the low (but detectable) thymic output of new TCR specificities in adult humans *(77)*. If an as yet ill-defined anergic state exists among these critical cells, understanding the subtle mechanisms by which antigen can stimulate functionally distinct kinds of differentiation may be critical to the design of effective therapeutic immunization.

ANATOMICAL DISTRIBUTION OF IMMUNE CELLS: RECRUITMENT TO INFLAMMATORY SITES AND REDISTRIBUTION

A final principle of the basic nature of T-cell-mediated immunity is the role of the anatomic distribution of immune cells in mediation of immune responses. First, unlike humoral responses in which the effector function of antibody is generally at a distant site from the antibody-producing cell, T-cell effector function is always localized to microenvironments directly associated with the active effector T-cell. The lytic function of cytotoxic T-lymphocytes (CTLs) takes place only in tight conjugates of the individual target cell and the CTLs, whereas cytokines are active only over short distances and act on other cells in the immediate tissue environment. In fact, a substantial portion of helper function for CTL formation is probably owing to the simple colocalization of activated CD4 and CD8 T-cells in the same tissue microenvironment caused by responses to the same antigenic entity, albeit to distinct peptides. This requirement for localized effector function results in the critical role of T-cell recirculation and recruitment to active inflammatory sites in the organization of in vivo T-cell-mediated immune responses. The development of a mononuclear infiltrate in a nonlymphoid tissue is the histopathologic hallmark of active T-cell immunity.

The ability to mobilize a sufficient number of T-cells to a local site is dependent on the constant recirculation of the low frequency of T-cells with a high-affinity TCR for a particular peptide/MHC epitope and the rapid recruitment of such cells. IFN-γ and TNF-α, as well as other cytokines produced by activated T-cells and macrophages, affect the local microvasculature, resulting in increased vascular permeability and the induction of vascular adhesion molecules. These adhesion molecules serve to facilitate recruitment of circulating T-cells into the microvascular bed surrounding the initial cytokine-producing cells. Although antigen-specific cells are preferentially accumulated in such inflammatory foci, most of the T-cells that accumulate in sites of inflammation do not have TCRs that bind with high avidity to available peptide/MHC complexes. Among the T-cells that are nonspecifically recruited to such sites are a few that reach a threshold of stimulation by the available peptide/MHC complexes and produce additional cytokines that amplify the nascent inflammatory focus. In addition, since T-cell activation occurs in such an inflammatory site bathed in cytokines such as IFN-γ and TNF-α, their pattern of antigen-activated differentiation is biased toward further production of these Th1-type cytokines. Control of the tempo of such iterative cycles of cellular recruitment and inflammatory cytokine production is probably the critical step in the overall intensity of T-cell-mediated immunity.

A corollary of these principles is that the population of T-cells in the blood may not be fully representative of T-cells that are actively involved in a tissue-localized immune response (Fig. 3). During periods of active T-cell immunity, such as localized responses to infectious agents in lymphoid tissue or responses such as solid organ transplant rejection, the blood is relatively depleted of antigen-reactive cells, owing to their sequestration in the local site of the active immune response. Although this is a relatively simple point, fundamental methodologic difficulties often produce subtle conceptual bias. To some extent, this conceptual focus on blood T-cells, simply because they are routinely available for analysis, is a contributor to the controversy concerning the interpretation

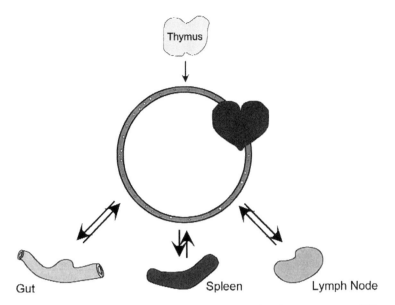

Fig. 3. The in vivo population of T-cells constantly recirculates to many different tissues. Local immune responses result in redistribution of T-cells to the site of immune activation and then nonhomogeneous distribution among body compartments.

of cellular changes after induction of HAART in HIV-1 infection. The initial proposal that the increase in blood CD4 T-cells after HAART was caused by an increase in total body T-cell number reflected the common use of the CD4 count (in blood) as a surrogate for total body T-cells. Although this relationship may be largely correct over the long-term natural history of HIV disease, short-term changes in blood lymphocyte numbers often reflect redistribution of cells between body compartments.

Some investigators proposed the alternative interpretation of a redistribution of cells early on *(78,79)*, but the controversy lingers despite any direct evidence that the total body number of T-cells rises rapidly in any circumstance. Recent studies focused on comparison of lymphoid tissue and blood specimens before and after induction of HAART strongly indicate the reciprocal relationship of blood and tissue lymphocytes and the resolution of lymphoid tissue inflammation coincident with resolution of active viral infection of these tissues *(80)*.

A similar line of reasoning cautions against overinterpretation of the relatively modest level of antigen-specific CTL effector function detected in blood T-cells during chronic HIV disease. Since the active infection exists primarily in the lymphoid tissue, the cells isolated from blood may have an inconsistent relationship with the level of active in vivo immunity during episodes of chronic infection. Together with the relatively difficult analytic procedure required to identify functional CTLs, tissue sequestration of active cells makes assessment of immunity using in vitro methodologies problematic. Ten years ago the failure to detect infectious virus in blood during prolonged asymptomatic chronic HIV infection led to the view of a dormant infection. The advent of sensitive viral RNA assays, together with evidence of rapid fall in viremia after induction of HAART, resulted in a conceptual shift: that there is rapid viral turnover throughout chronic infection. Similarly, the failure to detect robust immune responses during chronic HIV infection using assays of blood T-cells does not indicate that viral replication is not controlled by active immune clearance mechanisms.

SUMMARY

This chapter has attempted to incorporate some insights from our current understanding of cellular immunity into an understanding of the pathogenesis of infectious diseases, with a primary focus on HIV disease. The complexity of T-cell recognition, with subtle functional consequences of particular MHC restriction elements, local milieu of activation, and kinetic profile of antigen dose, results in complex interactions between the immune system and persistent infectious agents. The interaction of ideas derived from basic biologic studies and development of workable therapeutic interventions is most productive when both basic and clinical investigators develop two-way communication. Incorporation of basic insights into new hypotheses that can be directly tested in infected humans offers an additional feature for clinical trial design beyond the availability of novel agents. Furthermore, development of an effective therapeutic strategy is often the key element in resolving fundamental questions of disease mechanisms, since effective interventions must be modifying key mechanisms in disease pathogenesis.

REFERENCES

1. June CH, Ledbetter JA, Gillespie MM, Lindsten T, Thompson CB. T-cell proliferation involving the CD28 pathway is associated with cyclosporine-resistant interleukin 2 gene expression. Mol Cell Biol 1987; 7:4472–4481.
2. Thompson CB, Lindsten T, Ledbetter JA, et al. CD28 activation pathway regulates the production of multiple T-cell-derived lymphokines/cytokines. Proc Natl Acad Sci USA 1989; 86:1333–1337.
3. Fraser JD, Irving, BA, Crabtree GR, Weiss A. Regulation of interleukin-2 gene enhancer activity by the T cell accessory molecule CD28. Science 1991; 251:313–316.
4. Dustin ML, Springer TA. T-cell receptor cross-linking transiently stimulates adhesiveness through LFA-1. Nature 1989; 341:619–624.
5. Bierer BE, Sleckman BP, Ratnofsky SE, Burakoff SJ. The biologic roles of CD2, CD4, and CD8 in T-cell activation. Ann Rev Immunol 1989; 7:579.
6. Pingel JT, Thomas ML. Evidence that the leukocyte-common antigen is required for antigen-induced T lymphocyte proliferation. Cell 1989; 58:1055–1065.
7. Koretzky GA, Picus J, Thomas ML, Weiss A. Tyrosine phosphatase CD45 is essential for coupling T-cell antigen receptor to the phosphatidyl inositol pathway. Nature 1990; 346:66–68.
8. Trowbridge IS, Thomas ML. CD45: an emerging role as a protein tyrosine phosphatase required for lymphocyte activation and development. Annu Rev Immunol 1994; 12:85–116.
9. Kisielow P, Blüthmann H, Staerz UD, Steinmetz M, von Boehmer H. Tolerance in T cell receptor transgenic mice involves deletion of nonmature $CD4^+8^+$ thymocytes. Nature 1988; 333:742–746.
10. Kappler JW, Staerz U, White J, Marrack, P. Self-tolerance eliminates T cells specific for Mls-modified products of the major histocompatibility complex. Nature 1988; 332:35–40.
11. MacDonald HR, Lees RK, Schneider R, Zinkernagel RM, Hengartner H. Positive selection of CD4+ thymocytes controlled by MHC class II gene products. Nature 1988; 336:471–473.
12. Tough DF, Sprent J. Turnover of naive and memory phenotype T cells. J Exp Med 1994; 179:1127–1136.
13. Sprent J, Tough DF, Sun S. Factors controlling the turnover of T memory cells. Immunol

Rev 1997; 156:79–85.

14. Rocha B, Grandien A, Freitas AA. Anergy and exhaustion are independent mechanisms of peripheral T cell tolerance. J Exp Med 1995; 181:993–1003.

15. Tanchot C, Rocha B. The peripheral T-cell repertoire: independent homeostatic regulation of virgin and activated CD8+ T cell pools. Eur J Immunol 1995; 25:2127–2136.

16. Takeda S, Rodewald HR, Arakawa H, Bluethmann H, Shimizu T. MHC class II molecules are not required for survival of newly generated CD4+ T cells, but affect their long-term life span. Immunity 1996; 5:217–228.

17. Brocker T. Survival of mature CD4 T lymphocytes is dependent on major histocompatibility complex class II-expressing dendritic cells. J Exp Med 1997; 186:1223–1232.

18. Kirberg J, Berns A, von Boehmer H. Peripheral T-cell survival requires continual ligation of the T cell receptor to major histocompatibility complex-encoded molecules. J Exp Med 1997; 186:1269–1275.

19. Metz DP, Farber DL, Konig R. Bottomly K. Regulation of memory CD4 T cell adhesion by CD4-MHC class II interaction. J Immunol 1997; 159:2567–2573.

20. Tanchot C, Rocha B. Peripheral selection of T cell repertoires: the role of continuous thymus output. J Exp Med 1997; 186:1099–1106.

21. Buus S, Sette A, Colon SM, Miles C, Grey HM. The relation between major histocompatibility complex (MHC) restriction and the capacity of Ia to bind immunogenic peptides. Science 1987; 235:1353–1358.

22. Schaeffer EB, Sette A, Johnson DL, et al. Relative contribution of "determinant selection" and "holes in the T-cell repertoire" to T-cell responses. Proc Natl Acad Sci USA 1989; 86:4649–4653.

23. Kaslow RA, Carrington M, Apple R, et al. Influence of combinations of human major histocompatibility complex genes on the course of HIV-1 infection. Nat Med 1996; 2:405–411.

24. Saah, AJ, Hoover DR, Weng S, et al. Association of HLA profiles with early plasma viral load, CD4+ cell count and rate of progression to AIDS following acute HIV-1 infection. Multicenter AIDS Cohort Study. AIDS 1998; 12:2107–2113.

25. Carrington M, Nelson GW, Martin MP, et al. HLA and HIV-1: heterozygote advantage and B*35-Cw*04 disadvantage. Science 1999; 283:1748–1752.

26. Borrow P, Lewicki H, Hahn BH, Shaw GM, Oldstone MB. Virus-specific CD8+ cytotoxic T-lymphocyte activity associated with control of viremia in primary human immunodeficiency virus type 1 infection. J Virol 1994; 68:6103–6110.

27. Klenerman P, Phillips RE, Rinaldo CR, et al. Cytotoxic T lymphocytes and viral turnover in HIV type 1 infection. Proc Natl Acad Sci USA 1996; 93:15323–15328.

28. Borrow P, Lewicki H, Wei X, et al. Antiviral pressure exerted by HIV-1-specific cytotoxic T lymphocytes (CTLs) during primary infection demonstrated by rapid selection of CTL escape virus. Nat Med 1997; 3:205–211.

29. Ogg GS, Jin X, Bonhoeffer S, et al. Quantitation of HIV-1-specific cytotoxic T lymphocytes and plasma load of viral RNA. Science 1998; 279:2103–2106.

30. Jin X, Bauer DE, Tuttleton SE, et al. Dramatic rise in plasma viremia after CD8(+) T cell depletion in simian immunodeficiency virus-infected Macaques. J Exp Med 1999; 189:991–998.

31. Schmitz JE, Kuroda MJ, Santra S, et al. Control of viremia in simian immunodeficiency virus infection by CD8(+) lymphocytes. Science 1999; 283:857–860.

32. McKeithan TW. Kinetic proofreading in T-cell receptor signal transduction. Proc Natl Acad Sci USA 1995; 92:5042–5046.

33. Grakoui A, Bromley SK, Sumen C, et al. The immunological synapse: a molecular machine controlling T cell activation. Science 1999; 285:221–227.

34. Crabtree GR. Contingent genetic regulatory events in T lymphocyte activation. Science 1989; 243:355–361.

35. Kearney ER, Pape KA, Loh DY, Jenkins MK. Visualization of peptide-specific T cell immunity and peripheral tolerance in vivo. Immunity 1994; 1:327–339.

36. Weaver CT, Saparov A, Kraus LA, Rogers WO, Hockett RD, Bucy RP. Heterogeneity in the clonal T cell response. Implications for models of T cell activation and cytokine phenotype development. Immunol Res 1998; 17:279–302.

37. Bucy RP, Panoskaltsis-Mortari A, Huang GQ, et al. Heterogeneity of single cell cytokine gene expression in clonal T cell populations. J Exp Med 1994; 180:1251–1262.

38. Bucy RP, Karr L, Huang GQ, et al. Single-cell analysis of cytokine gene co-expression during naive CD4$^+$ T cell phenotype development. Proc Natl Acad Sci USA 1995; 92:7565–7569.

39. Rogers WO, Weaver CT, Kraus LA, Li J, Li L, Bucy RP. Visualization of antigen specific T cell activation and cytokine expression in vivo. J Immunol 1997; 158:649–657.

40. Hosken NA, Shibuya K, Heath AW, Murphy KM, O'Garra A. The effect of antigen dose on CD4+ T helper cell phenotype development in a T cell receptor-alpha beta-transgenic model. J Exp Med 1995; 182:1579–1584.

41. Itoh Y, Germain RN. Single cell analysis reveals regulated hierarchial T cell antigen receptor signaling thresholds and intraclonal heterogeneity for individual cytokine responses of CD4+ T cells. J Exp Med 1997; 186:757–766.

42. Swain SL, Weinberg AD, English M, Huston G. IL-4 directs the development of Th2-like helper effectors. J Immunol 1990; 145:3796–3806.

43. Hsieh, C-S, Heimberger AB, Gold JS, O'Garra A, Murphy KM. Differential regulation of T helper phenotype development by interleukins 4 and 10 in an $\alpha\beta$ T-cell-receptor transgenic system. Proc Natl Acad Sci USA 1993; 89:6065–6069.

44. Hsieh CS, Macatonia SE, Tripp CS, Wolf SF, O'Garra A, Murphy KM. Development of T$_H$ 1 CD4$^+$ T cells through IL-12 produced by *Listeria*-induced macrophages. Science 1993; 260:547–549.

45. Seder RA, Paul WE, Davis MM, de St Groth BF. The presence of interleukin 4 during in vitro priming determines the lymphokine-producing potential of CD4+ T cells from T cell receptor transgenic mice. J Exp Med 1992; 176:1091–1098.

46. Mosmann TR, Coffman RL. TH1 and TH2 cells: different patterns of lymphokine secretion lead to different functional properties. Annu Rev Immunol 1989; 7:145–173.

47. Croft M, Carter L, Swain SL, Dutton, RW. Generation of polarized antigen-specific CD8 effector populations: reciprocal action of interleukin (IL)-4 and IL-12 in promoting type 2 versus type 1 cytokine profiles. J Exp Med 1994; 180:1715–1728.

48. O'Garra A. Cytokines induce the development of functionally heterogeneous T helper cell subsets. Immunity 1998; 8:275–283.

49. Mosmann TR, Cherwinski H, Bond MW, Giedlin MA, Coffman RL. Two types of murine helper T cell clone. I. Definition according to profiles of lymphokine activities and secreted proteins. J Immunol 1986; 136:2348–2357.

50. Street NE, Mosmann TR. Functional diversity of T lymphocytes due to secretion of different cytokine patterns. FASEB J. 1991; 5:171–177.

51. Fiorentino DF, Bond MW, Mosmann TR. Two types of mouse T helper cell. IV. Th2 clones secrete a factor that inhibits cytokine production by Th1 clones. J Exp Med 1989; 170:2081–2095.

52. Gajewski TF, Fitch FW. Anti-proliferative effect of IFN gamma in immune regulation I. IFN gamma inhibits the proliferation of Th2 but not Th1 murine helper T lymphocyte clones. J Immunol 1988; 140:4245–4252.

53. Schreiber RD, Hicks LJ, Celada A, Buchmeier NA, Gray PW. Monoclonal antibodies to murine gamma-interferon which differentially modulate macrophage activation and antiviral activity. J Immunol 1985; 134:1609–1618.

54. Spitalny GL, Havell EA. Monoclonal antibody to murine gamma interferon inhibits lymphokine-induced antiviral and macrophage tumoricidal activities. J Exp Med 1984;

159:1560-1565.

55. Cher DJ, Mosmann TR. Two types of murine helper cell clone. II. Delayed-type hypersensitivity is mediated by T_H1 clones. J Immunol 1987; 138:3688–3694.

56. Fong TA, Mosmann TR. The role of IFN-gamma in delayed-type hypersensitivity mediated by Th1 clones. J Immunol 1989; 143:2887–2893.

57. DeKruyff RH, Ju ST, Hunt AJ, Mosmann TR, Umetsu DT. Induction of antigen-specific antibody responses in primed and unprimed B cells. Functional heterogeneity among Th1 and Th2 T-cell clones. J Immunol 1989; 142:2575–2582.

58. Croft M, Swain SL. B cell response to T helper cell subsets: II. Both the stage of T cell differentiation and the cytokines secreted determine the extent and nature of helper activity. J Immunol 1991; 147:3679–3689.

59. Fiorentino DF, Zlotnik A, Vieira P, et al. Il-10 acts on the antigen-presenting cell to inhibit cytokine production by Th1 cells. J Immunol 1991; 146:3444–3451.

60. Yamamura M, Uyemura K, Deans RJ, et al. Defining protective responses to pathogens: cytokine profiles in leprosy lesions. Science 1991; 254:277–279.

61. Henderson GS, Conray JT, Summar M, McCurley TL, Colley DG. In vivo molecular analysis of lymphokines involved in the murine immune response during *Schistosoma mansoni* infection. I. Il-4 mRNA, not IL-2 mRNA, is abundant in the granulomatous livers, mesenteric lymph nodes, and spleens of infected mice. J Immunol 1991; 147:992–997.

62. Holaday BJ, Sadick MD, Wang Z-E, et al. Reconstitution of *Leishmania* immunity in severe combined immunodeficient mice using Th1- and Th2-like cell lines. J Immunol 1991; 147:1653–1658.

63. Salgame P, Abrams JS, Clayberger C, et al. Differing lymphokine profiles of functional subsets of human CD4 and CD8 T-cell clones. Science 1991; 254:279–282.

64. Salgame P, Convit J, Bloom BR. Immunological suppression by human $CD8^+$ T cells is receptor dependent and HLA-DQ restricted. Proc Natl Acad Sci USA 1991; 88:2598–2602.

65. Sadick MD, Locksley RM, Tubbs C, Raff HV. Murine cutaneous leishmaniasis: resistance correlates with the capacity to generate interferon-gamma in response to *Leishmania* antigens in vitro. J Immunol 1986; 136:655–661.

66. Heinzel FP, Sadick MD, Holaday BJ, Coffman RL, Locksley RM. Reciprocal expression of interferon gamma or interleukin 4 during the resolution or progression of murine leishmaniasis. Evidence for expansion of distinct helper T cell subsets. J Exp Med 1989; 169:59–72.

67. Locksley RM, Heinzel FP, Holaday BJ, Mutha SS, Reiner SL, Sadick MD. Induction of Th1 and Th2 CD4+ subsets during murine *Leishmania* major infection. Res Immunol 1991; 142:28–32.

68. Coffman RL, Varkila K, Scott P, Chatelain R. Role of cytokines in the differentiation of $CD4^+$ T-cell subsets in vivo. Immunol Rev 1991; 123:189–207.

69. Kelso A. Th1 and Th2 subsets: paradigms lost? Immunol Today 1995; 16:374–379.

70. Miller A, Lider O, Roberts AB, Sporn MB, Weiner HL. Suppressor T cells generated by oral tolerization to myelin basic protein suppress both in vitro and in vivo immune responses by the release of transforming growth factor β after antigen-triggering. Proc Natl Acad Sci USA 1992; 89:421–425.

71. Chen Y, Kuchroo VK, Inobe J, Hafler DA, Weiner HL. Regulatory T cell clones induced by oral tolerance: suppression of autoimmune encephalomyelitis. Science 1994; 265:1237–1240.

72. Groux H, O'Garra A, Bigler M, et al. A CD4+ T-cell subset inhibits antigen-specific T-cell responses and prevents colitis. Nature 1997; 389:737–742.

73. Modlin RL, Kato H, Mehra V, et al. Genetically restricted suppressor T-cell clones derived from lepromatous leprosy lesions. Nature 1986; 322:459–461.

74. Bloom BR, Mehra V, Melancon Kaplan J, et al. Mechanisms of immunological unrespon-

siveness in the spectra of leprosy and leishmaniasis. Adv Exp Med Biol 1988; 239:263–278.

75. Guler ML, Gorham JD, Hsieh C-S, et al. Genetic susceptibility to *Leishmania:* IL-12 responsiveness in T_H1 cell development. Science 1996; 271:984–990.

76. Clerici M, Shearer GM. A TH1 → TH2 switch is a critical step in the etiology of HIV infection. Immunol Today 1993; 14:107–111.

77. Douek DC, McFarland RD, Keiser PH, et al. Changes in thymic function with age and during the treatment of HIV infection. Nature 1998; 396:690–695.

78. Sprent J, Tough D. HIV results in the frame. CD4+ cell turnover. Nature 1995; 375:194.

79. Mosier D. CD4+ cell turnover. Nature 1995; 375:193–194.

80. Bucy RP, Hockett RD, Derdeyn CA, et al. Initial increase in blood CD4+ lymphocytes after HIV antiretroviral therapy reflects redistribution from lymphoid tissues. J Clin Invest 1999; 103:1391–1398.

3

Immune Defense at Mucosal Surfaces

Prosper N. Boyaka and Jerry R. McGhee

INTRODUCTION

Mucosal immune responses include a major B-cell component characterized by surface IgA-positive ($SIgA^+$) B-cells that become plasma cells which produce polymeric IgA antibody (Ab). In addition, both T-helper (Th) cells and cytotoxic T-lymphocytes (CTLs) are induced in mucosa-associated lymphoreticular tissues (MALT) *(1)*. These B- and T-cell responses can be induced by pathogens in organized mucosal inductive sites. In fact, the host has evolved a sophisticated network of cells and molecules that maintain the homeostasis of exposed mucosal surfaces *(1,2)*. This system, termed MALT, is anatomically and functionally distinct from the systemic counterpart and is strategically located at the portal of entry of most microorganisms, including specific pathogens. Prior to the development of acquired immune responses, the mucosa are protected by innate defenses including the physical barrier provided by epithelial cells, secreted molecules with antibacterial activity, and the cytolytic activity of natural killer (NK) cells. However, effective protection against virulent mucosal pathogens requires prophylactic immune responses that can be achieved by mucosal vaccines, which, in contrast to systemic vaccines, can trigger both mucosal and systemic immunity. A major challenge for the development of mucosal vaccines will be to overcome the natural tendency of the host to suppress immune responses to orally administered antigens, a state commonly termed oral tolerance. In addition, effective protection against infectious agents will require the development of safe mucosal vaccines capable of promoting targeted immune responses.

THE COMMON MUCOSAL IMMUNE SYSTEM

The mucosal immune system can be divided into organized secondary lymphoid tissue (which allows antigen sampling, uptake, and presentation for initiation of the mucosal immune response) and more diffuse collections of lymphoid cells constituting mucosal effector sites *(2)*. It now well established that Peyer's patches, appendix, and solitary lymphoid nodules in the gastrointestinal (GI) tract constitute the inductive sites of the gut-associated lymphoreticular tissues (GALT). Similarly, the tonsils and adenoids may represent the nasal-associated lymphoreticular tissues (NALT) in the upper airway and aerodigestive tracts. Organized bronchus-associated lymphoreticular tissues

From: *Immunotherapy for Infectious Diseases*
Edited by: J. M. Jacobson © Humana Press Inc., Totowa, NJ

(BALT) *(3)* were also described at airway branches of experimental animals such as rabbits, rats, and guinea pigs, but these structures rarely occur in humans *(4)*. Collectively, GALT and NALT in humans and GALT, BALT, and NALT in experimental species are termed MALT. The mucosal effector tissues include the interstitial tissues of all exocrine glands, e.g., mammary, lacrymal, salivary, and sweat glands, as well as the lamina propria and the epithelium of the GI tract. In addition, lamina propria areas of the upper respiratory and genitourinary tracts are effector sites of this enormously large immune network. MALT is connected with effector sites through migratory patterns of lymphoid cells. Thus, immune effector cells initiated by encounter with antigen at one mucosal inductive site can migrate to distant mucosal effector sites, where they will exert their effector functions. The existence of this interconnected system of inductive and effector sites has been termed the common mucosal immune system (CMIS).

Mucosal Inductive Sites

Peyer's Patches of the GALT

The columnar epithelium that covers the MALT is infiltrated with B- and T-lymphocytes and antigen-presenting cells (APCs), which has led to the term follicle-associated epithelium (FAE). Soluble and particulate lumenal antigens are taken up by a microfold or M cell and delivered to adjacent APCs. M-cells have been described in human Peyer's patches, appendix, and tonsils *(5)*. These cells appear to be ideal for antigen uptake *(6)*. However, M-cells that only contain sparse numbers of lysosomes *(7)* probably do not degrade ingested antigens and thus are not classical APCs *(8)*. M-cells serve as the entry points for uptake; as such they actively ingest soluble proteins as well as particulate antigens, which can include viruses, bacteria, small parasites, and microspheres *(6,9–11)*. In addition to serving as a means of transport for lumenal antigens, the M-cells also provide an entry pathway for pathogens. A recent study suggested that lymphocytes and especially B-cells possess signaling molecules that induce M-cell differentiation of epithelial cells. In this study, mouse Peyer's patch T- and B-cells as well as a human B-cell line (Raji) induced Caco-2 cells to differentiate into M-like cells *(12)*.

Peyer's patches contain a dome region underneath the FAE, as well as underlying follicles that contain five or more germinal centers *(13)*. The dome region is characterized by the presence of T- and B-cells as well as both macrophages and dendritic cells (DCs). The presence of all three major APC types in the dome, e.g., memory B-cells, MØ and DCs make it likely that antigen uptake occurs immediately after release from M cells. Furthermore, Peyer's patch germinal centers differ from those in peripheral lymph nodes and spleen in that relatively high frequencies of SIgA$^+$ B-cells predominate *(14-17)*.

The regulation of Peyer's patch formation in mammals is only partially understood; nevertheless, recent studies suggest that interactions of membrane lymphotoxin (LT)/tumor necrosis factor (TNF) cytokines with LT-β receptor are of central importance in Peyer's patch development *(18,19)*. For example, injection of pregnant mice with lymphotoxin β-receptor Ig (LT-β-R-Ig) fusion protein resulted in loss of Peyer's patches *(19)* and most lymph nodes except the mesenteric lymph nodes. Recent studies with this model showed that Peyer's patches are not strictly required for the induction of mucosal S-IgA Ab responses and suggest a role for mesenteric lymph nodes as alternative inductive sites in the GI tract. Indeed, S-IgA Abs were induced when mice from LT-β-R-Ig-treated mothers were orally immunized with cholera toxin (CT) and a soluble protein antigen *(20)*. In contrast, neither systemic nor mucosal S-IgA Ab responses were seen after administration of the same oral vaccine regimen to TNF-α and LT-α double knockout mice that lack both Peyer's patches and mesenteric lymph nodes *(20)*. However, Peyer's patches appear to be crucial for the development of oral tolerance to protein antigens since mice from LT-β-R-Ig-treated mothers showed impaired induction of this type of tolerance *(21)*.

Other Mucosal Inductive Sites

The NALT includes the palatine, lingual, and nasopharyngeal tonsils, which collectively create a ring of tissue (Waldeyer's ring) that is strategically positioned at the entry of the digestive and respiratory tracts. These tissues possess structural features resembling both lymph nodes and Peyer's patches, including an FAE with M-cells in tonsillar crypts that are essential for selective antigen uptake. In addition, germinal centers containing B-cells, and professional APCs are also present. Direct unilateral injection of antigens (cholera toxin B subunit [CT-B] and tetanus toxoid [TT]) into the tonsil of human volunteers resulted in the induction of mucosal immune responses manifested by the appearance of antigen-specific IgG- and (to a lesser degree) IgA-producing cells in the noninjected tonsil *(22)*. These studies suggest that the tonsils may serve as an inductive site, analogous to Peyer's patches. Several recent nasal immunization studies have emphasized the importance of the NALT for induction of both mucosal and systemic immune responses that may exceed in magnitude those induced by oral immunization *(22–30)*.

Follicular structures analogous to Peyer's patches are also found in the large intestine, with especially pronounced accumulations in the rectum. In fact, monkeys immunized intrarectally with simian immunodeficiency virus (SIV) developed both T- and B-cell-mediated immune responses, including the induction of anti-SIV Abs in rectal washes and genital secretions *(31,32)*. Similarly, mice immunized intrarectally with CT or recombinant vaccinia virus expressing gp120 of SIV exhibited Abs responses in genital tract secretions as well as in serum; this immunization route was frequently superior to either the intragastric or intravaginal route *(33)*.

Homing of Effector Lymphocytes into Mucosal Compartments

Early studies in rabbits showed that GALT B-cells repopulated the gut with IgA plasma cells, suggesting a direct connection for B-cell migration between Peyer's patches and GI tract lamina propria *(34,35)*. Furthermore, orally immunized experimental animals possessed antigen-specific precursors of IgA plasma cells in GALT-associated mesenteric lymph nodes, which repopulated the lamina propria of the gut and the mammary, lacrymal, and salivary glands *(36–39)*. These studies, when combined with others showing that oral immunization led to S-IgA antibodies in multiple mucosal sites, served as the basis for suggesting a "common" mucosal immune system in humans *(40–42)*. Studies in recent years have unveiled molecular mechanisms involved in the migration of immune cells into the GI tract and, to a lesser extent, homing into other mucosal effector sites.

Lymphocyte Homing in the GI Tract

Naive lymphocytes enter mucosal or systemic lymphoid tissues from the blood through the endothelium via specialized high endothelial venules (HEVs) *(43)*. In GALT, HEV are present in the interfollicular zones rich in T-cells *(44)*. The mucosal addressin cell adhesion molecule-1 (MAdCAM-1) is the major addressin expressed by Peyer's patch HEV *(45)*. The major homing receptors expressed by lymphocytes are the integrins, which represent a large class of molecules characterized by a heterodimeric structure of α and β chains. In general, expression of the $\alpha 4$ chain paired with either $\beta 1$ or $\beta 7$ integrins differentiates between homing receptors for the skin or gut, respectively. Thus, the $\alpha 4 \beta 1$ pair allows binding to vascular cell adhesion molecule-1 (VCAM-1) and is associated with homing to inflamed sites and skin *(46,47)*. Pairing of $\alpha 4$ with $\beta 7$ represents the major integrin molecule responsible for lymphocyte binding to MAdCAM-1 expressed on HEVs in Peyer's patches *(48)*. A number of studies have now established that MAdCAM-1 is the major mucosal homing receptor ligand *(48-50)*. In addition to $\alpha 4 \beta 7$ integrin, L-selectin, which also binds to carbohydrate-decorated MAdCAM-1, is an important initial receptor for homing into GALT HEVs. Interestingly, L-selectin is expressed on all naive lymphocytes; however, memory T- and B-cells can be separated into $\alpha 4 \beta 7^{hi}$, L-selectin$^+$, and L-selectin$^-$ subsets *(51)*.

It is now clear that chemokines are directly involved in lymphocyte homing and that they trigger arrest and cell activation via specific Gsαi receptors *(52)*. For example, loss of secondary lymphoid tissue chemokine (SLC) results in lack of naive T-cell or dendritic cell migration into the spleen or Peyer's patches *(53)*. Furthermore, thymus-expressed chemokine (TECK) mediated human memory T-cell migration into the lamina propria of the GI tract. In fact, the gut homing $\alpha 4 \beta 7^{hi}$ T-cells expressed a TECK receptor, designated G-protein-coupled receptor-9-6, or CCR-9 *(54)*. Interestingly, human $\alpha E \beta 7^+$ as well as $\alpha 4 \beta 7^{hi}$ CD8 T-cells expressed CCR-9, suggesting that TECK-CCR-9 is also involved in lymphocyte homing and arrest of intraepithelial lymphocytes (IELs) into the GI tract epithelium *(54)*.

Lymphocyte Homing in NALT and Lung-Associated Tissues

Unlike Peyer's patch HEVs which are found in T-cell zones, murine NALT HEVs are found in B-cell zones and express, peripheral node addressin (PNAd) either alone or associated with MAdCAM-1 *(55)*. Furthermore, anti-L-selectin but not anti-MAdCAM-1 Abs blocked the binding of naive lymphocytes to NALT HEV, suggesting predominant roles for L-selectin and PNAd in the binding of naive lymphocytes to these HEVs *(55)*. In a rat model of antigen-induced lung inflammation, the percentage of activated T-cells expressing $\alpha 4$ was increased in the bronchial lumen compared with blood and lymph node T-cells after antigen challenge *(56)*. An interesting approach used to address the homing of human cells in the NALT was the analysis of tissue-specific adhesion molecules after systemic, enteric, or nasal immunization *(57)*. This study showed expression of L-selectin by most effector B-cells induced by systemic immunization, with only a small proportion expressing $\alpha 4 \beta 7$; the opposite was seen after enteric (oral or rectal) immunization. Interestingly, effector B-cells induced by intranasal immunization displayed a more promiscuous pattern of adhesion molecules, with a large majority of these cells expressing both L-selectin and $\alpha 4 \beta 7$ *(57)*.

IMMUNE RESPONSES IN MUCOSAL SURFACES

Mucosal Innate Immune Responses

In the mucosa, innate defense includes the physical barrier provided by epithelial cells and cilia movement, mucus production, secreted molecules with antibacterial activity, and the cytolytic activity of NK cells. Recent studies have demonstrated that a number of innate molecules produced at mucosal surfaces (including cytokines, chemokines, and defensins) can provide the necessary signals to enhance systemic or both systemic and mucosal immunity to antigens.

Barriere Function of Epithelial Cells

Mucosal surfaces are covered by a layer of epithelial cells that prevent the entry of exogenous antigens into the host. The physical protection of the largest mucosal surface, i.e., the GI tract, involves a monolayer of tightly joined absorptive epithelial cells termed enterocytes, which constitute a highly specialized selective barrier that allows the absorption of nutrients while preventing the entry of pathogens *(2)*. The barrier effect of intestinal epithelial cells is facilitated by the mucus blanket that covers these cells and prevents the penetration of microorganisms and the diffusion of molecules toward the intestinal surface. Mucus resembles glycoprotein and glycolipid receptors that occur on enterocyte membranes, tending to interfere with the attachment of microorganisms. The barrier effect of the epithelial surface is ensured by the continuous renewal of the epithelial cell layer. By this process, which results in complete renewal of the absorptive enterocyte layer every 2–3 days, damaged or infected enterocytes are replaced by crypt epithelial cells, which differentiate into enterocytes as they migrate toward the desquamation zone at the villus tip. The epithelia of other mucosal surfaces (including the oral cavity, pharynx, tonsils, urethra, and vagina) are made of stratified epithelial cells that lack tight junctions. However, the renewal of exposed epithelial cell layers by cells from subjacent layers and mucus secretion contribute to the permeability barrier effect on these surfaces as well.

Mucosal Antimicrobial Peptides

Epithelial cells also secrete antimicrobial peptides such as defensins, inflammatory cytokines, and chemokines, which contribute to mucosal innate immune responses. In this regard, the human intestinal α-defensins (HDs) HD-5 and HD-6 were identified in intestinal Paneth cells and in the human reproductive tract *(58)*. The α-Defensin are also secreted by tracheal epithelial cells, and they are homologous to peptides that function as mediators of nonoxidative microbial cell killing in human neutrophils (termed human neutrophil petide [HNPs]) *(59,60)*. The β-defensins, and in particular human β-defensin-1 (hBD-1), are expressed in the epithelial cells of the oral mucosa, trachea, and bronchi, as well as mammary and salivary glands in humans *(61-63)*. Human intestinal epithelial cells were reported to express hBD-1 constitutively, whereas hBD-2 was only seen in inflamed colon or after bacterial infection of a colonic epithelial cell line *(64)*. Secretory phospholipase A2 (S-PLA2) is an antimicrobial peptide present in granules of small intestinal Paneth cells and human polymorphonuclear neutrophils (PMNs). The S-PLA2 molecule is released by Paneth cells upon exposure to cholinergic agonists, bacteria, or lipopolysaccharide (LPS). High concentrations of

S-PLA2 are also found in human tears. In contrast to other PLA2 molecules produced by mammalian cells, the S-PLA2 preferentially removes bacterial phosphatidyl glycerol and phosphatidyl ethanolamine, a property that can explain the potent antimicrobial activity of S-PLA2 *(65,66)*. Other antimicrobials produced of mucosal surfaces include lysozyme, peroxidases, cathelin-associated peptides, and lactoferrin. In this regard, lactoferrin was recently reported to inhibit HIV-1 replication at the level of viral fusion/entry *(67)*.

Proinflammatory Cytokines and Chemokines

It is now well established that epithelial cells produce proinflammatory cytokines, including interleukin (IL)-1, IL-6, tumor necrosis factor-α (TNF-α), and granulocyte/macrophage colony-stimulating factor (GM-CSF) in response to pathogen invasion *(68,69)*. Interestingly, epithelial cells also express CxC and CC chemokines. For example, bacterial or parasitic (i.e., *Cryptosporidium parvum*) infections of intestinal epithelial cells were shown to upregulate expression and secretion of the CxC chemokines IL-8 and GRO-α *(70)*. Bacterial infection of intestinal epithelial cell lines was also reported to stimulate the expression of the CC chemokines monocyte chemotactic protein-1 (MCP-1), RANTES, and macrophage inflammatory protein-3α (MIP-3α) *(71,72)*, and freshly isolated colon epithelial cells produced an array of chemokines similar to the cell lines, as well as MIP-1α and MIP-1β *(71)*. More recently, inflammatory protein-10 (IP-10) and monokine inducible by interferon-γ (IFN-γ) (MIG), which are CxC chemokines that are known to attract CD4$^+$ T-cells, were detected in normal intestinal epithelial cells, and their expression was upregulated by infection with invasive bacteria or stimulation with proinflammatory cytokines *(73)*. Furthermore, γδ T-cell receptor-positive (TCR$^+$) (IELs) produce the C-type chemokine lymphotactin, which is chemotactic for T-cells and NK cells but not for monocytes, neutrophils, or dendritic cells *(74,75)*. Taken together, these studies clearly indicate that the mucosal epithelium has the potential to produce a large spectrum of C, CC, and CxC chemokines and that both epithelial cells and intestinal lymphocytes can contribute to these innate responses.

Mucosal Natural Killer Cells

NK cells are major players in the innate immune system, especially in the GI tract. NK cells occur in both the lamina propria and the intraepithelial compartment as large granular lymphocytes *(76,77)*. Studies performed on human IELs have shown that the αEβ7 integrin is the main surface molecule involved in the lysis process *(77)*. Significant increases in intestinal IEL NK cell activity were seen during the early phase of secondary infection of chickens with the *Eimeria* parasite *(78)*. Furthermore, nonspecific recruitment of cytotoxic effector cells into the intestinal mucosa of enteric virus-infected mice has been reported *(79)*. Humans with inherited deficiency of NK cells experience more severe herpesvirus infections *(80)*; however, these individuals clear the virus infection in a fashion comparable to that seen in immunocompetent subjects, suggesting that the role of NK cells may be to limit the extent of certain mucosal viral infections. Finally, NK cells are known to secrete interferon-γ (IFN-γ) and IL-4 after infection. Thus, mucosal NK cells could be major players in the cytokine environment that influences the development of effector T-cells.

Mucosal Adaptive Immune Responses

Cytokines In Mucosal Immunity

It is now well accepted that the functional diversity of the immune response is exemplified by an inverse relationship between antibody and cell-mediated immune responses. This dichotomy is due to Th cell subsets, which are classified as either Th1 or Th2 according to the pattern of cytokines produced *(81)*. Thus, Th1 cells produce IL-2, IFN-γ and lymphotoxin-α (LT-α, also known as TNF-β), LT-β and TNF-α, and Th2 cells produce IL-4, IL-5, IL-6, IL-9, IL 10, and IL-13. The cytokine environment plays a key role in the differentiation of both Th cell subsets from precursor Th0 cells. IL-2 is produced by Th0 cells upon antigen exposure and serves as an important growth factor. IL-12 induces NK cells to produce IFN-γ *(82,83)*, which, together with IL-12, triggers Th0 cells to differentiate along the Th1 pathway. Murine Th1-type responses are associated with development of cell-mediated immunity as manifested by delayed-type hypersensitivity (DTH) as well as by B-cell responses with characteristic IgG Ab subclass patterns.

For example, IFN-γ induces murine $\mu \rightarrow \gamma 2a$ switches *(84)* and production of complement-fixing IgG2a antibodies. On the other hand, IL-4 production induces Th0 $\rightarrow$ Th2-type development. The production of IL-4 by Th2 cells is supportive of B-cell switches from sIgM expression to SIgG1$^+$ and to sIgE$^+$ B-cells *(85–87)*. Furthermore, the Th2 cell subset is an effective helper phenotype for supporting the IgA isotype in addition to IgG1, IgG2b, and IgE responses in the mouse system. Both Th1 and Th2 cells are also quite sensitive to cross-regulation. IFN-γ produced by Th1 cells inhibits both Th2 cell proliferation and B-cell isotype switching stimulated by IL-4 *(88,89)*. Likewise, Th2 cells regulate Th1 cell effects by secreting IL-10, which inhibits IFN-γ secretion by Th1 cells. This decreased IFN-γ production allows development of Th2-type cells. It is also clear that Th1- and Th2-type cells express distinct patterns of chemokine receptors *(90,91)*. Thus, CCR5 and the CxC chemokine receptors CxCR3 and CxCR5 are preferentially expressed by human Th1 cell clones, whereas Th2 cells express CCR4 and to a lesser extent CCR3 *(91,92)*.

Studies in the last decade have shown that two Th2 cytokines, IL-5 and IL-6, are of particular importance for inducing SIgA$^+$ B-cells to differentiate into IgA-producing plasma cells *(93-95)*. In this regard, IL-6 induced strikingly high IgA responses in vitro in both mouse *(93–95)* and human *(96)* systems. However, the role of IL-6 in IgA responses in vivo remains to be demonstrated since both reduced *(97)* and normal IgA responses were reported in IL-6$^{-/-}$ mice *(98)*. IL-10 has also been shown to play an important role in the induction of IgA synthesis, especially in humans *(99-101)*. Finally, high frequencies of Th2 cells producing IL-5, IL-6, and IL-10 were shown in mucosal effector sites (e.g., the intestinal lamina propria and the salivary glands) where IgA responses predominate *(102,103)*.

Secretory IgA Antibodies

The S-IgA Abs constitute the predominant isotype present at mucosal surfaces, and they are the first Abs to come into contact with the microorganisms that have entered the host through the mucosae. Inhibition of microbial adherence is a critical initial step for the protection of the host and is mediated by both specific and nonspecific mechanisms. For instance, the agglutinating ability of S-IgA specific to capsular poly-saccharide of *Hemophilus influenzae* seems to be crucial for avoiding colonization by *H. influenzae (104)*. Finally, another nonspecific mechanism that inhibits microbial adherence is owing to the presence of carbohydrate chains on the S-IgA molecule that bind to bacteria or other antigens *(105–107)*. The S-IgA Abs have been shown to be effective at neutralizing viruses at different steps in the infectious process. In particu-lar, S-IgA specific for influenza hemagglutinin can interfere with the initial binding of influenza virus to target cells or with the internalization and the intracellular replica-tion of the virus *(108)*. The S-IgA can neutralize the catalytic activity of many enzymes of microbial origin (such as neuraminidase, hyaluronidase, glycosyltransferase and IgA-specific protease), as well as the toxic activity of bacterial enterotoxins (cholera toxin and the related heat-labile enterotoxin of *E. coli*). In vitro experiments employ-ing murine polarized epithelial cells have demonstrated that antibodies specific to rotavirus and hepatitis virus can neutralize the respective viruses inside the epithelial cells *(109,110)*, and evidence has been provided that similar mechanisms occur in vivo *(111)*. Similarly, it has been shown that transcytosis of primary HIV isolates is blocked by polymeric IgA specific to HIV envelope proteins *(112)*. These authors have shown that neutralization of HIV transcytosis occurs within the apical recycling endosome and that immune complexes are specifically recycled to the mucosal surface *(112)*.

It should be mentioned that S-IgA appears to be important in limiting inflammation at mucosal surfaces. In fact, IgA Abs are unable to activate complement and interfere with IgM- and IgG-mediated complement activation *(113,114)*. Furthermore, S-IgA inhibits phagocytosis, bactericidal activity, and chemotaxis by neutrophils, monocytes, and macrophages. In addition, IgA can downregulate the synthesis of TNF- α and IL-6 as well as enhance the production of IL-1R antagonists by LPS-activated human monocytes *(115,116)*.

Mucosal Cytotoxic T-Lymphocytes

There is a clear demarcation between inductive sites, which harbor precursor (p)CTLs, and effector sites, which include the lamina propria and the epithelial cells where activated $CD8^+$ CTLs function. it is now established that administration of virus into the GI tract results in a higher frequency of pCTL in Peyer's patches *(117,118)*. For example, reovirus localizes to T-cell regions and is clearly associated with increased $CD8^+$ pCTLs and memory B-cell responses *(119)*. Oral administration of *Vaccinia* to rats resulted in the induction of virus-specific CTLs in Peyer's patches and mesenteric lymph nodes *(120)*. These findings suggest that after enteric infection or immunization, antigen-stimulated CTLs are disseminated from Peyer's patches into mesenteric lymph nodes via the lymphatic drainage *(120)*. Furthermore, virus-specific CTLs are also gen-erated in mucosa-associated tissues by oral immunization with reovirus and rotavirus *(117,118)* and a high frequency of virus-specific CTLs is present in the Peyer's patches as early as 6 days after oral immunization. These studies suggest that oral immuniza-tion with live virus can induce antigen-specific CTLs in both mucosal inductive and effector tissues for mucosal responses and in systemic lymphoid tissues as well.

The vaginal infection model of rhesus macaques with SIV has been useful in stud-ies of immunity to SIV in the female reproductive tract *(121,122)*. Recent studies in this model have provided direct evidence that pCTLs occur in female macaque reproductive tissues and that infection with SIV induces CTL responses *(123)*. This important finding has now been extended to vaginal infection with an SIV/HIV-1 chimeric virus (SHIV) containing HIV-1 89.6 env gene *(124)*. Interestingly, all macaques resisted two challenges with virulent SIV, and functional, gag-specific CTLs were present in the peripheral blood *(124)*. Again, it should be emphasized that vaginal Abs were also induced; however, these results clearly indicate that mucosal CTL responses may be of importance in immunity to SIV infection. Recent work has shown that intranasal immunization with SIV/HIV components induces antibody responses in vaginal secretions (reviewed in ref. *125*). It should be noted that intranasal immunization of mice with HIV-1 T-cell epitopes and the mucosal adjuvant CT induced functional CTLs *(126)*. This evidence suggests that mucosal delivery of SIV/HIV components can induce mucosal CTLs that will contribute to immunity.

MUCOSAL ADJUVANTS AND DELIVERY SYSTEMS

Since immune effector cells initiated by triggering mucosal inductive sites can migrate to the systemic compartment and to distant mucosal sites, mucosal administration of vaccines represents an attractive strategy for provision of immunity in both the mucosal and systemic compartments. Unfortunately, probably because the mucosal surfaces are continuously exposed to a myriad of exogenous antigens, most protein antigens are poorly immunogenic when given mucosally. Furthermore, oral delivery of antigen can instead result in immunologic unresponsiveness (oral tolerance). Therefore, adjuvants or antigen delivery systems are needed to ensure the development of effective immune responses to mucosally delivered antigens. For reasons still to be elucidated, classic systemic adjuvants such as alum are unable to stimulate mucosal S-IgA Ab responses. Unlike many protein antigens, the bacterial enterotoxin CT is highly immunogenic when administered by mucosal routes *(127)*. Furthermore, CT and the related heat-labile toxin (LT)-I from *E. coli* are effective adjuvants that promote mucosal and systemic immune responses to coadministered antigens *(128–130)*. However, the toxicity of these molecules precludes their use in humans. Recombinant attenuated bacterial and viral vectors were found to be effective mucosal delivery systems for induction of mucosal immunity *(131,132)*. Again, however, toxicity issues will need to be addressed before their use in humans. Some of the strategies to develop safe mucosal vaccines are discussed below.

Nontoxic Enterotoxin Derivatives

Although CT and LT were identified as effective mucosal adjuvants, the enterotoxicity of these molecules has precluded their use in human vaccines. The main strategy undertaken to make these molecules more suitable for use in humans consisted of developing mutants that lack the adenosine diphosphate (ADP) ribosyl transferase activity of the native toxins. Other approaches include substitution of the B subunit by a B-cell targeting moiety and the covalent binding of protein antigens to CT-B or LT-B.

ADP-Ribosylation-Defective Mutants of CT and LT

Mutants defective in ADP-ribosyl transferase activity were generated by single amino acid substitutions in the ADP-ribosylation activity site of the A subunit of CT or LT or in the protease-sensitive loop of LT. In this regard, cholera toxin is a heterologous macromolecule consisting of two structurally and functionally separate A and B subunits *(133,134)*. The B subunit of CT consists of five identical 11.6-kD peptides that bind to GM1 gangliosides *(135)*. The binding of CT-B to GM1 ganglioside on epithelia allows the A subunit to reach the cytosol of target cells, where it binds to nicotinamide (N) ADP and catalyzes the ADP ribosylation of Gsα protein. The later guanosine triphosphate (GTP) binding protein activates adenyl cyclase with subsequent elevation of cyclic adenosine monophosphate (cAMP) in epithelial cells followed by secretion of water and chloride ions into the intestinal lumen *(136)*. The labile toxin from *E. coli* is closely related to CT, and the two enterotoxins share 80% amino acid sequence homology *(137)*. Although both CT and LT bind GM1 gangliosides, LT also exhibits an affinity for GM2 and asialo-GM1 *(134)*.

Two CT mutants were contructed by substitution of serine by phenylalanine at position 61 (CT-S61F) and glutamate by lysine at position 112 (CT-E112K) in the ADP-ribosyl transferase activity center of the CT gene from *Vibrio cholerae* 01 strain GP14. Similar substitutions in LT have been shown to inactivate ADP-ribosyl-transferase activity and enterotoxicity completely *(138,139)*. The levels of antigen-specific serum IgG and secretory IgA Abs induced by the mutants are comparable to those induced by wild-type CT and are significantly higher than those induced by recombinant CT-B *(140, 141)*. Furthermore, the mutant CT-E112K, like nCT, induces Th2-type responses through a preferential inhibition of Th1-type CD4$^+$ T-cells, and both nCT and mCTs enhanced the expression of costimulatory molecules of the B7 family and their corresponding receptors *(142,143)*. Mutations in other sites of the CT molecule were reported to induce nontoxic derivatives, but the adjuvant activity was also affected. For example, the CT-106S mCT, with a partial knockout of the ADP-ribosylating activity, exhibited an adjuvant activity lower that that of wild-type CT *(144)*.

Mutant LT molecules with either a residual ADP-ribosyltransferase activity (e.g., LT-72R) or totally devoid of such enzymatic activity (e.g., LT-7K and LT-63K) can function as mucosal adjuvants when intranasally administered to mice together with unrelated antigens *(26,145,146)*. When mLTs were tested as mucosal adjuvants, they generally induced mucosal and systemic Ab responses comparable to those of nLTs, although higher doses of mLT were often needed *(147)*. Since LT induces a mixed CD4$^+$ Th1- (i.e., IFN-γ) and Th2-type (i.e., IL-4, IL-5, IL-6, and IL-10) response *(148)*, one might envision the use of mutants of LT where both Th1- and Th2-type responses are desired.

Other CT and LT Derivatives

It has also been hypothesized that the strong toxic effect of CT and LT could be largely owing to their promiscuous binding to cells via their B subunits. This assumption led to the construction of a fusion protein consisting of CTA1 and two Ig binding domains (DD) of staphylococcal protein A, which binds IgG, IgE, IgA, and IgM *(149)*. The CTA1-DD fusion protein displayed adjuvant activity when given by the nasal route and promoted both mucosal and systemic immune responses *(149)*. More detailed analyses of CTA1-DD adjuvanticity have shown that this CT derivative promotes both T-cell-dependent and -independent responses and that both the ADP-ribosylation and Ig binding activities were required *(150,151)*.

Another approach used to develop nontoxic derivatives of CT consisted of genetically substituting the entire CT-A subunit, or the toxic CT-A1 portion, with a protein antigen. Thus, nasal or oral immunization with the chimeric fusion protein made of

CT-B/A2 and a *Streptococcus mutans* protein adhesin elicited antigen-specific mucosal and systemic immunity *(152)*. Similarly, nasal immunization with CT-B conjugated to a *Schistosoma mansoni* antigen protected infected animals from schistosomiasis *(153)*. It is important to note that mucosal administration of low doses of antigen coupled to CT-B was shown to induce tolerance *(154,155)*. Thus, caution is recommended when using antigen coupled to CT-B for induction of mucosal immunity or tolerance.

Cytokines and Chemokines as Mucosal Adjuvants

The use of cytokines and chemokines to enhance the immune responses to mucosal vaccines is an attractive strategy for several reasons. First, cytokines and chemokines act by often known mechanisms through specific interactions with corresponding receptors. Furthermore, whereas important adverse effects are often associated with large and repeated parenteral cytokine doses generally required for the effective targeting of tissues/organs, only low serum cytokine levels are achieved after mucosal delivery of these regulatory molecules *(156)*. Finally, cytokines/chemokines that influence the development of Th cell subsets can help promote targeted Th1-type responses for protection against intracellular pathogens or Th2-type responses required for protection against soluble antigens and toxins.

The cytokines IL-1, IL-6, and IL-12 were recently tested for their ability to enhance mucosal and systemic immune responses to nasal vaccines. A nasal vaccine of TT given with either IL-6 or IL-12 induced serum TT-specific IgG Ab responses that protected mice against lethal challenge with tetanus toxin, suggesting that both IL-6 and IL-12 can enhance protective systemic immunity to mucosal vaccines *(157)*. Furthermore, IL-12 but not IL-6 as an adjuvant induced high titers of S-IgA Ab responses in the GI tract, vaginal washes, and saliva *(157)*. In another system, mice nasally immunized with soluble influenza H1 and N1 proteins and IL-12 developed anti-influenza systemic and mucosal immunity, further demonstrating that nasal IL-12 does not require additional stimuli for induction of S-IgA Ab responses *(158)*. Nasal administration of protein antigens with IL-1 also enhanced systemic and mucosal immune responses to coadministered antigens *(159)*. As an illustration of the potential of regulatory cytokines to promote targeted immunity, IL-12 was shown to redirect CT-induced antigen-specific Th2-type responses toward the Th1-type when given by oral *(160)* or intranasal routes *(156)*. In addition, IL-12 could also promote both Th1- and Th2-type responses when administered by a separate mucosal route than a vaccine regimen containing CT as an adjuvant *(156)*.

As mentioned above, a number of innate molecules are secreted in mucosal epithelia. To test whether these molecules could provide signals to bridge the innate and adaptive mucosal immune systems, protein antigens were given nasally with α-defensins, (i.e., HNPs) *(161)*, lymphotactin *(162)*, or RANTES *(163)*. All of these vaccine regimens were found to promote systemic immune responses to the coadministered antigen *(161–163)*. Furthermore, whereas defensins failed to promote mucosal S-IgA Ab responses, significant S-IgA Abs were induced by the CC chemokine RANTES and the C chemokine lymphotactin *(161–163)*. The adjuvant activity of lymphotactin resulted in Th1- and Th2-type responses, whereas only Th1- and selected Th2-type cytokines were produced by RANTES-induced CD4$^+$ Th cells *(162,163)*.

Immunostimulating DNA Sequences and Saponin Derivatives

Immunostimulatory DNA Sequences

Bacterial but not eukaryotic DNA contain immunostimulatory sequences consisting of short palindromic nucleotides centered around a CpG dinucleotide core, e.g., 5'-purine-purine-CG-pyrimidine-pyrimidine-3' or CpG motifs *(164)*. It is now clear that CpG motifs can induce B-cell proliferation and Ig synthesis as well as cytokine secretion (i.e., IL-6, IFN-α, IFN-β, IFN-γ, IL-12, and IL-18) by a variety of immune cells *(165)*. Since CpG motifs create a cytokine microenvironment favoring Th1-type responses, they can be used as adjuvants to stimulate antigen-specific Th1-type responses or to redirect harmful allergic or Th2-dominated autoimmune responses. Indeed, coinjection of bacterial DNA or CpG motifs with a DNA vaccine or with a protein antigen promotes Th1-type responses even in mice with a preexisting Th2-type of immunity *(166,167)*. In addition, vaccination of mice with hen egg lysozyme (HEL) and a CpG oligonucleotide in incomplete Freund's adjuvant induced a Th1-type response comparable to that achieved by injecting HEL in complete Freund's adjuvant *(168)*. It has also been reported that CpG motifs can enhance systemic as well as mucosal immune responses when given intranasally to mice *(169)*. The observation that these CpG motifs can also function as mucosal adjuvants was confirmed by the finding that delivery to lungs of hepatitis B surface antigen (HBsAg) with CpG DNA resulted in high HBsAg-specific mucosal and systemic immune responses *(170)*.

Saponin Derivatives

Immunostimulating complexes (ISCOMs) are cage-like particules generated after addition of cholesterol to the Quil A from the bark of the *Quillaja saponaria* Molina tree *(171)*. Since antigens can be incorporated into ISCOMs, these particules represent good delivery systems for mucosal vaccines. In fact, ISCOMs are effective oral delivery systems that promote mucosal and systemic immunity *(172)*. It is believed that the cage-like structure of ISCOMs protects both the antigen and Quil A from degradation in the GI tract. However, ISCOMs appeared to be toxic after parenteral immunization of experimental animals. It is possible that ISCOMs are less toxic after oral delivery. This point will need to be carefully addressed before considering a broader use of ISCOMs.

QS-21 is a highly purified complex triterpene glycoside isolated from the bark of the *Quillaja saponaria* Molina tree *(173,174)*. This molecule promotes both humoral and cell-mediated immunity when added to systemic vaccine formulations *(175–177)* and is now being tested in several parenteral vaccine formulations *(173)*. QS-21 was reported to act as an adjuvant for both systemic and mucosal immunity to a nasally administered DNA vaccine *(178)*. More recently, it has been shown that QS-21 also acts as adjuvant when administered by the oral route *(179)*. Interestingly, low oral QS-21 doses promoted mucosal S-IgA Abs responses, whereas no S-IgA responses were induced by high oral QS-21 *(179)*. On the other hand, stronger Th1-type responses were seen after immunization with high oral QS-21 doses *(179)*.

CONCLUSIONS

The increasing numbers of bacteria that are resistant to antibiotic therapy and the inefficiency of antiviral drugs to resolve virus infections leave vaccines as the most promising immunoprophylactic approach against infectious diseases. Mucosal surfaces, which are the main portal of entry for exogenous pathogens, are protected by a first line of innate defenses provided by epithelial cells, NK cells, and IELs. Although regulation of these innate defenses is only partially understood, a growing body of evidence shows that mucosal innate factors can provide the necessary signals for the development of adaptive immunity. It is also clear that effective protection of mucosal surfaces can only be achieved by vaccines promoting both systemic and mucosal immunity. A number of mucosal adjuvants and delivery systems capable of inducing mucosal S-IgA Abs as well as systemic immunity have been identified. However, toxicity issues preclude their use in humans (i.e., native enterotoxin, as well as the complex saponin derivatives such as Quil A and recombinant bacterial and viral vectors). Safe mucosal adjuvants and vaccination strategies are being developed to induce targeted Th1- or Th2-type immunity for optimal protection against different pathogens.

REFERENCES

1. McGhee JR, Lamm ME, Strober W. Mucosal immune responses: an overview. In: Ogra PL, et al. (eds). Mucosal Immunology. San Diego: Academic, 1999, pp. 485–506.
2. McGhee JR, Kiyono H. The mucosal immune system. In: Paul WE (ed). Fundamental Immunology. Philadelphia: Lippincott-Raven, 1999, pp. 909–945.
3. Bienenstock J, McDermot MR, Clancy RL. Respiratory tract defenses: role of mucosal lymphoid tissues. In: Ogra PL, et al. (eds). Mucosal Immunology. San Diego: Academic, 1999, pp. 283–292.
4. Pabst R. Is BALT a major component of the human lung immune system? Immunol Today 1992; 13:119–122.
5. Owen RL, Jones AL. Epithelial cell specialization within human Peyer's patches: an ultrastructural study of intestinal lymphoid follicles. Gastroenterology 1974; 66:189–203.
6. Neutra MR, Frey A, Kraehenbuhl JP. Epithelial M cells: gateways for mucosal infection and immunization. Cell 1996; 86:345–348.
7. Owen RL, Apple RT, Bhalla DK. Morphometric and cytochemical analysis of lysosomes in rat Peyer's patch follicle epithelium: their reduction in volume fraction and acid phosphatase content in M cells compared to adjacent enterocytes. Anat Rec 1986; 216:521–527.
8. Neutra MR, Kreahenbuhl JP. Cellular and molecular basis for antigen transport across epithelial barriers. In: Ogra PL, et al. (eds). Mucosal Immunology. San Diego: Academic, 1999, pp. 110–114.
9. Wolf JL, Bye WA. The membranous epithelial (M) cell and the mucosal immune system. Ann Rev Medi 1984; 35:95–112.
10. Gebert A, Rothkotter HJ, Pabst R. M cells in Peyer's patches of the intestine. Int Rev Cytol 1996; 167:91–159.
11. Ermak TH, Dougherty EP, Bhagat HR, Kabok Z, Pappo J. Uptake and transport of copolymer biodegradable microspheres by rabbit Peyer's patch M cells. Cell Tissue Res 1995; 279:433–436.
12. Kerneis S, Bogdanova A, Kraehenbuhl JP, Pringault E. Conversion by Peyer's patch lymphocytes of human enterocytes into M cells that transport bacteria. Science 1997; 277:949–952.
13. Brandtzaeg P, Baklien K, Bjerke K, Rognum TO, Scott H, Valnes K. Nature and properties of the human gastrointestinal immune system. In: Miller K, Nicklin S (eds). Immunology of the Gastrointestinal Tract. Boca Raton, FL: CRC, 1987, pp. 1–85.
14. George A, Cebra JJ. Responses of single germinal-center B cells in T-cell-dependent microculture. Proc Natl Acad Sci USA 1991; 88:11–15.
15. Butcher EC, Rouse RV, Coffman RL, Nottenburg CN, Hardy RR, Weissman IL. Surface phenotype of Peyer's patch germinal center cells: implications for the role of germinal centers in B cell differentiation. J Immunol 1982; 129:2698–2707.

16. Lebman DA, Griffin PM, Cebra JJ. Relationship between expression of IgA by Peyer's patch cells and functional IgA memory cells. J Exp Med 1987; 166:1405–1418.

17. Weinstein PD, Cebra JJ. The preference for switching to IgA expression by Peyer's patch germinal center B cells is likely due to the intrinsic influence of their microenvironment. J Immunol 1991; 147:4126–4135.

18. Erickson SL, de Sauvage FJ, Kikly K, et al. Decreased sensitivity to tumour-necrosis factor but normal T-cell development in TNF receptor-2-deficient mice. Nature 1994; 372:560–563.

19. Rennert PD, Browning JL, Mebius R, Mackay F, Hochman PS. Surface lymphotoxin alpha/beta complex is required for the development of peripheral lymphoid organs. J Exp Med 1996; 184:1999–2006.

20. Yamamoto M, Rennert P, McGhee JR, et al. Alternate mucosal immune system: organized Peyer's patches are not required for IgA responses in the gastrointestinal tract. J Immunol 2000; 164:5184 5191.

21. Fujihashi K, Dohi T, Rennert PD, et al. Peyer's patches are required for oral tolerance to proteins. Proc Natl Acad Sci USA 2001; 98:3310–3315.

22. Quiding-Jarbrink M, Granstrom G, Nordstrom I, Holmgren J, Czerkinsky C. Induction of compartmentalized B-cell responses in human tonsils. Infect Immun 1995; 63:853–857.

23. Lubeck MD, Natuk RJ, Chengalvala M, et al. Immunogenicity of recombinant adenovirus-human immunodeficiency virus vaccines in chimpanzees following intranasal administration. AIDS Res Hum Retroviruses 1994;10:1443–1449.

24. Gallichan WS, Rosenthal KL. Specific secretory immune responses in the female genital tract following intranasal immunization with a recombinant adenovirus expressing glycoprotein B of herpes simplex virus. Vaccine 1995; 13:1589–1595.

25. Pal S, Peterson EM, de la Maza LM. Intranasal immunization induces long-term protection in mice against a *Chlamydia trachomatis* genital challenge. Infect Immun 1996; 64:5341–5348.

26. Di Tommaso A, Saletti G, Pizza M, et al. Induction of antigen-specific antibodies in vaginal secretions by using a nontoxic mutant of heat-labile enterotoxin as a mucosal adjuvant. Infect Immun 1996; 64:974–979.

27. Staats HF, Jackson RJ, Marinaro M, Takahashi I, Kiyono H, McGhee JR. Mucosal immunity to infection with implications for vaccine development. Curr Opin Immunol 1994; 6:572–583.

28. Russell MW, Moldoveanu Z, White PL, Sibert GJ, Mestecky J, Michalek SM. Salivary, nasal, genital, and systemic antibody responses in monkeys immunized intranasally with a bacterial protein antigen and the cholera toxin B subunit. Infect Immun 1996; 64:1272–1283.

29. Johansson EL, Rask C, Fredriksson M, Eriksson K, Czerkinsky C, Holmgren J. Antibodies and antibody-secreting cells in the female genital tract after vaginal or intranasal immunization with cholera toxin B subunit or conjugates. Infect Immun 1998; 66:514–520.

30. Bergquist C, Johansson EL, Lagergard T, Holmgren J, Rudin A. Intranasal vaccination of humans with recombinant cholera toxin B subunit induces systemic and local antibody responses in the upper respiratory tract and the vagina. Infect Immun 1997; 65:2676–2684.

31. Lehner T, Bergmeier LA, Panagiotidi C, et al. Induction of mucosal and systemic immunity to a recombinant simian immunodeficiency viral protein. Science 1992; 258:1365–1369.

32. Lehner T, Brookes R, Panagiotidi C, et al. T- and B-cell functions and epitope expression in nonhuman primates immunized with simian immunodeficiency virus antigen by the rectal route. Proc Natl Acad Sci USA 1993; 90:8638–8642.

33. Moldoveanu Z, Russell MW, Wu HY, Huang WQ, Compans RW, Mestecky J. Compartmentalization within the common mucosal immune system. Adv Exp Med Biol 1995; 371A:97–101.

34. Craig SW, Cebra JJ. Peyer's patches: an enriched source of precursors for IgA-producing immunocytes in the rabbit. J Exp Med 1971; 134:188–200.

35. Craig SW, Cebra JJ. Rabbit Peyer's patches, appendix, and popliteal lymph node B lymphocytes: a comparative analysis of their membrane immunoglobulin components and plasma cell precursor potential. J Immunol 1975; 114:492–502.

36. McDermott MR, Bienenstock J. Evidence for a common mucosal immunologic system. I. Migration of B immunoblasts into intestinal, respiratory, and genital tissues. J Immunol 1979; 122:1892–1898.

37. McWilliams M, Phillips-Quagliata JM, Lamm ME. Characteristics of mesenteric lymph node cells homing to gut-associated lymphoid tissue in syngeneic mice. J Immunol 1975; 115:54–58.

38. McWilliams M, Phillips-Quagliata JM, Lamm ME. Mesenteric lymph node B lymphoblasts which home to the small intestine are precommitted to IgA synthesis. J Exp Med 1977; 145:866–875.

39. Roux ME, McWilliams M, Phillips-Quagliata JM, Weisz-Carrington P, Lamm ME. Origin of IgA-secreting plasma cells in the mammary gland. J Exp Med 1977; 146:1311–1322.

40. Czerkinsky C, Prince SJ, Michalek SM, et al. IgA antibody-producing cells in peripheral blood after antigen ingestion: evidence for a common mucosal immune system in humans. Proc Natl Acad Sci USA 1987; 84:2449–2453.

41. Kantele A, Arvilommi H, Jokinen I. Specific immunoglobulin-secreting human blood cells after peroral vaccination against *Salmonella* typhi. J Infect Dis 1986; 153:1126–1131.

42. Quiding M, Nordstrom I, Kilander A, et al. Intestinal immune responses in humans. Oral cholera vaccination induces strong intestinal antibody responses and interferon-gamma production and evokes local immunological memory. J Clin Invest 1991; 88:143–148.

43. Kraal G, Mebius RE. High endothelial venules: lymphocyte traffic control and controlled traffic. Adv Immunol 1997; 65:347–395.

44. Butcher EC. Lymphocyte homing and intestinal immunity. In: Ogra PL, et al. (eds). Mucosal Immunology. San Diego: Academic, 1999, pp. 507–522.

45. Berlin C, Berg EL, Briskin MJ, et al. Alpha 4 beta 7 integrin mediates lymphocyte binding to the mucosal vascular addressin MAdCAM-1. Cell 1993; 74:185–195.

46. Bevilacqua MP. Endothelial-leukocyte adhesion molecules. Annu Rev Immunol 1993; 11:767–804.

47. Osborn L. Leukocyte adhesion to endothelium in inflammation. Cell 1990; 62:3–6.

48. Holzmann B, McIntyre BW, Weissman IL. Identification of a murine Peyer's patch—specific lymphocyte homing receptor as an integrin molecule with an alpha chain homologous to human VLA-4 alpha. Cell 1989; 56:37–46.

49. Bell RG, Issekutz T. Expression of a protective intestinal immune response can be inhibited at three distinct sites by treatment with anti-alpha 4 integrin. J Immunol 1993; 151: 4790–4802.

50. Hamann A, Andrew DP, Jablonski-Westrich D, Holzmann B, Butcher EC. Role of alpha 4-integrins in lymphocyte homing to mucosal tissues in vivo. J Immunol 1994; 152: 3282–3293.

51. Rott LS, Briskin MJ, Andrew DP, Berg EL, Butcher EC. A fundamental subdivision of circulating lymphocytes defined by adhesion to mucosal addressin cell adhesion molecule-1. Comparison with vascular cell adhesion molecule-1 and correlation with beta 7 integrins and memory differentiation. J Immunol 1996; 156:3727–3736.

52. Campbell JJ, Hedrick J, Zlotnik A, Siani MA, Thompson DA, Butcher EC. Chemokines and the arrest of lymphocytes rolling under flow conditions. Science 1998; 279:381–384.

53. Gunn MD, Kyuwa S, Tam C, et al. Mice lacking expression of secondary lymphoid organ chemokine have defects in lymphocyte homing and dendritic cell localization [see comments]. J Exp Med 1999; 189:451–460.

54. Zabel BA, Agace W, Campbell JJ, et al. Human G protein-coupled receptor GPR-9-6/CC chemokine receptor 9 is selectively expressed on intestinal homing T lymphocytes, mucosal lymphocytes, and thymocytes and is required for thymus-expressed chemokine-mediated chemotaxis. J Exp Med 1999; 190:1241–1256.

55. Csencsits KL, Jutila MA, Pascual DW. Nasal-associated lymphoid tissue: phenotypic and functional evidence for the primary role of peripheral node addressin in naive lymphocyte adhesion to high endothelial venules in a mucosal site. J Immunol 1999; 163:1382–1389.

56. Richards IM, Kolbasa KP, Hatfield CA, et al. Role of very late activation antigen-4 in the antigen-induced accumulation of eosinophils and lymphocytes in the lungs and airway lumen of sensitized brown Norway rats. Am J Respir Cell Mol Biol 1996; 15:172–183.

57. Quiding-Jabrink M, Nordstrom I, Granstrom G, et al. Differential expression of tissue-specific adhesion molecules on human circulating antibody-forming cells after systemic, enteric, and nasal immunizations. A molecular basis for the compartmentalization of effector B cell responses. J Clin Invest 1997; 99:1281–1286.

58. Quayle AJ, Porter EM, Nussbaum AA, et al. Gene expression, immunolocalization, and secretion of human defensin-5 in human female reproductive tract. Am J Pathol 1998; 152:1247–1258.

59. Porter EM, Liu L, Oren A, Anton PA, Ganz T. Localization of human intestinal defensin 5 in Paneth cell granules. Infect Immun 1997; 65:2389–2395.

60. Porter EM, van Dam E, Valore EV, Ganz T. Broad-spectrum antimicrobial activity of human intestinal defensin 5. Infect Immun 1997; 65:2396–3401.

61. Zhao C, Wang I, Lehrer RI. Widespread expression of beta-defensin hBD-1 in human secretory glands and epithelial cells. FEBS Lett 1996; 396:319–322.

62. Singh PK, Jia HP, Wiles K, et al. Production of beta-defensins by human airway epithelia. Proc Natl Acad Sci USA 1998; 95:14961–14966.

63. Mathews M, Jia HP, Guthmiller JM, et al. Production of beta-defensin antimicrobial peptides by the oral mucosa and salivary glands. Infect Immun 1999; 67:2740–2745.

64. O'Neil DA, Porter EM, Elewaut D, et al. Expression and regulation of the human beta-defensins hBD-1 and hBD-2 in intestinal epithelium. J Immunol 1999; 163:6718–6724.

65. Weinrauch Y, Elsbach P, Madsen LM, Foreman A, Weiss J. The potent anti-*Staphylococcus aureus* activity of a sterile rabbit inflammatory fluid is due to a 14-kD phospholipase A2. J Clin Invest 1996; 97:250–257.

66. Harwig SS, Tan L, Qu XD, Cho Y, Eisenhauer PB, Lehrer RI. Bactericidal properties of murine intestinal phospholipase A2. J Clin Invest 1995; 95:603–610.

67. Moriuchi M, Moriuchi H. A milk protein lactoferrin enhances human T cell leukemia virus type i and suppresses HIV-1 infection. J Immunol 2001; 166:4231–4236.

68. Jung HC, Eckmann L, Yang SK, et al. A distinct array of proinflammatory cytokines is expressed in human colon epithelial cells in response to bacterial invasion. J Clin Invest 1995; 95:55–65.

69. Mayer L, Blumberg RS. Antigen presentating cells: epithelial cells. In: Ogra PL, et al. (eds). Mucosal Immunology. San Diego: Academic, 1999, pp. 365–379.

70. Laurent F, Eckmann L, Savidge TC, et al. *Cryptosporidium parvum* infection of human intestinal epithelial cells induces the polarized secretion of C-X-C chemokines. Infect Immun 1997; 65:5067–5073.

71. Yang SK, Eckmann L, Panja A, Kagnoff MF. Differential and regulated expression of C-X-C, C-C, and C-chemokines by human colon epithelial cells. Gastroenterology 1997; 113:1214–1223.

72. Izadpanah A, Dwinell MB, Eckmann L, Varki NM, Kagnoff MF. Regulated MIP-3alpha/CCL20 production by human intestinal epithelium: mechanism for modulating mucosal immunity. Am J Physiol (Gastrointest Liver Physiol) 2001; 280:G710–G719.

73. Dwinell MB, Lugering N, Eckmann L, Kagnoff MF. Regulated production of interferon-inducible T-cell chemoattractants by human intestinal epithelial cells. Gastroenterology 2001; 120:49–59.

74. Boismenu R, Feng L, Xia YY, Chang JC, Havran WL. Chemokine expression by intraepithelial gamma delta T cells. Implications for the recruitment of inflammatory cells to damaged epithelia. J Immunol 1996; 157:985–992.

75. Hedrick JA, Saylor V, Figueroa D, et al. Lymphotactin is produced by NK cells and attracts both NK cells and T cells in vivo. J Immunol 1997; 158:1533–1540.

76. Tagliabue A, Befus AD, Clark DA, Bienenstock J. Characteristics of natural killer cells in the murine intestinal epithelium and lamina propria. J Exp Med 1982; 155:1785–1796.

77. Roberts AI, O'Connell SM, Biancone L, Brolin RE, Ebert EC. Spontaneous cytotoxicity of intestinal intraepithelial lymphocytes: clues to the mechanism. Clin Exp Immunol 1993; 94:527–532.

78. Lillehoj HS. Intestinal intraepithelial and splenic natural killer cell responses to Eimerian infections in inbred chickens. Infect Immun 1989; 57:1879–1884.

79. Carman PS, Ernst PB, Rosenthal KL, Clark DA, Befus AD, Bienenstock J. Intraepithelial leukocytes contain a unique subpopulation of NK-like cytotoxic cells active in the defense of gut epithelium to enteric murine coronavirus. J Immunol 1986; 136:1548–1553.

80. Biron CA, Byron KS, Sullivan JL. Severe herpesvirus infections in an adolescent without natural killer cells. N Engl J Med 1989; 320:1731–1735.

81. Mosmann TR, Coffman RL. TH1 and TH2 cells: different patterns of lymphokine secretion lead to different functional properties. Ann Rev Immunol 1989; 7:145–173.

82. Kobayashi M, Fitz L, Ryan M, et al. Identification and purification of natural killer cell stimulatory factor (NKSF), a cytokine with multiple biologic effects on human lymphocytes. J Exp Med 1989; 170:827–845.

83. Chan SH, Perussia B, Gupta JW, et al. Induction of interferon gamma production by natural killer cell stimulatory factor: characterization of the responder cells and synergy with other inducers. J Exp Med 1991; 173:869–879.

84. Snapper CM, Paul WE. Interferon-gamma and B cell stimulatory factor-1 reciprocally regulate Ig isotype production. Science 1987; 236:944–947.

85. Finkelman FD, Holmes J, Katona IM, et al. Lymphokine control of in vivo immunoglobulin isotype selection. Annu Rev Immunol 1990; 8:303–333.

86. Esser C, Radbruch A. Immunoglobulin class switching: molecular and cellular analysis. Annu Rev Immunol 1990; 8:717–735.

87. Coffman RL, Seymour BW, Lebman DA, et al. The role of helper T cell products in mouse B cell differentiation and isotype regulation. Immunol Rev 1998; 102:5–28.

88. Gajewski TF, Fitch FW. Anti-proliferative effect of IFN-gamma in immune regulation. I. IFN-gamma inhibits the proliferation of Th2 but not Th1 murine helper T lymphocyte clones. J Immunol 1988; 140:4245–4252.

89. Golding B. Cytokine regulation of humoral immune responses. Topics Vaccine Adjuvant Res 1991, pp. 37–45.

90. Bonecchi R, Bianchi G, Bordignon PP, et al. Differential expression of chemokine receptors and chemotactic responsiveness of type 1 T helper cells (Th1s) and Th2s. J Exp Med 1998; 187:129–134.

91. Sallusto F, Lenig D, Mackay CR, Lanzavecchia A. Flexible programs of chemokine receptor expression on human polarized T helper 1 and 2 lymphocytes. J Exp Med 1998; 187:875–883.

92. Imai T, Nagira M, Takagi S, et al. Selective recruitment of CCR4-bearing Th2 cells toward antigen-presenting cells by the CC chemokines thymus and activation-regulated chemokine and macrophage-derived chemokine. Int Immunol 1999; 11:81–88.

93. Beagley KW, Eldridge JH, Kiyono H, et al. Recombinant murine IL-5 induces high rate IgA synthesis in cycling IgA-positive Peyer's patch B cells. J Immunol 1988; 141:2035–2042.

94. Beagley KW, Eldridge JH, Lee F, et al. Interleukins and IgA synthesis. Human and murine interleukin 6 induce high rate IgA secretion in IgA-committed B cells. J Exp Med 1989; 169:2133–2148.

95. Beagley KW, Eldridge JH, Aicher WK, et al. Peyer's patch B cells with memory cell characteristics undergo terminal differentiation within 24 hours in response to interleukin-6. Cytokine 1991; 3:107–116.

96. Fujihashi K, McGhee JR, Lue C, et al. Human appendix B cells naturally express receptors for and respond to interleukin 6 with selective IgA1 and IgA2 synthesis. J Clin Invest 1991; 88:248–252.

97. Ramsay AJ, Husband AJ, Ramshaw IA, et al. The role of interleukin-6 in mucosal IgA antibody responses in vivo. Science 1994; 264:561–563.

98. Bromander AK, Ekman L, Kopf M, Nedrud JG, Lycke NY. IL-6-deficient mice exhibit normal mucosal IgA responses to local immunizations and *Helicobacter felis* infection. J Immunol 1996; 156:4290–4207.

99. Briere F, Bridon JM, Chevet D, et al. Interleukin 10 induces B lymphocytes from IgA-deficient patients to secrete IgA. J Clin Invest 1994; 94:97–104.

100. Defrance T, Vanbervliet B, Briere F, Durand I, Rousset F, Banchereau J. Interleukin 10 and transforming growth factor beta cooperate to induce anti-CD40-activated naive human B cells to secrete immunoglobulin A. J Exp Med 1992; 175:671–682.

101. Nonoyama S, Farrington M, Ishida H, Howard M, Ochs HD. Activated B cells from patients with common variable immunodeficiency proliferate and synthesize immunoglobulin. J Clin Invest 1993; 92:1282–1287.

102. Mega J, McGhee JR, Kiyono H. Cytokine- and Ig-producing T cells in mucosal effector tissues: analysis of IL-5- and IFN-gamma-producing T cells, T cell receptor expression, and IgA plasma cells from mouse salivary gland-associated tissues. J Immunol 1992; 148:2030-2039.

103. Taguchi T, McGhee JR, Coffman RL, et al. Analysis of Th1 and Th2 cells in murine gut-associated tissues. Frequencies of CD4+ and CD8+ T cells that secrete IFN-gamma and IL-5. J Immunol 1990; 145:68–77.

104. Kauppi-Korkeila M, van Alphen L, Madore D, Saarinen L, Kayhty H. Mechanism of antibody-mediated reduction of nasopharyngeal colonization by *Haemophilus influenzae* type b studied in an infant rat model. J Infect Dis 1996; 174:1337–1340.

105. Davin JC, Senterre J, Mahieu PR. The high lectin-binding capacity of human secretory IgA protects nonspecifically mucosae against environmental antigens. Biol Neonate 1991; 59:121–125.

106. Wold AE, Mestecky J, Tomana M, et al. Secretory immunoglobulin A carries oligosaccharide receptors for *Escherichia coli* type 1 fimbrial. Infect Immun 1990; 58:3073–3077.

107. Wold AE, Motas C, Svanborg C, Mestecky J. Lectin receptors on IgA isotypes. Scand J Immunol 1994; 39:195–201.

108. Armstrong SJ, Dimmock NJ. Neutralization of influenza virus by low concentrations of hemagglutinin-specific polymeric immunoglobulin A inhibits viral fusion activity, but activation of the ribonucleoprotein is also inhibited. J Virol 1992; 66:3823–3832.

109. Mazanec MB, Coudret CL, Fletcher DR. Intracellular neutralization of influenza virus by immunoglobulin A anti-hemagglutinin monoclonal antibodies. J Virol 1995; 69:1339–1343.

110. Mazanec MB, Kaetzel CS, Lamm ME, Fletcher D, Nedrud JG. Intracellular neutralization of virus by immunoglobulin A antibodies. Pro Natl Acad Sci USA 1992; 89:6901–6905.

111. Burns JW, Siadat-Pajouh M, Krishnaney AA, Greenberg HB. Protective effect of rotavirus VP6-specific IgA monoclonal antibodies that lack neutralizing activity. Science 1996; 272:104–107.

112. Bomsel M, Heyman M, Hocini H, et al. Intracellular neutralization of HIV transcytosis across tight epithelial barriers by anti-HIV envelope protein dIgA or IgM. Immunity 1998; 9:277–287.

113. Griffiss JM, Goroff DK. IgA blocks IgM and IgG-initiated immune lysis by separate molecular mechanisms. J Immunol 1983; 130:2882–2885.

114. Russell MW, Mansa B. Complement-fixing properties of human IgA antibodies. Alternative pathway complement activation by plastic-bound, but not specific antigen-bound, IgA. Scand J Immunol 1989; 30:175–183.

115. Wolf HM, Fischer MB, Puhringer H, Samstag A, Vogel E, Eibl MM. Human serum IgA downregulates the release of inflammatory cytokines (tumor necrosis factor-alpha, interleukin-6) in human monocytes. Blood 1994; 83:1278–1288.

116. Wolf HM, Hauber I, Gulle H, et al. Anti-inflammatory properties of human serum IgA: induction of IL-1 receptor antagonist and Fc alpha R (CD89)-mediated down-regulation of tumour necrosis factor-alpha (TNF-alpha) and IL-6 in human monocytes. Clin Exp Immunol 1996; 105:537–543.

117. Offit PA, Cunningham SL, Dudzik KI. Memory and distribution of virus-specific cytotoxic T lymphocytes (CTLs) and CTL precursors after rotavirus infection. J Virol 1991; 65:1318–1324.

118. London SD, Rubin DH, Cebra JJ. Gut mucosal immunization with reovirus serotype 1/L stimulates virus-specific cytotoxic T cell precursors as well as IgA memory cells in Peyer's patches. J Exp Med 1987; 165:830–847.

119. London SD, Cebra-Thomas JA, Rubin DH, Cebra JJ. CD8 lymphocyte subpopulations in Peyer's patches induced by reovirus serotype 1 infection. J Immunol 1990; 144:3187–3194.

120. Issekutz TB. The response of gut-associated T lymphocytes to intestinal viral immunization. J Immunol 1984; 133:2955–2960.

121. Marx PA, Compans RW, Gettie A, et al. Protection against vaginal SIV transmission with microencapsulated vaccine. Science 1993; 260:1323–1327.

122. Miller CJ, Alexander NJ, Sutjipto S, et al. Genital mucosal transmission of simian immunodeficiency virus: animal model for heterosexual transmission of human immunodeficiency virus. J Virol 1989; 63:4277–4284.

123. Lohman BL, Miller CJ, McChesney MB. Antiviral cytotoxic T lymphocytes in vaginal mucosa of simian immunodeficiency virus-infected rhesus macaques. J Immunol 1995; 155:5855–5860.

124. Miller CJ, McChesney MB, Lu X, et al. Rhesus macaques previously infected with simian/human immunodeficiency virus are protected from vaginal challenge with pathogenic SIVmac239. J Virol 1997; 71:1911–1921.

125. Miller CJ. Mucosal transmission of simian immunodeficiency virus. Curr Top Microbiol Immunol 1994; 188:107–122.

126. Porgador A, Staats HF, Faiola B, Gilboa E, Palker TJ. Intranasal immunization with CTL epitope peptides from HIV-1 or ovalbumin and the mucosal adjuvant cholera toxin induces peptide-specific CTLs and protection against tumor development in vivo. J Immunol 1997; 158:834–841.

127. Elson CO, Ealding W. Generalized systemic and mucosal immunity in mice after mucosal stimulation with cholera toxin. J Immunol 1984; 132:2736–2741.

128. Elson CO, Ealding W. Cholera toxin feeding did not induce oral tolerance in mice and abrogated oral tolerance to an unrelated protein antigen. J Immunol 1984; 133:2892–2897.

129. Clements JD, Hartzog NM, Lyon FL. Adjuvant activity of *Escherichia coli* heat-labile enterotoxin and effect on the induction of oral tolerance in mice to unrelated protein antigens. Vaccine 1988; 6:269–277.

130. Lycke N, Holmgren J. Strong adjuvant properties of cholera toxin on gut mucosal immune responses to orally presented antigens. Immunology 1986; 59:301–308.

131. VanCott JL, Staats HF, Pascual DW, et al. Regulation of mucosal and systemic antibody responses by T helper cell subsets, macrophages, and derived cytokines following oral immunization with live recombinant *Salmonella*. J Immunol 1996; 156:1504-1514.

132. Van Ginkel FW, Liu C, Simecka JW, et al. Intratracheal gene delivery with adenoviral vector induces elevated systemic IgG and mucosal IgA antibodies to adenovirus and beta-galactosidase. 1995; Hum Gene Ther 1995; 6:895–903.

133. Gill DM. The arrangement of subunits in cholera toxin. Biochemistry 1976; 15:1242–1248.
134. Spangler BD. Structure and function of cholera toxin and the related *Escherichia coli* heat-labile enterotoxin. Microbiol Rev 1992; 56:622–647.
135. Heyningen SV. Cholera toxin: interaction of subunits with ganglioside GM1. Science 1974; 183:656–657.
136. Field M, Rao MC, Chang EB. Intestinal electrolyte transport and diarrheal disease (1). N Engl J Med 1989; 321:800–806.
137. Dallas WS, Falkow S. Amino acid sequence homology between cholera toxin and *Escherichia coli* heat-labile toxin. Nature 1980; 288:499–501.
138. Tsuji T, Inoue T, Miyama A, Okamoto K, Honda T, Miwatani T. A single amino acid substitution in the A subunit of *Escherichia coli* enterotoxin results in a loss of its toxic activity. J Biol Chem 1990; 265:22520–22525.
139. Harford S, Dykes CW, Hobden AN, Read MJ, Halliday IJ. Inactivation of the *Escherichia coli* heat-labile enterotoxin by in vitro mutagenesis of the A-subunit gene. Eur J Biochem 1989; 183:311–316.
140. Yamamoto S, Takeda Y, Yamamoto M, et al. Mutants in the ADP-ribosyltransferase cleft of cholera toxin lack diarrheagenicity but retain adjuvanticity. J Exp Med 1997; 185:1203–1210.
141. Yamamoto S, Kiyono H, Yamamoto M, et al. A nontoxic mutant of cholera toxin elicits Th2-type responses for enhanced mucosal immunity. Pro Natl Acad Sci USA 1997; 94:5267–5272.
142. Yamamoto M, Kiyono H, Yamamoto S, et al. Direct effects on antigen-presenting cells and T lymphocytes explain the adjuvanticity of a nontoxic cholera toxin mutant. J Immunol 1999; 162:7015–7021.
143. Cong Y, Weaver CT, Elson CO. The mucosal adjuvanticity of cholera toxin involves enhancement of costimulatory activity by selective upregulation of B7.2 expression. J Immunol 1997; 159:5301–5308.
144. Douce G, Fontana M, Pizza M, Rappuoli R, Dougan G. Intranasal immunogenicity and adjuvanticity of site-directed mutant derivatives of cholera toxin. Infect Immun 1997; 65:2821–2828.
145. Douce G, Turcotte C, Cropley I, et al. Mutants of *Escherichia coli* heat-labile toxin lacking ADP-ribosyltransferase activity act as nontoxic, mucosal adjuvants. Proc Natl Acad Sci USA 1995; 92:1644–1648.
146. Giuliani MM, Del Giudice G, Giannelli V, et al. Mucosal adjuvanticity and immunogenicity of LTR72, a novel mutant of *Escherichia coli* heat-labile enterotoxin with partial knockout of ADP-ribosyltransferase activity. J Exp Med 1998; 187:1123–1132.
147. Rappuoli R, Pizza M, Douce G, Dougan G. Structure and mucosal adjuvanticity of cholera and *Escherichia coli* heat-labile enterotoxins. Immunol Today 1999; 20:493–500.
148. Takahashi I, Marinaro M, Kiyono H, et al. Mechanisms for mucosal immunogenicity and adjuvancy of *Escherichia coli* labile enterotoxin. J Infect Dis 1996; 173, no. 3: 627–635.
149. Agren LC, Ekman L, Lowenadler B, Lycke NY. Genetically engineered nontoxic vaccine adjuvant that combines B cell targeting with immunomodulation by cholera toxin A1 subunit. J Immunol 1997; 158:3936–3946.
150. Agren L, Sverremark E, Ekman L, et al. The ADP-ribosylating CTA1-DD adjuvant enhances T cell-dependent and independent responses by direct action on B cells involving anti-apoptotic Bcl-2- and germinal center-promoting effects. J Immunol 2000; 164:6276–6286.
151. Agren LC, Ekman L, Lowenadler B, Nedrud JG, Lycke NY. Adjuvanticity of the cholera toxin A1-based gene fusion protein, CTA1-DD, is critically dependent on the ADP-ribosyltransferase and Ig-binding activity. J Immunol 1999; 162:2432–2440.

152. Hajishengallis G, Hollingshead SK, Koga T, Russell MW. Mucosal immunization with a bacterial protein antigen genetically coupled to cholera toxin A2/B subunits. J Immunol 1995; 154:4322–4332.

153. Sun JB, Mielcarek N, Lakew M, et al. Intranasal administration of a *Schistosoma mansoni* glutathione S-transferase-cholera toxoid conjugate vaccine evokes antiparasitic and antipathological immunity in mice. J Immunol 1999; 163:1045–1052.

154. Sun JB, Rask C, Olsson T, Holmgren J, Czerkinsky C. Treatment of experimental autoimmune encephalomyelitis by feeding myelin basic protein conjugated to cholera toxin B subunit. Proc Natl Acad Sci USA 1996; 93:7196–7201.

155. Bergerot I, Ploix C, Petersen J, et al. A cholera toxoid-insulin conjugate as an oral vaccine against spontaneous autoimmune diabetes. Proc Natl Acad Sci USA 1997; 94:4610–4614.

156. Marinaro M, Boyaka PN, Jackson RJ, et al. Use of intranasal IL-12 to target predominantly Th1 responses to nasal and Th2 responses to oral vaccines given with cholera toxin. J Immunol 1999; 162:114–121.

157. Boyaka PN, Marinaro M, Jackson RJ, et al. IL-12 is an effective adjuvant for induction of mucosal immunity. J Immunol 1999; 162: 122–128.

158. Arulanandam BP, O'Toole M, Metzger DW. Intranasal interleukin-12 is a powerful adjuvant for protective mucosal immunity. J Infect Dis 1999; 180:940–949.

159. Staats HF, Ennis, Jr. FA. IL-1 is an effective adjuvant for mucosal and systemic immune responses when coadministered with protein immunogens. J Immunol 1999; 162:6141–6147.

160. Marinaro M, Boyaka PN, Finkelman FD, et al. Oral but not parenteral interleukin (IL)-12 redirects T helper 2 (Th2)-type responses to an oral vaccine without altering mucosal IgA responses. J Exp Med 1997; 185:415–427.

161. Lillard JW, Jr, Boyaka PN, Chertov O, Oppenheim JJ, McGhee JR. Mechanisms for induction of acquired host immunity by neutrophil peptide defensins. Proc Natl Acad Sci USA 1999; 96:651–656.

162. Lillard JW, Jr, Boyaka PN, Hedrick JA, Zlotnik A, McGhee JR. Lymphotactin acts as an innate mucosal adjuvant. J Immunol 1999; 162:1959–1965.

163. Lillard JW, Boyaka PN, Taub DD, McGhee JR. RANTES potentiates antigen-specific mucosal immune responses. J Immunol 2001; 166:162–169.

164. Krieg AM. CpG DNA: a pathogenic factor in systemic lupus erythematosus? J Clin Immunol 1995; 15:284–292.

165. Tighe H, Corr M, Roman M, Raz E. Gene vaccination: plasmid DNA is more than just a blueprint. Immunol Today 1998; 19:89–97.

166. Roman M, Martin-Orozco E, Goodman JS, et al. Immunostimulatory DNA sequences function as T helper-1-promoting adjuvants. Nat Med 1997; 3:849–854.

167. Klinman DM, Yi AK, Beaucage SL, Conover J, Krieg AM. CpG motifs present in bacteria DNA rapidly induce lymphocytes to secrete interleukin 6, interleukin 12, and interferon gamma. Proc Natl Acad Sci USA 1996; 93:2879–2883.

168. Chu RS, Targoni OS, Krieg AM, Lehmann PV, Harding CV. CpG oligodeoxynucleotides act as adjuvants that switch on T helper 1 (Th1) immunity. J Exp Med 1997; 186:1623–1631.

169. Moldoveanu Z, Love-Homan L, Huang WQ, Krieg AM. CpG DNA, a novel immune enhancer for systemic and mucosal immunization with influenza virus. Vaccine 1998; 16:1216–1224.

170. McCluskie MJ, Davis HL. CpG DNA is a potent enhancer of systemic and mucosal immune responses against hepatitis B surface antigen with intranasal administration to mice. J Immunol 1998; 161:4463–4466.

171. Elson CO, Dertzbaugh MT. Mucosal adjuvants. In: Ogra PL, et al. (eds). Mucosal Immunology. San Diego: Academic, 1999, pp. 817–838.

172. Mowat AM, Donachie AM, Reid G, Jarrett O. Immune-stimulating complexes containing Quil A and protein antigen prime class I MHC-restricted T lymphocytes in vivo and are immunogenic by the oral route. Immunology 1991; 72:317–322.
173. Kensil CR, Kammer R. QS-21: A water-soluble triterpene glycoside adjuvant. Expert Opin Invest Drugs 1998; 7:1475–1482.
174. Kensil CR, Patel U, Lennick M, and Marciani D. Separation and characterization of saponins with adjuvant activity from *Quillaja saponaria* Molina cortex. J Immunol 1991; 146:431–437.
175. Livingston P, Zhang S, Adluri S, et al. Tumor cell reactivity mediated by IgM antibodies in sera from melanoma patients vaccinated with GM2 ganglioside covalently linked to KLH is increased by IgG antibodies. Cancer Immunol Immunother 1997; 43:324–330.
176. Coughlin RT, Fattom A, Chu C, White AC, Winston S. Adjuvant activity of QS-21 for experimental *E. coli* 018 polysaccharide vaccines. Vaccine 1995. 13:17–21.
177. Newman MJ, Wu JY, Gardner BH, et al. Saponin adjuvant induction of ovalbumin-specific CD8+ cytotoxic T lymphocyte responses. J Immunol 1992; 148:2357–2362.
178. Sasaki S, Sumino K, Hamajima K, et al. Induction of systemic and mucosal immune responses to human immunodeficiency virus type 1 by a DNA vaccine formulated with QS-21 saponin adjuvant via intramuscular and intranasal routes. J Virol 1998; 72:4931–4939.
179. Boyaka PN, Marinaro M, Jackson RJ, et al. Oral QS-21 requires early IL-4 help for induction of mucosal and systemic immunity. J Immunol 2001; 166:2283–2290.

II
Molecular Basis for Immunotherapy

4

Production of Immunoglobulins and Monoclonal Antibodies Targeting Infectious Diseases

Renate Kunert and Hermann Katinger

INTRODUCTION

Infectious and parasitic diseases have been the major cause of death over the last centuries in developing countries. Similarly, in the past, viral and bacterial infections have killed tens of thousands of people in the large cities of Europe. The first success in overcoming the mortality related to infectious diseases was derived from observations that the serum from cows infected with smallpox protected against human poxviruses. In 1800, Jenner was the first to apply experimental inoculations of cowpox to human volunteers. Vaccination against smallpox, beginning in the 19th century, quickly restricted the disease in Europe and North America.

The basis of immunotherapy was established in Berlin at the Robert Koch Institute of Hygiene. In 1890, Emil von Behring and Shibasabura Kitasato published a landmark article showing that serum from actively immunized animals could neutralize toxic concentrations of toxin in other animals. They could also successfully cure children of diphtheria with horse antisera. Serotherapy was established as a treatment against diphtheria as well as tetanus toxin.

After the principles of serotherapy were evident the doors were open for further applications. The major problem arising from this first generation of passive serotherapy was anaphylactoid reaction. Stepwise technologic improvements such as precipitation of the immunoglobulins from sera reduced these problems. The γ-globulins are now a group of safe drugs that are prepared from either healthy donors, vaccinated volunteers, or even reconvalescent donors by applying sophisticated manufacturing technologies. Both basic research and broad clinical applications of immunoglobulins over decades have provided us with a good knowledge base for technologic and application improvements. The advantages of antibody-based prevention strategies and therapies include versatility, low toxicity, pathogen specificity, enhancement of immune function, and favorable pharmacokinetics; the disadvantages include high cost, limited usefulness against mixed infections, and the need for early and precise microbiologic diagnosis (1). Hospital infections and resistance to antibiotics generate serious problems that need to be solved. The combination of antibody therapy with other therapeutic drugs is still a widely unexplored field of new forms of treatment (2).

From: *Immunotherapy for Infectious Diseases*
Edited by: J. M. Jacobson © Humana Press Inc., Totowa, NJ

IMMUNOGLOBULINS

Immunoglobulins (Igs) are part of the adaptive immune system and basically fulfill two major biologic functions related to the variable and constant regions of the antibody molecule common to all immunoglobulins (Fig.1). The first function, carried out by the variable region, is the recognition and specific binding to antigens, either soluble antigens such as toxins, or solid antigens such as viruses or microorganisms. The constant region of the molecule mediates various effector functions and subclasses of immunoglobulins.

Antibodies (Ab) or immunoglobulins are glycoproteins generated in all mammals. A cascade of immunoglobulins is produced upon stimulation with a foreign immunogenic antigen. During the maturation of the immunologic cascade, five distinct immunoglobulin classes can evolve, IgG, IgA, IgM, IgD, and IgE, which differ in size as well as amino acid and carbohydrate composition of the heavy chains. Figure 2 shows the monomeric and oligomeric structures of IgG, IgA, and IgM. The different regions of the basic Ig monomere are described in Figure 1. IgG is a monomeric protein representing approx. 70% of the antibody pool in the human serum. IgM molecules are the first antibodies to be expressed in the course of an immunogenic response to an antigen. The pentameric structure of IgM is stabilized by a peptide structure called the joining (J) chain. The dimeric structure of IgA is an immunologic barrier in seromucosal secretions. IgD acts in conjunction with antigen-triggered lymphocyte differentiation. IgE is displayed on the surface membrane of basophilic and mast cells and is often associated with allergic symptoms.

Humoral Immune Response and the Cellular Basis of Immune Response

Primary contact of invading antigens with the cells of the immune system either triggers tolerance or induces an immune reaction. The form of antigen presentation determines whether a cell-mediated or an antibody response is elicited. The antigen moves to the local lymph nodes, where it is endocytosed by antigen-presenting cells (APCs) and presented together with class II major histocompatibility complex (MHC) molecules on the surface of the cells. The degradation and transport through the endoplasmatic reticulum is mediated by class I MHC molecules. Many additional ligands and receptors like CD40/CD40 ligand or interleukin (IL)-2/IL-2 receptor support the interaction of T- and T/B-cell collaboration. T-helper cells cooperate with B-cells to induce antibody production.

B-Cell Development

B-cell development starts in the fetal liver, before the bone marrow becomes the dominant hematopoietic organ. Pre-B-cells begin differentiating and proliferating in response to signals of local stromal cells. As shown in Figure 3 in more detail, pre-B-cells rearrange their heavy-chain variable-region gene segments and express signal transduction receptors for further development. After also rearranging the gene segments of the light chain, the premature IgM B-cells migrate from the bone marrow to the secondary lymphoid tissue, where antigen contact and cytokine interaction with T-helper cells take place. Further differentiation to plasma cells prepares them for subclass switch and expression of high quantities of soluble immunoglobulins.

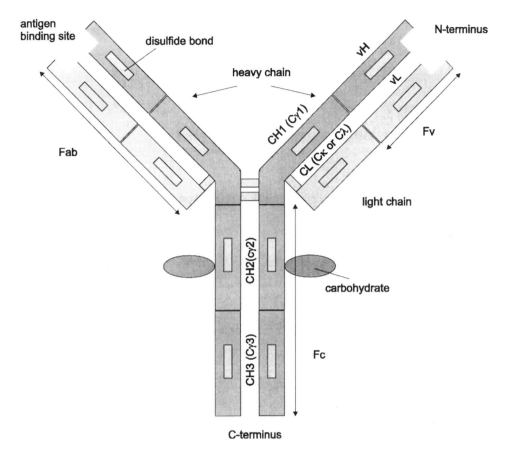

Fig. 1. The basic structure of IgG. The variable regions of heavy and light chains are on the amino-terminal end of the peptide chains. The constant region of IgG is divided into three structurally discrete regions: C_H1, C_H2, and C_H3. These globular regions are stabilized by disulfide bonds and are called domains. The variable domain binds to the antigen; the constant regions are responsible for different effector mechanisms.

Antibodies: Structure and Function

Constant Region

Immunoglobulins consist of two identical heavy-chain/light-chain heterodimers. The constant region of the heavy chain determines the class affiliation. Figure 1 shows a schematic diagram of an IgG1 molecule with the different peptide regions, carbohydrate moieties, and disulfide bonds. The carboxy-terminal half of the light chain (C_L; constant light chain) is constant except for certain allotypic and isotypic variations, whereas the amino-terminal half shows sequence variability and is known as V_L (variable light chain). The two subtypes of light chains ($C\kappa$ and $C\lambda$) can be combined with any heavy chain type (μ δ, γ, α, or ϵ) and are bound to one heavy chain via an intramolecular cystein-derived SH-group. Every light chain has two intrachain disulfide bonds, forming so-called loops, one in the variable and one in the constant region. The constant part of the heavy chains γ, α, and δ can be divided into three domains, each generating loops spanning about 60–70 amino acids ($C\gamma1$, $C\gamma2$, and $C\gamma3$). Thus,

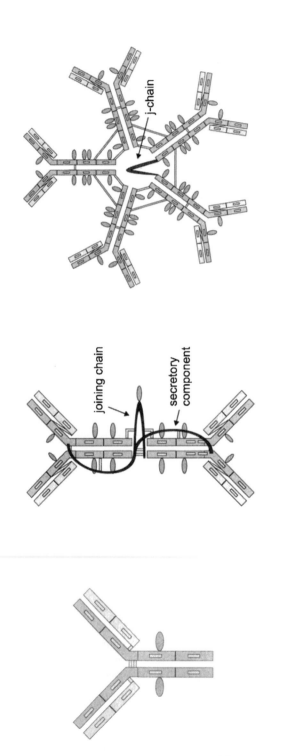

Monomeric structure of IgG1.

Human secretory IgA traveles through the epithelium aided by the secretory component. The two heavy chains are bound via j-chain like in IgM.

Human serum IgMs consist of five immunoglobulin molecules stabilized by disulfide bonds cross linking adjacent Cμ3 and Cμ4 of different units and the J-chain.

Fig. 2. Monomeric, dimeric, and pentameric structure of IgG and soluble IgA with secretory component and pentameric IgM. **(Left)** Monomeric structure of IgG1. **(Middle)** Human secretory IgA travels through the epithelium aided by the J chain as in IgM. **(Right)** Human serum IgMs consist of five immunoglobulin molecules stabilized by disulfide bonds cross linking adjacent Cμ3 and Cμ4 of different units and the J chain.

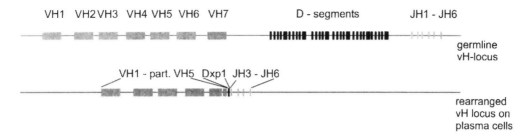

Fig. 3. Rearrangement of VH, D, and JH regions during B-cell development. Chromosomal rearrangement of the human variable region heavy chain locus on chromosome 14. One of approx 40 D segments is linked to one of six J regions; in a second recombination step, one V_H region is rearranged in front of the newly generated D-J_H locus.

the heavy chain displays four sections, V_H, C_H1, C_H2, and C_H3, defined by homologies in the secondary and tertiary structure through similar loops. μ and ϵ chains contain an additional domain after C_H1 so that $C\mu3$ is homologous to $C\gamma2$.

Effector Functions

In vivo the humoral response to foreign antigens takes place in a complex environment of body fluids in which various constituents such as plasma proteins, enzymes, and the complement system may contribute functions. On formation of the antigen-antibody complex, different defense mechanisms may be activated, which are summarized in Fig. 4. In some cases the penetration of cells by bacterial toxins or viral agents can be prevented by generating antigen-antibody complexes. This mechanism is called neutralization and represents a passive protection mechanism. Neutralization of an antigen or blockade of a ligand-receptor interaction does not require additional effector functions or domains. Depending on the effective valency of the target antigen, neutralization can function with monovalent single chains as well as bivalent antigen binding fragments (Fab) or whole immunoglobulin molecules.

If effector functions mediated via the constant fragment (Fc) specific receptors are involved in defending the invading agents, we speak of sterilizing immunity, meaning that the target antigen is actively attacked. The most important effector function is the activation of the complement system. The initiating step after antigen fixation is the binding of $C\gamma$, $C\gamma1$, or $C\gamma3$ to the C1q complement component. Partial cleavage of different complement proteins activates the complement cascade, and three major steps can be initiated: activation of immune mediators, cytolysis of target cells, or phagocytosis of the antigen. Another mechanism of antibody action is antibody-dependent cell-mediated cytotoxicity) (ADCC). Infected cells, which are recognized and opsonized by specific antibodies, can be lysed by natural killer cells, the classical K-cells.

Variable Region

The variable regions of the heavy and light chains jointly form the antigen binding domain of the immunoglobulin. The three-dimensional structure is generated by the three α-helical domains of the complementary determining regions (CDRs) on both heavy and light chains, which are stabilized by relatively conserved framework segments (FR) forming β-sheet structures. The different regions on the variable part of the heavy and light chains are determined by variable (V) diversity (D), and joining (J)

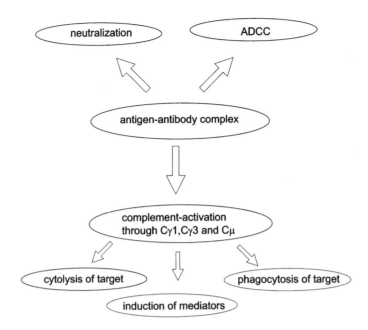

Fig. 4. Humoral defense of invading antigens. ADCC, antibody-dependent cellular cytotoxicity.

genomic segments rearranged on the RNA transcripts. The rearranged V_L and V_H mRNAs are then translated as variable regions, as shown in Fig. 5. In the light chain, FR1, FR2, and FR3, as well as CDR1, CDR2, and a part of CDR3 are determined by the genomic variable segment (V_L). The C terminus of CDR3 and the FR4 are translated from the genomic J segment. The variability of V_H is enhanced by an additional D segment that forms the CDR3 loop and generates more diversity.

The affinity of binding to the antigen is determined by multiple noncovalent bonds, whereby the forces depend on the distance between the interacting groups. To ensure maximun versatility of humoral immunity against a maximum number of antigens, the number of potential antibodies in humans must be high. This is achieved by additional mechanisms of genetic recombinations.

Genetic Basis of Antibody Diversity

Antibody V_Ls are genetically determined by the V and J segments; V_Hs are formed by the recombination of V, D, and J segments on the chromosome. Figure 3 shows an unrearranged and a rearranged human HC locus. Seven families of V_H gene segments provide about 50 V_H regions. More than 30 D segments and 6 J_H regions can be rearranged. In vivo recombination of gene segments for heavy and light chain variable regions during B-cell maturation allows the generation of specific antibodies directed against numerous antigens from a limited pool of genes. Splicing allows the combination of any of the genetic segments of V, D, and J with each other owing to recombinases. During B-cell differentiation, chromosomal rearrangement of heavy-chain V-D-J and light-chain V-J takes place. To generate a maximum of different antibodies, the immune system acquired additional mechanisms that increased the diversity of the

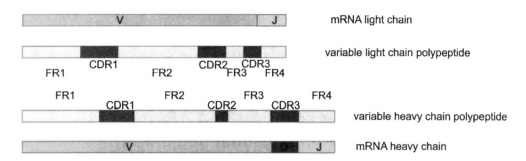

Fig. 5. mRNA of variable regions and corresponding polypeptides vH and vL. mRNAs of antibodies are composed of V-(D)-J regions. These are translated as vH and vL, characterized by relatively conserved FR regions and antigen-binding complementary determing regions (CDRs).

Table 1
Generation of Immunoglobulin Diversity by Independent Mechanisms

Multiple germline V, D, and J genes
Different V-J light chain and V-D-J heavy chain recombinations
Recombinational inaccuracies
Somatic point mutations
Assorted heavy and light chains

resulting antibody assortment through the combination of heavy and light chains, somatic point mutations, and recombinational accuracy. Table 1 summarizes these five mechanisms that allow the generation of a repertoire of at least 10^8 different antibodies, sufficient to recognize most antigens invading the body. Modern DNA recombination technologies learned to copy these naturally occurring principles for the design of artificial antibody molecules.

IN VIVO APPLICATION OF ANTIBODIES

Immunoglobulins for Therapeutic Applications

Immunoglobulins in the form of injectable polyclonal gammaglobulins, so-called intramuscular immunoglobulin (IMIG) and intravenous immunoglobulin (IVIG) preparations, have been used since 1944. In IVIG preparations, antibody oligomers must be elimimated, to avoid spontaneous complement activation. The associated side effects (adverse reactions) of the first generation of serotherapy were overcome by Cohn fractionation technology *(3)*. IVIG is prepared from pools of serum collected from large numbers of healthy donors. Cohn-Oncley cold ethanol fractionation is based on the principle that proteins can specifically precipitate in a certain environment, according to size, charge, and other physicochemical properties. This technology is used by several manufacturers to separate the γ-globulin fraction from other serum proteins. Subsequent biochemical steps downstream of the Cohn fraction are applied and may include ion exchange chromatography, ultrafiltration, enzymatic digestion, manipulation of pH, and salt concentration; these vary with the manufacturer. These procedures remove proteins and other contaminants and minimize the concentration of aggregates that increase the risk of anaphylactoid and other adverse reactions in recipients. Various technologies such as heat treatment (pasteurization) or treatment with solvent/detergent safely inactivate enveloped viruses and contribute to product safety. Nonenveloped viral contaminants are more difficult to inactivate. Nevertheless, careful control of plasma donations, combined with modern production technology, has established a high degree of safety for such products even if plasma donations are included from infected individuals.

In the last 50 years, an increasing number of diseases and patients have been treated with immunoglobulins. Mild adverse reactions (headache, flushing, backache, and nausea) are often associated with fast infusion rates. Only rarely are hematologic, neurologic, or renal adverse effects seen with high doses of IVIG.

Generally, antibodies can be used in different applications for prevention, diagnosis, or treatment of diseases. As summarized in Table 2, depending on the intended purpose, immunoglobulins can be generated by different production systems and in different molecular forms.

Usually the mammalian immune system is used to generate antibodies of particular specificities. As shown in Figure 6, antigen-induced humoral immune response leads to a predetermined spectrum of specific antibodies, which can be rescued for various methods of in vitro production, for permanent or transient B-cell immortalization, or for gene isolation. Once the ability to produce antibodies is preserved in an immortal hybridoma cell line or the genes are accessible in a transiently immortalized B-cell-transformed by Epstein-Barr virus (EBV), a broad network of technologies for stable expression can be applied (see Fig. 7 for an overview). In the following chapters these technologies and techniques are described in more detail.

IVIG from Healthy Donors

IVIGs are used in replacement therapy in patients with primary and secondary immunodeficiency in the prevention of bacterial infections *(4)*. HIV-infected children are also treated since they are immunocompromised *(5)*. In clinical experience, these γ-globulins have proved to be powerful agents in reducing the rate of serious bacterial infections *(6)*. Other applications, such as after bone marrow transplantations to prevent graft-versus-host disease, or immune thrombocytopenic purpura have been reported *(7)*. In addition, IVIG is now also being tested for the treatment of multiple myeloma *(8,9)* and recurrent spontaneous abortion *(10)*.

Hyperimmune Sera

Hyperimmune sera are produced from plasma donations of actively vaccinated, reconvalescent or infected donors. They are available for prevention of disease or treatment of various viruses and pathogens; they can help with acute diseases and can protect patients for a limited period.

A commonly used hyperimmune serum is the anti-Rh (D) immunoglobulin administered after Rh-D-incompatible child delivery or abortion or in circumstances that might result in maternal exposure to fetal blood of an unknown type *(11)*. Although the mechanism of action is not well understood, it is believed that the anti-Rh-D immunoglobulin interacts directly with the Rh-D antigens, thereby preventing the interaction between the antigens and the maternal immune system. The appropriate use of

Table 2
Summary of Favorable Functions of Antibodies for In Vivo Application

Purpose	Favorable functions	Preferred type of antibody	Favorable expression system
In vivo imaging of tumors for diagnostic purpose	Specific recognition and binding, rapid serum clearance	Fab, Fv	*E. coli*, yeast, others
Target agent for immunotoxins	High specificity, rapid serum clearance	Bispecific antibodies or fragments, conjugated antibodies	*E. coli*, chemical modification.
Neutralization of toxins after accident	High affinity	Fab, or whole antibody	*E. coli* or others
Prevention of infection	Specific recognition of infective target epitopes; also functional in mucosa	IgG, IgA, IgM	Mammalian cells as CHO, NSO, BHK, hybridoma
Treatment of manifest infections or diseases; long-term high-dose repeat treatment	As mentioned before plus: neutralization such as complement and ADCC, no ADE	IgG, IgA, IgM	Mammalian cells at high expression levels and low costs

Abbreviations: ADCC, antibody-dependent cellular cytotoxicity; ADE, antibody-dependent enhancement.

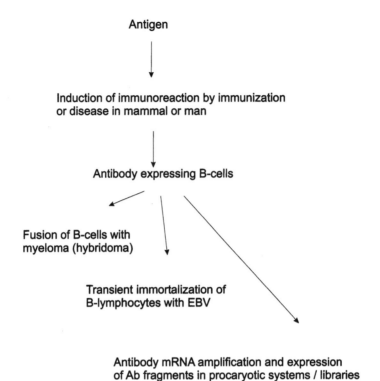

Fig. 6. Different ways of preserving the humoral immune reaction. EBV, Epstein-Barr virus.

anti-Rh-D immunoglobulin has reduced the prevalence of Rh isoimmunization in the United States and Canada by 96% since the 1940s; interestingly, it only received U.S. Food and Drug Administration (FDA) licensing approval in 1968.

Hyperimmune sera against different viruses, such as varicella-zoster virus, hepatitis B virus, cytomegalovirus (CMV), and respiratory syncytial virus (RSV) are used either after accidental exposure or to treat high-risk groups, such as immunocompromised patients.

Polyclonal human hyperimmunoglobulins are used to prevent lower RSV disease in high-risk children under 24 months of age *(12)*. Theses infants suffer from bronchopulmonary dysplasia or chronic lung disease or have a history of premature birth *(13)*. CMV immunoglobulin is used to attenuate primary CMV disease associated with renal transplantation if CMV-seronegative patients receive a kidney from a CMV-seropositive donor. When used prophylactically in renal allograft recipients, CMV-IGIV has been shown to reduce the incidence of virologically confirmed CMV-associated syndromes *(14,15)*.

Hepatitis B immunoglobulin (HBIG) has been shown to decrease the rate of recurrence after liver transplantation for hepatitis B *(16)*. Antibodies to the hepatitis B surface antigen (anti-HBs) are collected from individuals who have been hyperimmunized with hepatitis B vaccine. Varicella-zoster immunoglobulin (VZIG) is a prophylactic agent against chickenpox in immunocompromised children and is used in the prevention of postnatal chickenpox after intrauterine exposure and in immunocompromised

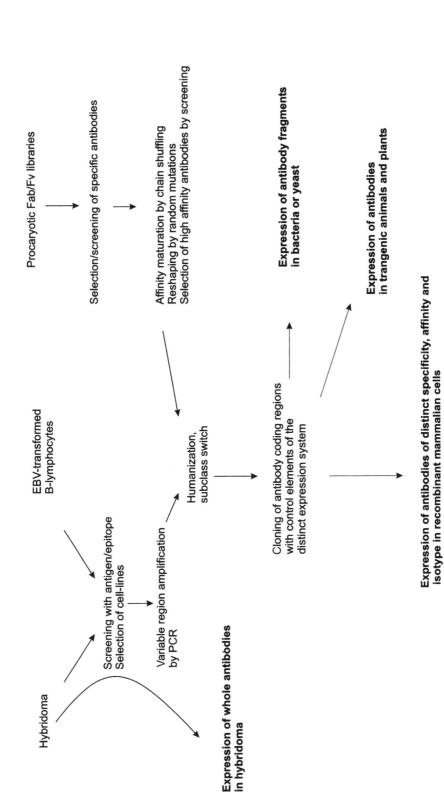

Fig. 7. Technologies for stable expression of human monoclonal antibodies. EBV, Epstein-Barr virus; PCR, polymerase chain reaction.

persons of any age *(17,18)*. Different preparations of hyperimmune sera are also available against rabies for application after rabies exposure *(19,20)*. Anti-thymocyte globulin is extensively used in the treatment and prophylaxis of rejection episodes in renal transplantations *(21)*. Furthermore, these preparations are used in different bone marrow recipients *(22)* and non-Hodgkin's lymphomas *(23)* to reduce CD3-bearing lymphocytes.

Other kinds of hyperimmune sera are the antitoxins and antitoxoids. With digoxin, the antibody Fab fragments are prepared by immunizing sheep with digoxin coupled to serum albumin as an adjuvant. Digoxin-immune Fab is then purified from sheep blood and used in the neutralization of digitalis toxin *(24,25)*. The protein was approved by the FDA in 1986.

Problems Concerning Naturally Occurring Antibodies:
Non-ADE-Inducing Monoclonal Antibodies

Because of their polyclonality, it is expected that antisera have the entire set of effector functions. Polyclonal antisera can prevent viral infections by different means. Binding of antibody to virus-infected cells can trigger phagocytosis or ADCC or can induce lysis via complement activation. However, a major question concerning the general utility of polyclonal human hyperimmune sera was raised by the discovery of antibody-dependent enhancement (ADE) in various viral infections through the binding of the Fc to FcγRI+ and FcγRII+ cells *(26)*. Although the exact mechanisms of the ADE phenomenon have not been determined, it is assumed that the virus/antibody complex on the Fc receptor triggers signals that are relevant for increased cell infectivity. It is also hypothesized that the virus/antibody complex is internalized via Fc/receptor interaction and thus promotes increased infectivity. As found with different Flaviviriadeae like dengue, yellow fever, Wesselsbron, West Nile, and tick-borne encephalitis viruses ADE can modify cell susceptibility through virus-reactive antibodies *(27,28)*.

Especially in asymptomatic HIV-1 patients, such antibodies with enhancing properties on homologous and heterologous HIV-1 isolates have been found *(29)*, and up to 95% of sera of HIV-infected persons revealed ADE *(30)*. In other studies the phenomenon of ADE could be assigned to distinct monoclonal antibodies *(31,32)*. These findings raise worries both for the establishment of a vaccine against HIV as well as for the therapy of HIV-1 with HIVIG. Alternatively, these risks could be reduced by using monoclonal antibodies as tools for mapping of non-ADE epitopes in vaccine design or by using non-ADE-inducing monoclonal antibodies (or characterized cocktails) for immunotherapy.

Monoclonal Antibodies in Therapy

Currently many "small synthetic molecules" are synthesized as drugs, which more or less specifically inhibit the activity of targets such as enzymes or block ligand/receptor-mediated pathways. This category of small-molecule drugs is often highly efficient in the treatment of particular diseases and is relatively cheap to manufacture. However, short half-lives as well as undesired and more or less severe adverse effects are observed. More recently highly specific monoclonal antibodies have been established, which will allow the pursuit of comparable therapeutic strategies with the expectation of increased half-life and reduced toxicity. Some of these antibodies have been successfully applied in human clinical trials and have received FDA marketing approval. In addition to their binding specificity, antibodies are able to confer important effector functions. In the following section we describe some cases in which experience in the use of therapeutic antibodies has been compiled.

Sepsis Syndrome

Sepsis syndrome, or systemic inflammatory response syndrome, is a clinical feature that occurs with serious systemic infections from Gram-negative bacteria or viruses. The stereotypical picture of septic shock occurs after trauma, hemorrhage, pancreatitis, and immune-mediated tissue injury. Many of the features of sepsis can be mimicked by certain cytokines, such as tumor necrosis factor (TNF) or IL-1. These individual cytokines or cellular mediators have been the targets in clinical trials. A range of different antibodies and antibody-based products has been tested that neutralize TNF *(33)* and prevent mortality in animal models of sepsis. Other interesting antibodies are directed against IL-8 *(34),* complement proteins, intercellular adhesion molecule (ICAM-1) *(35),* and E-selectin *(36),* which also cause neutrophil-mediated damage.

Another strategy is to block the cause of sepsis, namely, the effects of endotoxins of Gram-negative bacteria. Unfortunately, initial trials have not demonstrated a single antibody that was able to prevent or cure sepsis *(37–39).*

Infectious Diseases

A successful strategy for defending different viral infections requires the establishment of antibodies against protective epitopes. The identification of such epitopes is the most important step in efficient antibody development. The envelope glycoproteins of bacteria and viruses present such immunoreactive structures. The characterization of corresponding antibodies has confirmed their role for humoral protection. Usually, the most efficient neutralizing and protective antibodies are generated by the mammalian humoral immune system upon natural infection, probably because during primary infection complex oligomeric antigenic structures are presented in their native form.

However, the humoral immune defense of the infected host can be misled by its own defensive activity. The destruction of the infective pathogen may result in the circulation of antigenic debris that in no way represents the antigenic pressure of the original infection. In such a case the humoral immune response is induced to produce antibodies against epitopes that are irrelevant or even unfavorable. Mutation frequency of the infective agent is another mechanism for evading the humoral immune response. Infectious agents such as RNA viruses display the highest mutational frequencies. Monoclonal antibodies have been developed against a variety of infections including HVZ, CMV, herpes simplex virus, papillomavirus, hepatitis B virus, and HIV. Up to now the only one used for human therapy is a monoclonal antibody against RSV envelope glycoprotein *(40,41).*

Antibodies Against HIV

The humoral immune response to HIV-1 has been intensively studied. Considerable understanding of many details of the viral infective routes via receptor- and coreceptor-mediated mechanisms has been established. However, we are still far from a complete understanding of the role of antibodies in the prevention of primary infection and their role in the control of viremia during the chronic phases of infection. There is evidence that so-called neutralizing antibodies are not detectable during the acute phase of virus clearance after primary infection of seronaive individuals, whereas cellular immune responses are clearly found *(42,43)*.

During the chronic phase of HIV-1 infection, serum antibodies capable of neutralizing primary virus isolates in vitro are detectable. Long-term survivors apparently tend to have higher levels of those neutralizing antibodies than so-called fast progressors *(44)*. There is also evidence that the presence of maternal neutralizing antibodies correlates with reduced transmission of HIV-1 to the neonate. Indirect epidemiologic evidence suggests that mucosal virus transmission plays a major role during intrapartum infection of the infant *(45)*.

Nevertheless, the putative roles of neutralizing antibodies in prevention of infection or their beneficial contribution to the control of established viremia and disease progression remain to be established in clinical trials rather than by academic reasoning. The observation that HIV-1 appears to escape from neutralizing antibodies in vivo cannot be clarified by simple in vitro neutralization tests, which are inappropriate to simulate the complex in vivo dynamics of the battle between the immune system and a highly adaptive virus. Standard in vitro neutralization tests, even when done with primary virus isolates passaged on primary cells, do not reflect the complex interactive in vivo background matrix. Interactions with the complement system, antibody-mediated cellular immune responses, and other important in vivo derived and profound accessory factors are neglected.

It is well established that during the chronic phase of viremia the virus alters its (co)receptor tropism, and therefore neutralizing antibodies recognizing different epitopes (either so-called linear, structural, or complex epitopes) might be useful in prevention of infection or (therapeutic) control of viremia in different phases of progression. It is also established that viruses shedd in vivo are loaded with various cytoplasmatic and envelope proteins as well as with components contributed from the plasma of the host *(46)*. Little is known about the contribution of those host factors to either increased, or reduced or altered infectivity of the virus and its sensitivity to neutralizing antibodies in vitro or in vivo. At least it has become evident that the glycoprotein complex of HIV-1 isolates propagated in peripheral blood mononuclear cells (PBMCs) differs from that of T-cell line-adapted (TCLA) HIV-1 strains in various respects. The so-called primary HIV-1 isolates are generally less sensitive to neutralization by antibodies directed to certain domains on the gp120 envelope such as the CD4 binding domain and the V3 loop. It has even been noted that neutralizing monoclonal antibodies directed against these domains and also polyclonal HIV-1-specific antibodies derived from human donors (HIVIG) may enhance virus entry. One may even speculate that ADE is a strategy common to closely related lentivirus such as HIV-1, HIV-2, and simian immunodeficiency virus (SIV) in order to escape from neutralizing antibodies *(47)*.

On the other hand, it has been shown in extensive studies that the human monoclonal antibody 2F5 *(48)*, which binds to a conserved epitope on the ectodomain of the HIV-1 envelope protein gp41, is capable of inhibiting virus entry and shows no ADE phenomena. This antibody is obviously blocking an essential step in the process of virus entry of both TCLA- and PBMC-derived viruses *(49)*. One might therefore conclude that such types of neutralizing monoclonal antibodies and combinations thereof, which do not mediate ADE phenomena, may represent the most suitable candidates for passive immune intervention.

Nevertheless, as long as a clear relationship between in vitro observations and their in vivo relevance has not been established, animal models appropriate for studying the putative benefits of immune interventions with antibodies are probably more informative than results obtained from in vitro tests. However, none of the established animal models (the HIV-1/chimpanzee model, the simian/human immunodeficiency virus [SHIV]/macaque model, and the HIV/human severe combined immunodeficiency [hu-SCID] mouse model) perfectly simulates the complex HIV/human situation. Probably the SHIV/macaque model is the most suitable animal model available at present. It represents a versatile tool to investigate important mechanisms of intervention in the dynamics of HIV infection, phatogenesis, and prophylaxis. SIV infection of macaques mimics the natural course of HIV-1 infection in humans in terms of clinical signs *(50)*. SIV-HIV-1 chimeric viruses (SHIVs) were constructed that harbor HIV-1 *env, tat,* and *rev* genes in the SIV backbone. Some of these SHIV variants replicate in macaque PBMCs, infect monkeys, and cause AIDS in infected animals *(51–53)*. Thus the SHIV/macaque model represents an almost perfect animal model to study the protective effects of immune intervention with passively administered human antibodies.

Recent studies with passively infused MAbs either in single doses or in combination with polyclonal HIVIG have shown promising and protective phenomena in SHIV/macaque models. The antibodies 2F5, 2G12, and polyclonal HIVIG (all of IgG1 subtypes), when infused in combination or alone 24 hours prior to vaginal (mucosal) challenge with SHIV 89.6PD, were either completely protective against infection or against disease progression, whereas all control animals displayed high levels of plasma viremia and rapid CD4 cell decline *(54)*.

Compared with prior experiments applying intravenous challenge with the same virus and the same antibodies *(55)*, the data suggest greater protection upon vaginal (mucosal) challenge. Similar protective phenomena were observed in a maternal HIV-1 transmission model using SHIV vpu$^+$ for mucosal challenge and a combination of the human monoclonal antibodies 2F5, 2G12, and F105 for passive immunization. Four pregnant macaques were treated with the triple combination of antibodies approx. 1 week before section. All four dams were protected against intravenous challenge after delivery. The infants received the MAbs after birth and were challenged orally (mucosally) shortly thereafter. No evidence of infection in any infant was found during 6 month of follow-up *(56)*. In another small study, two chimpanzees were given the human anti-gp41 antibody 2F5 and challenged with the primary antibody HIV-5016. Compared with the controls, both passively immunized animals exhibited a significant delay in plasma viremia of approx. 4 months. Obviously the viremia returned with clearance of the antibody. One animal had a reduced viral load in plasma through 1 year of follow-up *(57)*.

The MAbs 2F5 and 2G12 are currently being tested in a phase I clinical trial to establish safety and pharmacokinetics. Seven healthy human HIV-1-positive volunteers have so far been infused with repeated single infusions of both MAbs, amounting to an accumulated dose of 14 g within a 4-week treatment period. No signs of any adverse effects, and, so far also no signs of escape mutants against neutralization, have been observed (Katinger et al., unpublished data). The MAbs 2F5 and 2G12 combined with the MAb b12 have also been investigated in an hu-PBL-SCID mouse model, to investigate their effects on the control of established HIV-1 infection *(58)*. In this experiment, undetectable levels of plasma viremia were seen in only one of three animals, whereas selected various escape mutants were found in the other two animals. There is, however, some criticism with respect to the conclusion that these neutralizing antibodies had a limited effect on the control of established HIV-1 infection in vivo. The weak point in these experiments was that none of the single antibodies applied neutralized the challenge virus potently in in vitro experiments.

Summarizing all the in vitro and animal model in vivo data available, one may conclude that specifically selected combinations of passively administered monoclonal antibodies have a high potential for the prevention of primary (mucosal) HIV-1 infection. We even dare to express our view that passive immune therapy could replace the current treatment of infants with inhibitors such as nucleoside analogs and nonnucleoside reverse transcriptase inhibitors and protease inhibitors.

Considering all the facts known from animal and human trials, there are various indications that antibodies might also contribute beneficially to the control of established HIV-1 infection. Although immune intervention with passively administered antibody combinations alone is probably not sufficient to control a full-blown viremia combination with existing inhibitors such as highly active antiretroviral therapy (HAART) would be compellingly logical. The current small-molecular inhibitors prevent virus replication inside the infected cell, whereas non-ADE-neutralizing antibodies prevent virus entry into the cell. Thus the therapeutic combination of antibodies with existing inhibitors could combine complementary interventive mechanisms. Furthermore, antibodies could additionally contribute to virus elimination by virus agglutination and by sterilizing immune mechanisms via complement activation and ADCC. One might also speculate that antibodies alone could control a low viremia once the peak viral load is brought down to the limits of polymerase chain reaction (PCR) detectability after combination treatment with the small-molecule inhibitors. If that was the case, patients could afford periodic interruptions of the triple therapy in order to recuperate from painful adverse effects while they are protected by well-tolerated antibodies. Nobody knows the answer as long as there is no evidence from clinical trials.

Rheumatoid Arthritis

The progressive destruction of bone joints in rhematoid arthritis is mediated by activated T-cells, macrophages, modified fibroblasts, and other inflammatory cells that deliver potent inflammatory mediators, cytokines, and proteases. Emerging clinical benefits are observed in antibody therapy directed toward the regulatory and effector cells of the immune system and their cytokines. The clinical response seen with anti-TNF antibodies *(59)* has confirmed the pivotal role of TNF in the process of disease *(60)*. Interventions directed towards T- and B-lymphocytes include antibodies against CD3, CD4, CD5, CD7, CD25 (IL-2 receptor), and CD52 (CAMPATH-1), depleting activated T-cells by binding to the cell surface *(61)*. Clinical trials with nondepleting anti-CD4 antibodies showed suppression of synovitis, but the state of improvement of disease is unknown *(62)*.

Cancer

Immunotherapy was and still is a central topic in tumor therapy. Cell surface antigens of tumor cells are targets for therapeutic attachment with antibody fragments—derivates and whole molecules. Most of the antibodies used today are directed against surface molecules of tumor cells and serve as diagnostic agents as they are coupled with radioisotopes such as ^{111}In or [99]Tc. Two MAbs have been applied in therapeutic use. Anti-HER2 MAbs are directed against a member of the human growth factor receptor family and inhibits the expansion of breast cancer cells in tumors with HER2 overexpression *(63)*. Another MAb with therapeutic significance is directed against the cell surface protein CD20 *(64)*. Patients with non-Hodgkin's lymphoma and chronic lymphocyte leukemia are thus depleted of lymphocytes and platelets *(65)*. A promising set of strategies employs radioisotopes or toxins that are attached to the antibodies as a means of targeting cytotoxicity ("the magic bullet" concept).

Immunosuppression and Transplation

The MAb OKT3 was pioneered with the idea of using antibodies in the field of immunosuppression and organ transplantation. The murine monoclonal antibody OKT3 *(66)* has been used since 1986 to improve graft survival and also to reduce the dose of toxic drugs such as cyclosporin. The main disadvantage of this anti-CD3 antibody is its murine origin and its significant immune response *(67)*. Another target for immunosuppression in organ transplantation is CD25, the IL-2 receptor *(68)*. Such antibodies are directed against activated T-cells and reduce acute rejection episodes in combination with cyclosporin and steroids *(69)*. Anti-TNF antibodies have also shown some encouraging activities *(70,71)* in the suppression of immune response after organ transplantations. The main drawback of immunosuppression strategies is the risk of unwanted infections after broad immunosuppression and massive release of proinflammatory cytokines *(72)*.

Cardiovascular diseases

Disorders of the cardiovascular system are often related to platelet aggregation or coagulation, causing arterial reocclusion or venous thrombosis. An anti-integrin MAb received marketing approval in 1994 and is directed against adhesion molecules involved in the final common pathway for platelet aggregation. The antibody Fab fragment is a chimeric human/mouse molecule and binds to the integrin GPIIb/IIIa *(73,74)*. Other antibodies reactive in cardiovascular system diseases are directed against von Willebrand factor *(75)* and tissue factor.

APPROACHES AND TECHNIQUES
FOR ESTABLISHING HUMAN MONOCLONAL ANTIBODIES

Today a broad variety of techniques to establish monoclonal antibodies are available. Through the use of cell immortalization and cell culture technologies, it was possible to isolate and grow antibody-expressing B-lymphocytes of rodent as well as human origin. Molecular engineering made it possible to express antibodies and their derivates in various host systems. Nevertheless, most MAbs used today were initially established through the humoral immune system from vaccinated or naturally infected mammals, in combination with B-cell immortalization techniques. Once the functions of those antibodies were established, the encoding genes were accessible for manipulation and expression in a host system of choice.

Immortalization of Human B-lymphocytes: Hybridoma Technology

The human immune system is a preferred source of antibody-producing B-lymphocytes. Vaccinated persons, infected, and/or reconvalescent patients represent an ideal source of antigen-primed B-lymphocytes either as a gene donor or for direct immortalization.

Different procedures have been established to immortalize lymphocytes as vehicles for the production of unlimited amounts of monoclonal antibodies. The first report describing the immortalization of human antibody-expressing B-lymphocytes with a distinct specificity with EBV was published by Steinitz et al. *(76)*.

Although the immortalization of B-lymphocytes is a rather easy technique to perform, an intrinsic problem is retaining stable antibody production in culture for prolonged periods. The transformation of peripheral B-lymphocytes from an antigen-primed donor with EBV generates expanded lymphocytes or even immortalized lymphocytes. Generally 2–3 weeks after virus infection transformants producing specific antibodies can be detected in the supernatant. However, with continued growth of the culture, specific antibody levels invariably fall and become undetectable after 3–4 months—probably owing to the overgrowth of the culture with nonproducing cells. Therefore EBV transformation is usually applied as a tool to enrich human antibody-producing B-lymphocytes for functional screening and as a means of amplifying the genes of interest. Somatic cell hybridization for the creation of antibodies with predetermined specificity was first described in 1975 *(77)*. This technology—the hybridoma technology—revolutionized immunology by allowing production of monoclonal antibodies of virtually any specificity. The hybridoma technology—first established with rodent species—was initially not used for the production of human MAbs. The application of hybridoma technology to create human antibodies suffered from the variable and often low fusion frequency of hybrids. Furthermore, the isolation and amplification of antibody-producing B-cells prior to fusion was one of the most critical points. In the following sections the main issues of immortalization of high-producing hybridoma cells will be addressed.

Source of Lymphocytes Capable of Cell Fusion and MAb Production

After immortalization of lymphoblastoid B-cells, the yield of antibody-secreting hybridomas very much depends on the status of the immunologic differentiation of the B-lymphocytes prior to cell fusion. In the rodent system, an optimized scheme of immunization can be applied, leading to the enrichment of antigen-stimulated B-lymphoblasts in the spleen, which are activated to enter mitosis concurrently with the fusion partner used for immortalization. By contrast, it is almost impossible to obtain human spleen B-lymphocytes from antigen-primed donors. Usually only PBLs of vaccinated or reconvalescent donors are available. Because of the lack of accessibility to surgically removed tonsils or spleen cells, alternative techniques have been developed to stimulate naive lymphocytes with the desired antigen outside human body.

In Vitro Antigen Priming

Techniques of in vitro antigen priming of B-cells are commonly refered to as in vitro immunization. Many protocols for in vitro immunization have been established *(78,79)*. Those include the purification of the lymphocyte population by inactivation or irradiation of T-suppressor cells and retaining T-helper cells and macrophages. After the antigen priming step *(80)*, the B-cells are amplified by incubation with B-cell mitogens such as *Staphylococcus aureus* Cowan I (SAC) and stimulated with lymphokines to secrete immunoglobulins. Often phytohemagglutinin is added to activate T-helper cells secreting the B-cell lymphokines. After screening of the supernatants for antibody production, the B-lymphocytes are fused. In vitro immunization procedures for B-cells producing high-affinity IgG have also been described *(81)*. However, none of these complex techniques have achieved widespread industrial application.

Amplification of human B-lymphocytes

Especially for the immortalization of human B-lymphocytes, very small amounts of cells are often available. The enrichment of the desired population of human B-lymphocytes prior to immortalization can be achieved by two methods. Peripheral B-lymphocytes expressing the receptor for EBV *(82)* can be immortalized by EBV transformation. Only a subset of 20% of the total B-cell population is actually immortalized *(83,84),* whereas a large fraction of activated antibody-producing plasma cells is resistant to transformation *(85)*. These findings and the fact that fully differentiated plasma cells lack the receptor for EBV indicate an increasing resistance of high-specificity, antibody-producing B-cells to EBV transformation as these mature into plasma cells following antigen or mitogen stimulation.

The second method for enrichment of primed B-lymphocytes uses growth factors (IL-4, IL-6, IL-14), mitogens such as plant mitogens (pokeweed mitogen), bacterial products (SAC), and chemical compounds such as phorbol myristate acetate or different antigens (tetanus toxoid, *Candida albicans*). This method needs no viral agents, and the cells are subsequently immortalized by fusion. Alternatively, primed B-lymphocytes can be enriched in the cell population by catching the cells with surface-bound, antigen-specific antibody *(86)*.

Fusion Partners for the Generation of Hybridomas

Several laboratories are still engaged in developing human myelomas or lymphoblastoid cells capable of establishing human hybridomas that stably produce human MAbs with a high yield *(87,88)*. However, only a few myeloma cell lines have been established that are capable of generating human-human hybridomas. Generally, these cell lines show low growth rates with doubling times of 40–60 hours. They also often tend to become senescent, possibly because of their nearly normal diploid chromosomal content *(89,90)*. The fusion of human lymphocytes with non-human fusion partners generates xenohybridomas preferentially segregating human chromosomes. Since the chromosomal constitution of intraspecific human hybrids is much more stable, human fusion partners for hybrid generation are preferable.

HUMAN FUSION PARTNERS

Plasmacytomas are differentiated human lymphoid neoplasias characterized in vivo by myeloma protein expression and in vitro by immunoglobuline synthesis *(91)*. These cell lines are very difficult to establish in continuous cell culture. Lymphoblastoid cell lines (LCLs) as fusion partners were taken into consideration because of the paucity of human myeloma cell lines *(92)*. LCLs are established from malignant or normal hematopoietic tissue and are easily maintained in tissue culture. Most of the cell lines described for human fusion are of lymphoblastoid origin. A comparison of different properties like hybridization frequency, yield of antigen-specific hybridomas, cloning efficiencies, growth rate, and clone stability shows no significant advantages of LCLs or plasmacytomas as fusion partners. The limitation of LCLs seems to be the sustained level of human MAb production in these hybrids. Cell morphology obviously correlates with the amount of antibody being produced; abundant rough endoplasmatic reticulum correlates with higher specific expression.

HUMAN/MOUSE HYBRID MYELOMAS AS FUSION PARTNERS

Human/mouse heteromyeloma cell lines efficient for human B-cell immortalization have been described by different authors *(93)*. The CB-F7 cell line was derived from xenogeneic somatic cell hybridization between normal human B-lymphocytes and the murine hypoxanthine/aminopterine/thymidine (HAT)-sensitive P3X63Ag8/653 cell line *(94)*. It displays rapid cell growth, high cloning efficiency, and a hybridizing efficiency of 2–6 clones/10^5 seeded lymphocytes. CB-F7 is ouabain-resistant and is therefore suitable for fusion with EBV-transformed lymphoblastoid cell lines, which, as human cells, are not resistant to ouabain. Several human monoclonal antibodies directed against HIV-1 were expressd from CB-F7 hybrids *(95)*.

Selection Screening and Stabilization for Antibody-Producing Hybridomas

After cell fusion, the primary hybrids contain a pool of primary transformants. These are mostly generated by random fusion events. In these inhomogenous cell pools, only a limited number of hybrids have the capacity to express antibodies of particular specificities. Furthermore, during fusion of the two karyons, the chromosomes capable of antibody expression may be lost. Therefore screening must be combined with an efficient selection system that eliminates all lymphocyte/lymphocyte and myeloma/myeloma primary hybrids. The HAT selection system is usually applied *(96)*, in which only hybrids fused between myelomas and lymphocytes can survive. Since only a minor fraction of the lymphocytes are antibody-producing B-lymphocytes, efficient screening procedures for antibody-secreting hybridomas are essential. Using, for example, human peripheral blood as a source of lymphocytes, it is often not possible to get more than 5×10^7 lymphocytes with approximately 10% B-cells. Calculating a fusion frequency of 1×10^{-4}, the fusion of 5×10^7 lymphocytes will yield approx. 5000 surviving hybrids containing only 500 B-cell hybridomas.

The first screening step is performed after 2 weeks when hybrids are starting to grow exponentially in the selective HAT medium. The surviving cell pool is then further stabilized by repeated subcloning with limited dilution techniques. Other immunologic methods have been established to screen the hybridoma supernatant, either with immunomagnetic catcher beads *(97)* or by dot immunobinding assay *(98,99)*. Repeated subcloning after every screening step is necessary to ensure that specific, high-producing subclones are selected. To establish monoclonal cell lines capable of large-scale industrial manufacture, an extensive stabilization procedure is essential. The stabilization procedure, by limiting dilution plating, can be assumed to be finished if at least 90% of the subclones show comparable IgG production as well as constant productivity over a period of 50–100 passages.

Recombinant Antibodies

In vivo application of murine MAbs shows reduced half-lives and induces human anti-mouse antibodies (HAMAs). Biochemical or recombinant engineering techniques are used to create more or less chimeric or humanized antibodies. Various methods can be used to generate functional antibody fragments or to replace regions of the protein backbone. To replace the murine Fc part of mouse-derived antibodies, the immunoglobulin molecule can be cleaved proteolytically by applying enzymes such as papain or pepsin. The smaller fragments can be separated chromatographically. According to the specificity of enzymes applied, Fab and/or $F(ab)_2$ fragments are generated. The $F(ab)_2$

fragments can then be chemically linked to a variety of substances including plant and bacterial toxins, enzymes, radionuclides, or cytotoxic drugs. Such modifications may be useful tools for the imaging of or to attack cancer cells if antibodies recognizing specific surface marker proteins are available.

Recombinant DNA techniques allow expression of hybrid molecules in different recombinant cell systems. Especially in human therapy, human/mouse hybrid antibodies are essential tools in overcoming the problems of interspecies reactions. Mouse MAbs that have undergone Fc replacement are described as chimeric antibodies. Humanization of antibodies is achieved by transferring the antigen-specific binding regions and single-framework amino acids of a mouse antibody into a human antibody backbone.

Chimeric Antibodies

Chimeric antibodies are generated biochemically or genetically by combining variable regions of mouse antibodies with human constant regions. Such recombined antibody cDNAs have been successfully expressed in different host cell lines. These expression systems use transcription of heavy- and light-chain cDNAs under the control of strong viral or cellular promoters and RNA processing elements in standard eukaryotic expression vectors. Such a hybrid chimeric antibody molecule contains less than 10% of mouse-derived sequences coupled to approx. 90% sequences of human origin, usually retaining 100% of the functional binding properties of the parental progenitor.

Humanized Antibodies (CDR-Grafted Antibodies)

To improve therapeutic benefit, humanization of antibodies has become essential. It was observed that not only rodent antibodies induced an immune response in patients, but also chimeric antibodies switched within the Fc region also induced the generation of HAMAs.

Humanized antibodies are chimeric molecules with only the six hypervariable loops of the original non-human antibody transfered into human framework regions (Fig. 5). Essentially, powerful techniques have been developed for the generation of antibodies that are nearly capable of substituting for the mammaliam immune system. The simplest way of performing humanization is to graft the complementary determining regions (CDRs) on human framework (FR) regions. The relative importance of at least single residues of the FR regions is determined by conformational adjustment of the CDRs after interaction with antigen. The first humanized monoclonal antibody of clinical relevance was CAMPATH-1 *(100)*. Humanization experiments with the murine anti-human CD3 mAb OKT3 made it evident that distinct amino acids in the FR regions contribute to the affinity of antibodies. A CDR-grafted version of OKT3 incorporating only the CDRs from OKT3 was found to be functionally inactive *(101)*.

Phage Antibody Libraries

The intact humoral immune system of the mammal represents the most potent library of antibodies. In vivo, after antigen contact the most suitable antibodies are selected, affinity-matured, and amplified in plasma cells. Screening and isolation of high-affinity human MAbs can be imitated by phage techniques and has been thoroughly reviewed *(102–104)*. Essentially, human V_H and V_L chains can be amplified from B-cell populations and cloned into the genome of phages. Fv or F(ab) fragments are expressed as soluble or fusion proteins, thus allowing linkage of genotypic and phenotypic properties of one antibody on each single phage particle. Phages are easy to handle and can be propagated in *E. coli*. A single phage library consists of at least 10^8 clones, each expressing one antibody attached to solid surfaces. Phages presenting antibody fragments of particular specificity can be selected from the library by a panning technique on surfaces on which the antigen of interest is immobilized. Afterward, low-affinity antibodies from such libraries can be randomly mutated by PCR under imperfect conditions yielding higher affinity variants. This procedure is called in vitro affinity maturation *(105)*. Several high-affinity antibodies, some of potential clinical interest, have been developed from such libraries *(106)*.

Host Cell Lines for Monoclonal Antibody Production

The choice of the proper expression system for antibody production depends very much on the intended use of the antibody. *E. coli* is an option for most of the nonglycosylated forms of antibody fragments. Mainly single-chain Fv fragments or their fusion proteins are expressed in *E. coli*, intracellularly or in the periplasmic space. High-level expression in *E. coli* tends to generate inclusion bodies in which the antibody fragments are accumulated at rather high purity but in a denatured form. Refolding to activate the protein is required. Different factors influence the protein folding, stability, and export of the antibodies *(107)*. *E. coli* can be grown in very large volumes and at high cell densities in simple defined media and with tightly controlled transcriptional regulation.

Yeasts such as *Saccharomyces cerevisiae* and *Pichia pastoris* have been tested as hosts, but little real progress has been described as yet *(108,109)*.

Attempts have been made to develop alternative production systems. The use of insect cells as a production vehicle is based on infection with recombinant baculoviruses; expression titers of around 30 mg/L are given *(110)*. The glycosylation pattern of such cells differs from that of mammalian cells. They process the so-called high-mannose type of glycosylation *(111–113)*.

The milk of transgenic animals has been reported to yield as much as 4 g IgG/L. The cloning of transgenic animals will probably open a new era of recombinant protein production. However, aspects of product quality assessment are still a serious concern.

Another novel approach for the production of antibodies is the use of transgenic plants as a production system *(114)*. Transgenic tobacco plants *(Nicotiana tabacum)* were first used to show stable accumulation of recombinant antibody in the seed *(115)*. Antibody production in a transgenic crop bears a potential of nearly unlimited mass production at low cost *(116)*. The expression and accumulation of up to 280 mg of secretory IgA antibodies per corn cob have been reported. Furthermore, corn is provided with the repertoire of housekeeping genes necessary to properly process complicated protein structures such as soluble IgA (sIgA) into their functional form.

Up to now antibodies for therapeutic application have been produced in mammalian cell culture. Generally, these are considered to confer proper posttranslational processing in order to achieve optimal induction of antibody effector functions *(117)*, pharmacokinetics, and biodistribution in patients. A variety of different mammalian cell lines are used, most commonly hybridomas. Hybridomas are easily grown in suspension in serum-free media, and, as long as rodent antibodies are acceptable, hybridomas are a common vehicle for antibody production. Human/mouse heteromyelomas are more complicated for mass production.

Most high-affinity MAbs are of rodent origin and it is often important to create chimeric or CDR-grafted antibodies, as described above. If molecular engineering technologies for antibody production are applied, the choice of the most suitable host cell line is essential. Criteria such as experience in the technologic use of a certain cell host, as well as the potential of posttranslational protein modifications, are also important.

Usually Chinese hamster ovary (CHO), myeloma cells (NSO and Sp2/0), baby hamster kidney cells (BHK), and monkey kidney cells (COS) are used. CHO cells and NSO have been used to express both full-length antibodies *(118,119)* and antibody fragments *(120)*. COS cells are usually only used for transient expression, often with low expression titers in preparative amounts for preliminary characterizations *(121)* to study different antibody constructs including whole molecules, F(ab) fragments, and bifunctional chimeric antibodies. The following characteristics are the main criteria for selecting a cell line for industrial production:

1. Posttranslational modifications of the MAb that do not elicit an immune response in patients
2. Production of high antibody titers
3. Stable production of the protein with consistent quality in serum-free media.

CHO, NSO, and BHK cells have been frequently used to express human glycoproteins. They obviously have the ability to modify, fold and secrete proteins comparable to that of the human in vivo situation. NSO and CHO cells are high-yielding expression systems with advantageous technologic properties. After processing for optimization, product titers up to 1 g/L for both cell lines have been described. In vitro tests of antibodies expressed in both cell lines gave identical results with respect to their functionality *(122,123)*. Antibodies are nontoxic for the host cell. Therefore permanent expression is possible.

Selection of a Stable Recombinant Cell Line

Recombinant cell lines expressing MAbs are provided with foreign cDNA, encoding the distinct heavy- and light-chain genes. The cDNAs are integrated into the host chromosome by mechanisms that so far have not been completely unravelled. There is, however, evidence that any cotransfected cDNAs underly comparable mechanisms of genomic integration. This phenomenon is purposely employed to create and select high-producing cells by cotransfecting selection or amplification marker genes together with the genes of interest. Different selection genes and amplification systems are available to obtain recombinant high producers in various hosts.

The goal of the selection procedure is always to amplify expression of the genes of interest in the transfected mammalian host cell line. Different systems can be used to select for high expression, so-called dominant markers and auxotrophic (also termed recessive) markers. Usually both systems are used in combination. Dominant selection markers generally combine the growth in the presence of an efficient drug substance, so that only clones with corresponding drug resistances will survive. The most widely used dominant selection markers are resistances against antibiotics. Auxotrophic or recessive marker systems make use of naturally or intentionally introduced deficiencies in metabolic pathways of the host cell. The resulting auxotrophy requires that the missing metabolite or a related agent be added to the growth medium or that genes capable of supplementing the metabolic deficit be introduced into the host. For example, many mammalian cell lines are glutamine auxotrophs, i.e., they require glutamine as an essential supplement in the growth medium.

The glutamine auxotrophic phenotype is also compensated for by transfection of the glutamine synthetase (GS) gene together with the antibody genes. Growing the cells in glutamine-free media thus ensures both the survival of the transfected host cell and stable antibody expression. The copy number of the gene encoding GS synchronously with the antibody genes can be further amplified by a gradually increasing addition of analogs inhibiting the activity of GS. Those cells that acquire increasing copies of the GS gene will survive and also coamplify the antibody genes. Thus high-expression cell clones are selected. This amplification system was shown to work very efficiently with the NSO cell line *(124)*.

Another widely used marker system is the dihydrofolate reductase (DHFR) system. DHFR converts folate to tetrahydrofolate, which is a critical metabolite in amino acid and purine synthesis. CHO cells lacking endogenous DHFR have been generated *(125)* by means of mutation and selection. CHO DHFR⁻ cells require supplemention with adenosine, desoxyadenosine, and thymidine in the growth medium. Transfection of an exogenous DHFR gene together with the antibody genes and omitting said supplements form the basis for selecting recombinant cells expressing DHFR and antibodies. A further amplification of the respective gene copy numbers can be achieved by a selection of surviving cells in the presence of methotrexate (MTX), which is an inhibitor of DHFR. High-producing recombinant cell clones can be selected by a stepwise increase of the MTX concentration. The DHFR marker/MTX selection system can also generally be used as a dominant marker. In this case an exogenous mutant DHFR with lower MTX affinity and sensitivity is used for transfection into DHFR-positive host cells. Thus the action of endogenous DHFR becomes negligible, and the transfectant cells survive in the presence of higher concentrations of MTX *(126,127)*.

Subsequent to the selection procedure, single high-expression cell clones are isolated. Various techniques have been established that are more or less labor-intensive. Fluorescence-activated cell sorting can be helpful *(128)*. The limiting dilution method in microtiter plates is very useful in obtaining cell clones of monoclonal origin. The assumption that monoclonality can be reached after only one round of subcloning is rather theoretical *(129,130)*. Repeated subcloning and intensive screening is necessary to establish stable, high-producing cell lines for industrial manufacture.

INDUSTRIAL PRODUCTION OF MONOCLONAL ANTIBODIES

Monoclonal antibodies for the prevention or therapy of infectious diseases are administered in doses of up to several milligrams per kilogram of body weight. Other biopharmaceuticals such as tissue plasminogen activator and erythropoietin, which are also manufactured by comparable recombinant technologies, are applied in only nanogram or microgram ranges per kilogram body weight. In other words, a beneficial antibody treatment dose requires an amount of at least a 1000-fold more of the recombinant protein. This simple comparison clearly shows the challenge and the necessity for the development of cost-effective manufacturing technologies. In fact, marketing and manufacturing costs as well as quality assurance have been the driving forces behind the major process improvements in mammalian cell technologies in the last few years. The manufacture of antibodies in transgenic animals or plants might be expected in the future, but quality considerations exist at the present time.

Large-Scale Production In Vitro

Figure 8 shows a typical flow diagram of the process of large-scale MAb manufacture. The manufacturing process attempts to obtain the highest possible product quality and safety, consistently produced at low costs in high amounts. A few manufacturing facilities have been established that allow production of several hundred kilograms of purified antibody a year.

Very important for the success of the entire manufacturing process is the availability of cloned cells that express the antibody stably at high levels. Commercial manufacturers usually do not publish detailed data describing levels of expression. According to the experience of the authors, cell clones, either hybridomas or recombinant cells such as CHO, can be established displaying specific expression rates in the range of 10–50 μg of antibody per 10^6 cells per day. As described previously, the establishment of these cell clones requires several subcloning and/or gene amplification steps.

The first logical step is the adaptation of the cloned cells to serum-free growth media. Again, commercial manufacturers do not publish the exact composition of media. Nevertheless, serum-free and even protein-free growth media have been empirically optimized that are also free of raw materials from animal origin, to avoid potential risks of contamination. Often enzymatically digested plant extracts are used as supplements to improve the growth-promoting quality of serum-free media *(131)*. These growth media are generally considered safe and are relatively inexpensive (approximately $1/L) when produced in large scale. Compounding of media is usually done by specialized companies that also certify the quality.

Once the cloned cells are adapted to a certain medium, an extensive program of stability testing is necessary to ensure that the cells are expressing the antibody in consistent quality and quantity over a certain number of passages. The number of passages in stability testing depends on the final production scale envisaged. If we assume that X cell passages are needed to reach the final production harvest, extension of stability testing to approximately $1.5 \times X$ cell passages is recommended, to ensure process consistency. It is therefore also recommended to perform the adaptation and stability testing of the cloned cells in a bioreactor that most closely simulates the physical environment of the bioreactor that will be used for the manufacturing process.

Once fully adapted and stable cell clones are obtained, a master cell bank (MCB) is established in accordance with the principles of good laboratory practice and good manufacturing practice. Usually, a working cell bank (WCB) is also established concomitantly from the master cells. The combination of MCB and WCB ensures a practically unlimited source of cells of identical quality for the manufacturing process. Each new production lot of product is then inoculated from the WCB and used for production up to passage level X. Full characterization of the MCB and the WCB is mandatory. The characterization includes a series of investigations that establish and define cell identity and safety in a clearly traceable and reproducible manner. These cells and the manufacturing process define the final drug with respect to all its characteristics *(132)*. In addition, various quality control tests are conducted on each batch of the biologic drug before

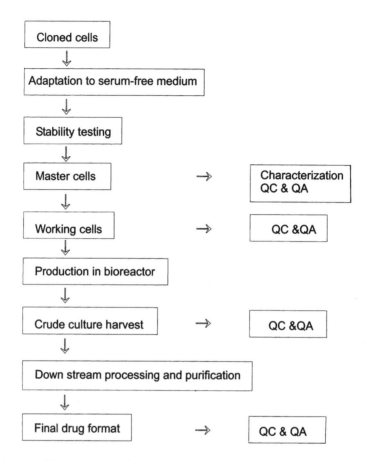

Fig. 8. Scheme of large-scale manufacture of antibodies. QC, quality control; QA, quality assurance.

release for sale or clinical testing. Manufacturing consistency must be proved in so-called consecutive lots, and changes in the established manufacturing process are only allowed under strict change control, validation, and approval by the licensing authority (depending on the status of the drug and the nature of the change). To establish maximum safety, controls are introduced at various process steps. For example, to control potential contaminations (such as viruses), samples from the crude culture harvest are tested since the chance finding of contaminants, if any, is highest at this particular step of the process.

Production in a Bioreactor

A great variety of devices for in vitro cultivation of animal cells have been developed. The choice of a proper bioreactor depends on the following criteria:

1. Cell type: in suspension or adherent to growth-supporting solid matrices
2. Cell culture method: batch, batch-fed, semicontinuous, or re-fed batch, continuously perfused
3. Scale of production.

Some common characteristics of animal cells that determine the design of in vitro cultivation systems (i.e., design of bioreactor and culture method) are low growth rates, sensitivity to shear stress, direct sparging, and ammonia. Designing large-scale cultivation systems is the art of determining the optimal compromise between engineering and reactor performance in order to avoid chemical or physical stress on the cells and to allow mass transfer to and from the cells. Such a compromise is easily achieved for small bioreactor units. However, if production units for manufacturing several hundred kilogram quantities per year are necessary, most of the currently used small-scale production devices are no longer useful. Only a few bioreactor configurations are applicable to large-scale, mass cell propagation and biologic manufacture. If the suspension type of cell culture is used for production, both the stirred tank reactor, the air lift reactor, and the packed bed reactor *(133)* can be used for large scale. If the adherent type of cell culture is necessary, the fluidized bed reactor is a good choice *(134)*.

It should be noted at this point that the standard cell lines such as hybridomas and NSO are preferentially grown in suspension, whereas CHO and BHK cells can be grown and propagated in both versions, adherent and in suspension. If the stirred tank reactor is used for animal cells, axial flow impellers with large blades are preferable, as they lead to good mixing with low mechanical shear forces. For aeration, direct sparging of air can be applied. Both reactor types (the airlift and the stirred tank reactors) have been used for up to 10,000-L working volume in animal cell suspension culture. Batch-, batch-fed, and continuous culture methods can be applied. Although the airlift reactor performance is optimal, with a constant filling volume slight modifications of the inner draft tube also allow its use with variable filling for batch-fed culture *(135)*. In batch culture the average cell densities are in the range of $1–4 \times 10^6$ cells/mL, whereas batch-fed culture allows a slight increase in cell density and maintenance in a productive state for longer time. Thus, increased yields of antibody in the culture supernatant are achieved. The batch-fed culture is defined by the increase of osmolarity due to the feed of substrates and by the accumulation of metabolites such as lactate and ammonia *(136,137)*.

On the basis of ultrafiltration principles, devices have been developed that give the reactor a kind of kidney function to remove low-molecular-weight metabolites and ammonia, while the large biomolecules are retained. Thus cell viability and density are improved and the yield of product is increased. Other possibilities to increase productivity are found with devices that allow continous perfusion with fresh media and cell retention in the reactor. Various unit operations such as ultrasonic devices *(138)*, special filters *(139)*, cartrifuges, or backlooping of cells into the reactor can increase cell retention. Such high-density continuous perfused systems can accumulate cell densities beyond 10^8 cells/mL *(140)*. Depending on the expression rate of the production cells and the cultivation methods applied, antibody titers above 1 g/L crude culture harvest can be accumulated.

Downstream Processing and Purification

Antibodies are applied therapeutically in high doses and at high concentrations. The process steps downstream from the bioreactor must therefore establish a product of the highest possible purity. Furthermore, the single process steps must allow safe sanitization procedures since downstream processing usually cannot be performed under sterile conditions. In addition to the purification of the antibody from impurities contained in the matrix of the culture supernatant, the downstream process steps have to be designed and validated to remove and inactivate potential viral contaminations.

A typical downstream processing procedure usually starts with removal of the cells and cell debris from the crude culture supernatant. Cell sedimentation combined with filtration or centrifugation are generally applied. The following process steps usually include a series of chromatographic columns containing different matrices, each of which contribute complementary separation principles to the entire purification process. Ideally, purification begins with a high-capacity antibody capture step based on the principle of affinity chromatography. Affinity ligands capable of reversible and specific binding of the antibody such as protein A result in an enormous reduction in volume as well as high concentration and purity of antibody. Additionally, they allow washing of the product with detergent and incubation with enzymes such as DNAses while the antibody is still bound to the matrix in the column. Last but not least, such procedures result in a robust inactivation and removal of potential virus contaminations achieved by a one-step unit operation *(141)*. Further purification steps after affinity chromatography usually apply ion-exchange principles that remove residual impurities, DNA, and ligands bleeding into the buffer from the first step. As for general safety cautions, the bulk purified antibody should be treated with one of the virus inactivation technologies routinely used in γ-globulin manufacture. The final drug format usually contains excipients useful for the stabilization and shelf life of the antibody.

ACKNOWLEDGMENTS

We thank Rudolf Bliem for helpful suggestions and critical review of the manuscript.

REFERENCES

1. Casadevall A. Antibody-based therapies for emerging infectious diseases. Emerging Infect Dis 1996; 2:200–208.
2. Schanz U, Hügle T, Gmür J. Additional inhibitory effects of intravenous immunoglobulins in combination with cyclosporine A on human T lymphocyte alloproliferative response in vitro [see comments]. Transplantation, 1996; 61:1736–1740.
3. Cohn EJ, Strong LE, Hughes WL, et al. Preparation and properties of of serum and plasma proteins. IV. A system for the separation into fractions of the protein and lipoprotein components of biological tissues and fluids. J Am Chem Soc 1946; 68:459–475.
4. Brenner B. Clinical experience with Octagam, a solvent detergent (SD) virus inactivated intravenous gammaglobulin. Clin Exp Rheumatol 1996; 14(suppl 15):S115–S119.
5. Crow ME. Intravenous immune globulin for prevention of bacterial infections in pediatric AIDS patients. Am J Health System Pharm 1995; 52:803–811.
6. Haywood CT, McGeer A, Low DE. Clinical experience with 20 cases of group A streptococcus necrotizing fasciitis and myonecrosis: 1995 to 1997. Plast Reconstr Surg 1999; 103:1567–1573.
7. Tarantino MD, et al. Treatment of childhood acute immune thrombocytopenic purpura with anti-D immune globulin or pooled immune globulin [see comments]. J Pediatr 1999; 134:21–26.
8. Chapel HM, Lee M, Hargreaves R, et al. Randomised trial of intravenous immunoglobulin as prophylaxis against infection in plateau-phase multiple myeloma. The UK Group for Immunoglobulin replacement therapy in multiple myeloma [see comments]. Lancet 1994; 343:1059–1063.
9. Chapel HM, Lee M. The use of intravenous immune globulin in multiple myeloma. Clin Exp Immunol 1994; 97(suppl 1):21–24.
10. Harris EN, Pierangeli SS. Utilization of intravenous immunoglobulin therapy to treat recurrent pregnancy loss in the antiphospholipid syndrome: a review. Scand J Rheumatol Suppl 1998; 107:97–102.
11. Mittendorf R, Williams MA. Rho(D) immunoglobulin (RhoGAM): how it came into being [see comments]. Obstet Gynecol 1991; 77:301–303.

12. Ottolini MG, Hemming VG. Prevention and treatment recommendations for respiratory syncytial virus infection. Background and clinical experience 40 years after discovery. Drugs 1997; 54:867–884.

13. Welliver RC. Respiratory syncytial virus immunoglobulin and monoclonal antibodies in the prevention and treatment of respiratory syncytial virus infection. Semin Perinatol 1998; 22:87–95.

14. Snydman DR. Use of immune globulin to prevent symptomatic cytomegalovirus disease in transplant recipients—a meta-analysis [letter; comment]. Clin Transplant 1995;. 9:490–491.

15. Snydman DR. Antiviral antibodies in transplantation. Transplant Proc 1995; 27(5 suppl 1):10–12.

16. Nymann T, et al. Prevention of hepatitis B recurrence with indefinite hepatitis B immune globulin (HBIG) prophylaxis after liver transplantation. Clin Transplant 1996; 10:663–667.

17. Chen PY, et al. Varicella-zoster virus infection in children with malignancy. Chung-Hua I Hsueh Tsa Chih [Chin Med J] 1994; 54:417–423.

18. Tarlow MJ, Walters S. Chickenpox in childhood. A review prepared for the UK Advisory Group on Chickenpox on behalf of the British Society for the Study of Infection. J Infect 1998; 36(suppl 1):39–47.

19. Lang J, et al. Suppressant effect of human or equine rabies immunoglobulins on the immunogenicity of post-exposure rabies vaccination under the 2-1-1 regimen: a field trial in Indonesia. MAS054 Clinical Investigator Group. Bull WHO 1998; 76:491–495.

20. Lang J, et al. Evaluation of the safety, immunogenicity, and pharmacokinetic profile of a new, highly purified, heat-treated equine rabies immunoglobulin, administered either alone or in association with a purified, Vero-cell rabies vaccine. Acta Trop 1998; 70:317–333.

21. Theodorakis J, et al. Aggressive treatment of the first acute rejection episode using first-line anti-lymphocytic preparation reduces further acute rejection episodes after human kidney transplantation. Transplant Int 1998; 11(suppl 1):S86–S89.

22. Eiermann TH, Lambrecht P, Zander AR. Monitoring anti-thymocyte globulin (ATG) in bone marrow recipients. Bone Marrow Transplant 1999; 23:779–781.

23. Fisher RI, et al. Objective regressions of T- and B-cell lymphomas in patients following treatment with anti-thymocyte globulin. Cancer Res 1982; 42:2465–2469.

24. Safadi R, et al. Beneficial effect of digoxin-specific Fab antibody fragments in oleander intoxication. Arch Intern Med 1995; 155:2121–2125.

25. Varriale P, Mossavi A. Rapid reversal of digitalis delirium using digoxin immune Fab therapy. Clin Cardiol 1995; 18:351–352.

26. Littaua R, Kurane I, Ennis FA. Human IgG Fc receptor II mediates antibody-dependent enhancement of dengue virus infection. J Immunol 1990; 144:3183–3186.

27. Morens DM, Halstead SB. Measurement of antibody-dependent infection enhancement of four dengue virus serotypes by monoclonal and polyclonal antibodies. J Gen Virol 1990; 71:2909–2914.

28. Morens DM. Antibody-dependent enhancement of infection and the pathogenesis of viral disease. Clin Infect Dis 1994; 19:500–512.

29. Auewarakul P, et al. Analysis of neutralizing and enhancing antibodies to human immunodeficiency virus type 1 primary isolates in plasma of individuals infected with env genetic subtype B and E viruses in Thailand. Viral Immunol 1996; 9:175–185.

30. Burke DS. Human HIV vaccine trials: does antibody-dependent enhancement pose a genuine risk? Perspect Biol Med 1992; 35:511–530.

31. Stamatatos L, et al. Binding of antibodies to virion-associated gp120 molecules of primary-like human immunodeficiency virus type 1 (HIV-1) isolates: effect on HIV-1 infection of macrophages and peripheral blood mononuclear cells. Virology 1997; 229:360–369.

32. Lee S, et al. Enhancement of human immunodeficiency virus type 1 envelope-mediated fusion by a CD4-gp120 complex-specific monoclonal antibody. J Virol 1997; 71:6037–6043.

33. Abraham E, et al. Double-blind randomised controlled trial of monoclonal antibody to human tumour necrosis factor in treatment of septic shock. NORASEPT II Study Group [see comments]. Lancet 1998; 351:929–933.

34. Mulligan MS, et al. Inhibition of lung inflammatory reactions in rats by an anti-human IL-8 antibody. J Immunol 1993; 150:5585–5595.

35. Mündi Y, et al. Inhibition of tumor necrosis factor production and ICAM-1 expression by pentoxifylline: beneficial effects in sepsis syndrome. Res Exp Med 1995; 195:297–307.

36. Owens R, et al. The in vivo and in vitro characterisation of an engineered human antibody to E-selectin. Immunotechnology 1997; 3:107–116.

37. Chmel H. Role of monoclonal antibody therapy in the treatment of infectious disease. Am J Hosp Pharm 1990; 47(11 suppl 3):S11–S15.

38. Chmel H. Monoclonal antibody therapy. Compr Ther 1990; 16:12–16.

39. Finch RG. Design of clinical trials in sepsis: problems and pitfalls. J Antimicrob Chemother 1998; 41(suppl A):95–102.

40. Meissner HC, et al. Safety and pharmacokinetics of an intramuscular monoclonal antibody (SB 209763) against respiratory syncytial virus (RSV) in infants and young children at risk for severe RSV disease. Antimicrob Agents Chemother 1999; 43:1183–1188.

41. Meissner HC, et al. Immunoprophylaxis with palivizumab, a humanized respiratory syncytial virus monoclonal antibody, for prevention of respiratory syncytial virus infection in high risk infants: a consensus opinion. Pediatr Infect Dis J 1999; 18:223–231.

42. Moore JP, et al. Development of the anti-gp120 antibody response during seroconversion to human immunodeficiency virus type 1. J Virol 1994; 68:5142–5155.

43. Koup RA, et al. Temporal association of cellular immune responses with the initial control of viremia in primary human immunodeficiency virus type 1 syndrome. J Virol 1994; 68:4650–4655.

44. Cao Y, et al. Virologic and immunologic characterization of long-term survivors of human immunodeficiency virus type 1 infection [see comments]. N Engl J Med 1995; 332: 201–208.

45. Mofenson L, Wilfert C. The challenge of HIV infection in infants, children and adolescents. In: Pediatric AIDS, 3rd ed. Baltimore, MD: Williams & Wilkins, 1998, pp. 487–513.

46. Stoiber H, et al. Inhibition of HIV-1 infection in vitro by monoclonal antibodies to the complement receptor type 3 (CR3): an accessory role for CR3 during virus entry? Mol Immunol 1997; 34:855–863.

47. Kostrikis LG, et al. Quantitative analysis of serum neutralization of human immunodeficiency virus type 1 from subtypes A, B, C, D, E, F, and I: lack of direct correlation between neutralization serotypes and genetic subtypes and evidence for prevalent serum-dependent infectivity enhancement. J Virol 1996; 70:445–458.

48. Muster T, et al. A conserved neutralizing epitope on gp41 of human immunodeficiency virus type 1. J Virol 1993; 67:6642–6647.

49. Schutten M, et al. Modulation of primary human immunodeficiency virus type 1 envelope glycoprotein-mediated entry by human antibodies. J Gen Virol 1997; 78:999–1006.

50. Franchini G, et al. Sequence of simian immunodeficiency virus and its relationship to the human immunodeficiency viruses. Nature 1987; 328:539–543.

51. Dunn CS, et al. High viral load and CD4 lymphopenia in rhesus and cynomolgus macaques infected by a chimeric primate lentivirus constructed using the env, rev, tat, and vpu genes from HIV-1 Lai. Virology 1996; 223:351–361.

52. Reimann KA, et al. A chimeric simian/human immunodeficiency virus expressing a primary patient human immunodeficiency virus type 1 isolate env causes an AIDS-like disease after in vivo passage in rhesus monkeys. J Virol 1996; 70:6922–6928.

53. Shibata R, et al. Infection and pathogenicity of chimeric simian-human immunodeficiency viruses in macaques: determinants of high virus loads and CD4 cell killing. J Infect Dis 1997; 176:362–373.

54. Mascola JR, et al. Protection of macaques against vaginal transmission of a pathogenic HIV-1/SIV chimeric virus by passive infusion of neutralizing antibodies. Nat Med 2000; 2:207–210.

55. Mascola JR, et al. Protection of Macaques against pathogenic simian/human immunodeficiency virus 89.6PD by passive transfer of neutralizing antibodies. J Virol 1999; 73:4009–4018.

56. Baba TW, et al. Human neutralizing monoclonal antibodies of the IgG1 subtype protect against mucosal simian-human immunodeficiency virus infection. Nat Med 2000; 6:1–7.

57. Conley AJ, et al. The consequence of passive administration of an anti-human immunodeficiency virus type 1 neutralizing monoclonal antibody before challenge of chimpanzees with a primary virus isolate. J Virol 1996; 70:6751–6758.

58. Poignard P, et al. Neutralizing antibodies have limited effects on the control of established HIV-1 infection in vivo. Immunity 1999; 10:431–438.

59. Kavanaugh AF. Anti-tumor necrosis factor-alpha monoclonal antibody therapy for rheumatoid arthritis. Rheum Dis Clin North Am 1998; 24:593–614.

60. Wendling D, et al. A randomized, double blind, placebo controlled multicenter trial of murine anti-CD4 monoclonal antibody therapy in rheumatoid arthritis. J Rheumatol 1998; 25:1457–1461.

61. Vitali C, Sciuto M, Bombardieri S. Immunotherapy in rheumatoid arthritis: a review. Int J Artific Organs 1993; 16(suppl 5):196–200.

62. Choy EH, et al. The pharmacokinetics and human anti-mouse antibody response in rheumatoid arthritis patients treated with a chimeric anti-CD4 monoclonal antibody [letter]. Br J Rheumatol 1998; 37:801–802.

63. Goldenberg MM. Trastuzumab, a recombinant DNA-derived humanized monoclonal antibody, a novel agent for the treatment of metastatic breast cancer. Clin Ther 1999; 21:309–318.

64. McLaughlin P, et al. Clinical status and optimal use of rituximab for B-cell lymphomas. Oncology 1998; 12:1763–1769; discussion 1769–1770, 1775–1777.

65. Jensen M, et al. Rapid tumor lysis in a patient with B-cell chronic lymphocytic leukemia and lymphocytosis treated with an anti-CD20 monoclonal antibody (IDEC-C2B8, rituximab). Ann Hematol 1998; 77:89–91.

66. Cosimi AB. Clinical development of Orthoclone OKT3. Transplant Proc 1987; 19(2 suppl 1):7–16.

67. Cahn JY, et al. Treatment of acute graft-versus-host disease with methylprednisolone and cyclosporine with or without an anti-interleukin-2 receptor monoclonal antibody. A multicenter phase III study. Transplantation 1995; 60:939–942.

68. Kovarik J, et al. Disposition and immunodynamics of basiliximab in liver allograft recipients. Clin Pharmacol Ther 1998; 64:66–72.

69. Blaise D, et al. Prevention of acute GVHD by in vivo use of anti-interleukin-2 receptor monoclonal antibody (33B3.1): a feasibility trial in 15 patients. Bone Marrow Transplant 1991; 8:105–111.

70. Heslop HE, et al. In vivo induction of gamma interferon and tumor necrosis factor by interleukin-2 infusion following intensive chemotherapy or autologous marrow transplantation. Blood 1989; 74:1374–1380.

71. Racadot E, et al. Sequential use of three monoclonal antibodies in corticosteroid-resistant acute GVHD: a multicentric pilot study including 15 patients. Bone Marrow Transplant 1995; 15:669–677.

72. Abbs IC, et al. Sparing of first dose effect of monovalent anti-CD3 antibody used in allograft rejection is associated with diminished release of pro-inflammatory cytokines. Ther Immunol 1994; 1:325–331.
73. Pereira H, et al. [Abciximab (ReoPro) in primary angioplasty]. Revi Port Cardiol 1998; 17:903–907.
74. Bailey SR, O'Leary E, Chilton R. Angioscopic evaluation of site-specific administration of ReoPro [see comments]. Cathet Cardiovasc Diagn 1997; 42:181–184.
75. Blann AD, Miller JP, McCollum CN. von Willebrand factor and soluble E-selectin in the prediction of cardiovascular disease progression in hyperlipidaemia. Atherosclerosis 1997; 132:151–156.
76. Steinitz M, et al. EB virus-induced B lymphocyte cell lines producing specific antibody. Nature 1977; 269:420–422.
77. Köhler G, Milstein C. Continuous cultures of fused cells secreting antibody of predefined specificity. Nature 1975; 256:495–497.
78. Ohlin M, et al. Human monoclonal antibodies against a recombinant HIV envelope antigen produced by primary in vitro immunization. Characterization and epitope mapping. Immunology 1989; 68:325–331.
79. Borrebaeck CA, Danielsson L, Müller SA. Human monoclonal antibodies produced by primary in vitro immunization of peripheral blood lymphocytes. Proc Natl Acad Sci USA 1988; 85:3995–3999.
80. Zafiropoulos A, et al. Induction of antigen-specific isotype switching by in vitro immunization of human naive B lymphocytes. J Immunol Methods 1997; 200;181–190.
81. Dueñas M, et al. In vitro immunization of naive human B cells yields high affinity immunoglobulin G antibodies as illustrated by phage display. Immunology 1996; 89:1–7.
82. Fresen KO, Hausen H. Establishment of EBNA-expressing cell lines by infection of Epstein-Barr virus (EBV)-genome-negative human lymphoma cells with different EBV strains. Int J Cancer 1976; 17:161–166.
83. Henderson E, et al. Efficiency of transformation of lymphocytes by Epstein-Barr virus. Virology 1977; 76:152–163.
84. Katsuki T, et al. Identification of the target cells in human B lymphocytes for transformation by Epstein-Barr virus. Virology 1977; 83:287–294.
85. Aman P, Ehlin-Henriksson B, Klein G. Epstein-Barr virus susceptibility of normal human B lymphocyte populations. J Exp Med 1984; 159:208–220.
86. Tomita M, Tsong TY. Selective production of hybridoma cells: antigenic-based preselection of B lymphocytes for electrofusion with myeloma cells. Biochim Biophys Acta 1990; 1055:199–206.
87. Shirahata S, Katakura Y, Teruya K. Cell hybridization, hybridomas, and human hybridomas. Methods Cell Biol 1998; 57:111–145.
88. Jahn, S, et al. Strategies in the development of human monoclonal antibodies. Dev Biol Stand 1990; 71:3–7.
89. Stanbridge EJ. Cell fusion, genetic cartography, and malignancy [letter]. Lancet 1976; 1:525.
90. Stanbridge EJ. Suppression of malignancy in human cells. Nature 1976; 260:17–20.
91. Kawahara H, et al. A new human fusion partner, HK-128, for making human-human hybridomas producing monoclonal IgG antibodies. Cytotechnology 1990; 4:139–143.
92. Rioux JD, et al. Molecular characterization of the GM 4672 human lymphoblastoid cell line and analysis of its use as a fusion partner in the generation of human-human hybridoma autoantibodies. Hum Antibodies Hybridomas 1993; 4:107–114.
93. Hirata Y, Sugawara I. Characterization of mouse-human hybridoma as a useful fusion partner for the establishment of mouse-human-human hybridoma secreting anti-tetanus toxoid human monoclonal antibody of IgM or IgG class. Microbiol Immunol 1987; 31:231–245.

94. Grunow R, et al. The high efficiency, human B cell immortalizing heteromyeloma CB-F7. Production of human monoclonal antibodies to human immunodeficiency virus. J Immunol Methods 1988; 106:257–265.

95. Buchacher A, et al. Generation of human monoclonal antibodies against HIV-1 proteins; electrofusion and Epstein-Barr virus transformation for peripheral blood lymphocyte immortalization. AIDS Res Hum Retroviruses 1994; 10:359–369.

96. Szybalski W. Use of the HPRT gene and the HAT selection technique in DNA-mediated transformation of mammalian cells: first steps toward developing hybridoma techniques and gene therapy. Bioessays 1992; 14:495–500.

97. Li X, Abdi K, Mentzer SJ. Hybridoma screening using an amplified fluorescence micro-assay to quantify immunoglobulin concentration. Hybridoma 1995; 14:75–78.

98. Bakkali L, et al. A rapid and sensitive chemiluminescence dot-immunobinding assay for screening hybridoma supernatants. J Immunol Methods 1994; 170:177–184.

99. Steinitz M, Rosen A, Klein G. An improved dot immunobinding assay for screening hybridoma supernatants. Non-purified antigen immobilized on nitrocellulose paper discs. J Immunol Methods 1991; 136:119–123.

100. Riechmann L, et al. Reshaping human antibodies for therapy. Nature 1988; 332:323–327.

101. Adair JR, et al. Humanization of the murine anti-human CD3 monoclonal antibody OKT3. Hum Antibodies Hybridomas 1994; 5:41–47.

102. Burton DR, Barbas CFR. Human antibodies from combinatorial libraries. Adv Immunol 1994; 57:191–280.

103. Hoogenboom HR. Mix and match: building manifold binding sites [news; comment]. Nature Biotechnol 1997; 15:125–126.

104. Winter G, Harris WJ. Humanized antibodies. Immunol Today 1993; 14:243–246.

105. Low NM, Holliger PH, Winter G. Mimicking somatic hypermutation: affinity maturation of antibodies displayed on bacteriophage using a bacterial mutator strain. J Mol Biol 1996; 260:359–368.

106. Burton DR, Barbas CFR. Human monoclonal antibodies: recent achievements. Hosp Pract 1994; 29:111–119.

107. Knappik A, Plöckthun A. Engineered turns of a recombinant antibody improve its in vivo folding. Protein Eng 1995; 8:81–89.

108. Pennell CA, Eldin P. In vitro production of recombinant antibody fragments in Pichia pastoris. Res Immunol 1998; 149:599–603.

109. Verma R, Boleti E, George AJ. Antibody engineering: comparison of bacterial, yeast, insect and mammalian expression systems. J Immunol Methods 1998; 216:165–181.

110. Tan W, Lam PH. Expression and purification of a secreted functional mouse/human chimaeric antibody against bacterial endotoxin in baculovirus-infected insect cells. Biotechnol Appl Biochem 1999; 30:59–64.

111. Carayannopoulos L, Max EE, Capra JD. Recombinant human IgA expressed in insect cells. Proc Natl Acad Sci USA 1994; 91:8348–8352.

112. Hasemann CA, Capra JD. High-level production of a functional immunoglobulin heterodimer in a baculovirus expression system. Proc Natl Acad Sci USA 1990; 87:3942–3946.

113. Nesbit M, et al. Production of a functional monoclonal antibody recognizing human colorectal carcinoma cells from a baculovirus expression system. J Immunol Methods 1992; 151:201–208.

114. Ma JK, et al. Generation and assembly of secretory antibodies in plants [see comments]. Science 1995; 268:716–719.

115. Fiedler U, Conrad U. High-level production and long-term storage of engineered antibodies in transgenic tobacco seeds. Biotechnology (NY) 1995; 13:1090–1093.

116. Zeitlin L, et al. A humanized monoclonal antibody produced in transgenic plants for immunoprotection of the vagina against genital herpes. Nat Biotechnol 1998; 16: 1361–1364.

117. Wright A, Morrison SL. Effect of altered CH2-associated carbohydrate structure on the functional properties and in vivo fate of chimeric mouse-human immunoglobulin G1. J Exp Med 1994; 180:1087–1096.
118. Page MJ, Sydenham MA. High level expression of the humanized monoclonal antibody Campath-1H in Chinese hamster ovary cells. Biotechnology (NY) 1991; 9:64–68.
119. Kunert R, et al. Stable recombinant expression of the anti HIV-1 monoclonal antibody 2F5 after IgG3/IgG1 subclass switch in CHO-cells. Biotechnol Bioeng 2000; 67:97–103.
120. Dorai H, et al. Mammalian cell expression of single-chain Fv (sFv) antibody proteins and their C-terminal fusions with interleukin-2 and other effector domains. Biotechnology (NY) 1994; 12:890–897.
121. Wurm F, Bernard A. Large-scale transient expression in mammalian cells for recombinant protein production. Curr Opin Biotechnol 1999; 10:156–159.
122. Peakman TC, et al. Comparison of expression of a humanized monoclonal antibody in mouse NSO myeloma cells and Chinese hamster ovary cells. Hum Antibodies Hybridomas 1994; 5:65–74.
123. Ray N, Rivera R, Gupta R. Large scale production of humanized monoclonal antibody expressed in a GS-NSO cell line antibody. In: Carrondo MJT, Moreira JLP (eds). Animal Cell Technology: From Vaccines to Genetic Medicine. Kluwer: Academic Publishers, 1997, pp. 235–241.
124. Bebbington CR, et al. High-level expression of a recombinant antibody from myeloma cells using a glutamine synthetase gene as an amplifiable selectable marker. Biotechnology 1992; 10:169–175.
125. Urlaub G, Chasin LA. Isolation of Chinese hamster cell mutants deficient in dihydrofolate reductase activity. Proc Natl Acad Sci USA 1980; 77:4216–4220.
126. Simonsen CC, Levinson AD. Isolation and expression of an altered mouse dihydrofolate reductase cDNA. Proc Natl Acad Sci USA 1983; 80:2495–2499.
127. McIvor RS, Simonsen CC. Isolation and characterization of a variant dihydrofolate reductase cDNA from methotrexate-resistant murine L5178Y cells. Nucleic Acids Res 1990; 18:7025–7032.
128. Borth N, et al. Analysis of changes during subclone development and ageing of human antibody-producing heterohybridoma cells by northern blot and flow cytometry. J Biotechnol 1999; 67:57–66.
129. Coller HA, Coller BS. Poisson statistical analysis of repetitive subcloning by the limiting dilution technique as a way of assessing hybridoma monoclonality. Methods Enzymol 1986; 121:412–417.
130. Underwood PA, Bean PA. Hazards of the limiting-dilution method of cloning hybridomas. J Immunol Methods 1988; 107:119–128.
131. Merten OW. Safety issues of animal products used in serum-free media. Dev Biol Stand 1999; 99:167–180.
132. Bliem R. Impact of research and development on validation, GMP and registration of biopharmaceuticals. Pharm Eng 1995; May/June:48–54.
133. Bliem R, et al. Antibody production in packed bed reactors using serum-free and protein-free medium. Cytotechnology 1990; 4:279–283.
134. Reiter M, et al. Modular integrated fluidized bed bioreactor technology. Biotechnology, 1991; 9:1100–1102.
135. Bliem R, Konopitzky K, Katinger H. Industrial animal cell reactor systems: aspects of selection and evaluation. Adv Biochem Eng Biotechnol 1991; 44:1–26.
136. Xie L, Wang DI. Integrated approaches to the design of media and feeding strategies for fed-batch cultures of animal cells. Trends Biotechnol 1997; 15:109–113.
137. Ryu JS, Lee GM. Application of hypoosmolar medium to fed-batch culture of hybridoma cells for improvement of culture longevity. Biotechnol Bioeng 1999; 62:120–123.

138. Gaida T, et al. Selective retention of viable cells in ultrasonic resonance field devices. Biotechnol Prog 1996; 12:73–76.
139. Banik GG, Heath CA. Partial and total cell retention in a filtration-based homogeneous perfusion reactor. Biotechnol Prog 1995; 11:584–588.
140. Bliem R, et al. Performance characteristics of mammalian cell culture process operating continuously with protein-free medium. Appl Biochem Biotechnol 1990; 26:217–229.
141. Amersham PB. Evaluating virus removal/inactivation in a process to purify anti-HIV-1 human monoclonal antibody by expanded bed adsorption with STREAMLINE rProteinA. Application note, 1998.

5

Dendritic Cells

*Their Role in the Immune Response to Infectious Organisms and
Their Potential Use in Therapeutic Vaccination*

Smriti K. Kundu-Raychaudhuri and Edgar G. Engleman

INTRODUCTION

The ability of the immune system to recognize and eliminate infectious agents has been well established. As detailed in the other chapters of this monograph, both humoral and cellular immune responses contribute to the elimination of infection. Over the past decade, our own research has focused on a critical component of the cell-mediated immune system, bone marrow-derived dendritic cells (DCs). At least two distinct populations of such DC have been described, including the classical and more numerous myeloid DC and the recently described plasmacytoid or Interferon-α secreting DC. Most studies of DC completed in the past two decades have not distinguished between these two populations, but because myeloid DC account for approx 90% of DC obtained from sources such as blood and lymphoid organs, the functions attributed to DC mainly reflect myeloid DC activity. Unless otherwise indicated, this report summarizes our current understanding of the functions of myeloid DC.

DCs are extremely potent antigen-presenting cells (APCs) that initiate immune responses to pathogens by taking up, processing, and presenting antigens to T-cells. Present in all tissues except the brain, DCs serve as sentinels for the immune system and (particularly in the skin, mucosal sites, and lung) are among the earliest cell populations to come into contact with invading organisms. When activated by antigen and "danger signals," DCs in peripheral tissues carry antigens via the lymphatic system into the T-cell regions of draining lymph nodes, where they stimulate primary and memory T-cell responses *(1)*. DCs are also central to the development of antibody responses because of the requisite role of activated helper T-cells in the differentiation of B-cells *(2,3)*. Through their activation of helper and cytolytic T-cells and the subsequent interaction of T-helper cells with B-cells, DCs dictate both the nature and potency of the immune response.

DCs are in effect nature's adjuvant. They are not only capable of inducing antigen-specific helper and cytotoxic T-cell responses, they also produce a cytokine, interleukin-12 (IL-12), and chemokines such as RANTES and fractalkine. IL-12 skews the T-cell response

From: *Immunotherapy for Infectious Diseases*
Edited by: J. M. Jacobson © Humana Press Inc., Totowa, NJ

toward production of interferon-γ (IFN-γ), a key immune effector molecule *(4)*. RANTES is a chemokine that attracts both naïve and memory T-cells *(5)*. Fractalkine has unique properties as both an adhesion molecule and a chemokine for DCs and T-cells *(6)*. Thus, RANTES and fractalkine help to increase DC/T-cell conjugate formation and, in turn, T-cell activation.

Exposure of DCs to foreign antigens does not on its own result in the efficient induction of IL-12 production *(7)*. In general, IL-12-inducing factors ("danger signals") such as lipopolysaccharide, immunostimulatory DNA sequences, double-stranded RNA, or products of activated T-cells such as CD40 ligand and IFN-γ are required to "super activate" DCs. These factors not only induce IL-12 synthesis by DCs but, in addition, trigger the development of an activated DC phenotype (increased surface expression of MHC antigens, costimulatory molecules, and adhesion molecules) such that the cells become far more efficient at antigen presentation. Importantly, most of these stimuli are products of infectious organisms. Of particular interest is the recent observation that certain immunostimulatory DNA sequences (so-called CpG-containing oligonucleotides) found principally in bacterial DNA are extraordinarily potent stimulators of the immune system *(8)*. At least part of this stimulatory effect appears to be owing to direct activation of DC by these sequences *(9)*. Most recently, double-stranded RNA from influenza virus has been reported to activate DCs in a manner somewhat analogous to that mediated by CpG-containing oligonucleotides *(10)*. Whether or not other viral RNAs also activate DCs is not yet known.

As noted above, IL-12 is an important mediator of DC function, and abnormal production of this cytokine during infection can be associated with a poor clinical outcome. Abnormalities in IL-12 production by APCs have been reported in a variety of infections, including *Leishmania major, Trypanosoma cruzi,* influenza virus, and HIV infection *(11–16)*. Addition of IL-12 to T-cells in vitro restores recall responses to antigen *(17)*. Genetic differences in cytokine-mediated responses may also influence disease progression following infection. For example, the genetic background of T-lymphocytes affects the development of the Th phenotype, resulting in either resistance or susceptibility of different mouse strains to pathogens such as *Leishmania major (18)*. Almost certainly, genetic differences contribute to the variable response to pathogens commonly observed in clinical practice. In this regard, Holland et al. *(19)* have reported rare patients who have refractory disseminated nontuberculosis mycobacterial infections without HIV infection and have abnormal IL-12 regulation. IFN-γ has been used successfully in combination with antimycobacterials in the treatment of these patients *(19)*.

DENDRITIC CELLS IN HIV INFECTION

The induction of antigen-specific immune responses is certainly the most pertinent function of DCs, and this function has been amply demonstrated. DCs exposed to infectious influenza virus or influenza nucleoprotein peptide, sendai, herpes simplex, Moloney leukemia virus, or HIV induce both proliferative and antiviral CTL responses, in vitro, in mouse and human systems *(20–23)*. In our earliest studies of human DCs, we demonstrated that these cells, but not monocytes or B-cells, can sensitize naïve T-cells to soluble protein antigens, enabling the generation of antigen-specific CD4+ helper and CD8+ cytotoxic T-lymphocyte (CTL) lines, in vitro *(24,25)*. Nonetheless, several organisms infect DCs and/or otherwise compromise DC function and presumably gain a significant survival advantage by doing so.

The role of DC in HIV infection and spread is controversial. A number of studies suggest that HIV takes advantage of the antigen-presenting and lymph node-homing properties of DCs. Thus, the initiation of most cases of HIV infection involves passage of the virus through mucous membranes, a process that is enhanced by local tissue damage and inflammation. DCs are believed to be the first cells to interact with HIV at these sites *(26)*, where they can be infected and become latent and/or persistent sources of infectious virus *(27,28)*. When these cells interact with CD4+ T-cells, either in the draining lymphoid organs or before migration at sites of inflammation, they can efficiently transfer infection *(28–31)*. Immature DCs in peripheral blood that migrate to mucosal sites have been posited to be the initial targets of HIV-1 infection, preferentially via R5 viruses. Freshly isolated peripheral blood DCs (DC precursors) have the highest number of CCR5 antibody binding sites based on quantitative fluorescence-activated cell sorting analysis. Downregulation of CCR5 and upregulation of CXCR4 occur with maturation of DCs. Mature cells express more CXCR4 receptors and are more susceptible to HIV R4 infection. However, different strains of HIV are often found in DCs and T-cells purified from the blood of AIDS patients, and there is no close correlation between infection levels in DCs and T-cells (32). These observations indicate that many strains may not be trafficking between DCs and T-cells. Finally, the possibility exists that myeloid and plasmacytoid DC differ in their susceptibility to HIV infection.

Despite their putative role in facilitating initial HIV infection, as APCs, DCs play important roles in both innate and acquired immunity to HIV infection. Plasmacytoid DC are important in innate immunity by producing IFN-α upon HIV exposure that partially inhibit viral replication. These cells also induce Th1 immunity *(33,34)*. Myeloid DC induce both primary and recall HIV-specific helper T-cell and CTL responses that kill virus-infected target cells *(20,35–37)*. There are controversial reports of defective antigen presentation by DCs to T-cells in HIV-infected patients *(38–45)*. Moreover, as HIV-infected patients progress to AIDS, there is progressive deterioration in the ability to generate functional DCs from precursors in the blood and bone marrow. Nonetheless, CTL epitopes of HIV induce both primary and secondary immune responses *(20,35)*, and such epitopes are candidates for use in vaccines. Exposure of DCs to these epitopes followed by administration of antigen-loaded DCs in vivo can also initiate primary CTL responses *(46)*. DCs loaded with HIV antigens can initiate both CD4+ and CD8+ T-cell-mediated immune responses, which have the potential to suppress viral load *(46,47)*. DCs also express macrophage inflammatory protein (MIP)-1α, MIP-1β, and RANTES, which could block virus coreceptor expression and protect otherwise susceptible cells from infection *(48,49)*. We have shown that DCs from HIV-infected persons with CD4+ T-cells > 400/mm³ can induce HIV-specific CTLs in vitro *(20)*. Most importantly, in a recent clinical trial, infusion of HIV antigen-pulsed DCs in HIV-infected patients was shown to be safe and immunogenic (see below and ref. *46*).

DENDRITIC CELLS IN OTHER (NON-HIV) INFECTIONS

Trypanosoma cruzi, the etiologic agent of Chagas' disease, infects humans and animals and induces natural killer (NK) cells, T-cells, and macrophages to secrete cytokines such as IFN-γ and tumor necrosis factor-α (TNF-α), which in turn control the disease.

However, infection of immature DCs with *T. cruzi* profoundly inhibits the ability of DCs to produce IL-12 and TNF-α. Moreover, infection of such cells prevents their maturation. Thus, by altering DC function, *T. cruzi* may escape the host immune responses, leading to persistent infection *(50,51)*.

Leishmania major appears to infect both macrophages and DCs. However, DC are the sole source of IL-12 production following infection with *Leishmania* organisms. The likely explanation for this phenomenon is that whereas both life cycle stages (promastigotes and amastigotes) infect macrophages, only amastigotes can infect DCs and do so without inhibiting IL-12 production by the cells. In contrast, infected macrophages do not produce IL-12 *(52)*.

During *Toxoplasma gondii* infection, host immunity is mediated by CTLs as well as IFN-γ, which is induced by IL-12. DCs stimulated with *T. gondii* tachyzoites or soluble antigens derived from this organism fail to produce IL-12. However, when DCs are cocultured with T-cells from *Toxoplasma*-seropositive individuals, they produce IL-12. These observations demonstrate that signals from contact between primed lymphocytes and DCs are essential for the induction of immunity to this parasite *(53)*.

Several viruses have evolved mechanisms that compromise the ability of DCs to mount an immune defense. DCs infected by measles virus are reported to lose their immunostimulatory functions and become immunosuppressive *(54)!* Human cytomegalovirus (CMV), a ubiquitous pathogen that is normally benign in healthy individuals, is a serious cause of morbidity and mortality in immunocompromised hosts. This virus and its closely related immune murine counterpart employ many diverse strategies to avoid detection by the host immune system. Among these are their ability to interfere with MHC class I and II expression on APCs *(55)*. Both human and murine CMV infect APCs, including macrophages and DCs, downregulate IFN-γ, and induce IL-10 production, leading to decreased expression of MHC class I and II, which in turn causes immunosuppression.

Human papillomavirus (HPV) is causally associated with cancer of the urogenital tract *(56)*. HPV-associated proliferative skin lesions expressing abundant viral protein can persist for years in immunocompetent subjects, a property that distinguishes HPV infection from that of the lytic RNA viruses. The fact that no antibody to viral capsid proteins is detectable for 6–12 months following infection confirms the idea that HPV infection does not generate a conventional immune response. One mechanism by which this virus may suppress the generation of immunity appears to be related to their infection of Langerhans cells (DCs of the epidermis). Thus, Langherhans cells expressing the E7 protein of papillomavirus have been shown to be poor stimulators of E7-specific T-cells. Precisely how HPV inhibits DC function is unknown.

Chlamydia trachomatis is a common cause of sexually transmitted diseases and a leading cause of preventable blindness worldwide *(57)*. Host defense against chlamydial infection is mediated by both cellular and humoral immune responses *(58)*. Ex vivo DCs pulsed with killed or live chlamydiae and reinfused into mice have been reported to induce strong protective immunity to vaginal infection *(59,60)*. Similar protective effects have been observed for *Borrelia bergdorfei,* lymphocytic choriomeningitis, *Toxoplasma, Leishmania major,* and equine herpesvirus.

As noted earlier, double-stranded RNA from *influenza virus* can increase the ability of DCs to process and present antigen. Presumably this is responsible for the observation that infection with influenza virus results in activation of DCs to such an extent that the cells are capable of activating CD8+ T-cells directly, bypassing the usual requirement for CD4+ T-cell help *(61)*.

CTLs are thought to contribute to *hepatitis B virus* (HBV) clearance by killing infected hepatocytes and by secreting antiviral cytokines *(62)*. HBV transgenic mice that are immunologically tolerant to HBV-encoded antigens represent a model of chronic HBV infection suitable for use in the development of therapeutic immunization strategies. Using this model, investigators have recently shown that antigen presentation by DCs can break tolerance and trigger an antiviral CTL response *(63)*.

In general, bacterial products processed by DCs are presented in the context of MHC class I and II molecules on the cell surface to T-cells. In addition to classical MHC molecules, DC express CD1, a molecule related in structure to MHC molecules that is involved in presenting non-protein antigens to T-cells. In this regard, the presence of CD1+ DCs at sites of *Mycobacterium leprae* infection has been associated with an improved clinical outcome *(64)*. Moreover, recent studies indicate that human DCs can present *Mycobacterium tuberculosis* antigens to CD1-restricted T-cells in vitro *(65)*.

Taken together, these results suggest that DCs play a critical role in the induction of protective immunity against a variety of infectious organisms. On the other hand, several organisms have evolved mechanisms to inhibit the ability of DCs and other APCs to process and present antigens, thereby hindering the development of protective immunity. Useful reviews of this topic have appeared *(54,66)*.

ONTOGENY AND PHENOTYPIC
IDENTIFICATION OF DENDRITIC CELLS

The same attributes that make DCs potent APCs make them ideal vehicles to deliver pathogen- or tumor-associated antigens for immunotherapy or prophylaxis. As noted above, antigen-pulsed DCs have been shown to confer protection against infection in numerous animal models. Alternatively, DCs might be used to deliver immune-modulating and antimicrobial cytokines and chemokines such as IL-12, IFN-γ, RANTES, and fractalkine to sites of infection or inflammation in vivo *(67–72)*. A potential advantage of this approach is the ability to target the delivery of immunomodulatory products to sites of DC/T-cell engagement where they will exert maximal effects and minimal systemic toxicity. Before considering how this might be accomplished, it is necessary to review our current knowledge of the life cycle of DCs, including the changes in their phenotype that occur with maturation and activation and the molecules that mediate their interactions with T-cells.

DC precursors are derived from CD34+ hematopoietic progenitor cells. These precursors migrate from the bone marrow and circulate in the blood to specific sites in the body, where they mature and act as sentinels for the immune system *(73)*. This trafficking to the tissues is directed by expression on DCs of the chemokine receptors CCR1, CCR5, and CCR6 as well as adhesion molecules such as the CD62P-ligand *(74–76)*. Tissue-resident DCs, including Langerhans cells in the skin, hepatic DCs in portal triads, mucosal DCs and lung DCs, take up, process, and present antigens to T-cells in the context of MHC class I and II molecules. The DCs present in peripheral tissues are efficient at taking up and processing antigen (microbial proteins or apoptotic bodies *[77,78]*) but not at presenting them to T-cells. Antigen-independent "danger" signals such as lipopolysaccharide (LPS), interferon (IFN)-α and -γ, IL-1β, and immunostimulatory DNA sequences present in many bacteria are required for DC activation, which is accompanied by dramatically increased expression of MHC class I and II molecules, costimulatory molecules, and other molecules (for example, adhesion molecules) that contribute to DC-mediated T-cell activation *(79)*. Once activated, DCs leave the tissues and migrate via the afferent lymphatics to the T-cell-rich paracortex of the draining lymph nodes, drawn by the chemokines MIP-3β and secondary lymphoid-tissue chemokine (SLC) through upregulation of their chemokine receptor CCR7 *(80,81)*. Activated DCs secrete chemokines, e.g., RANTES, that attract naïve and memory T-cells for priming *(82)*. They also secrete IL-7 and IL-12, which induce T-cell proliferation and B-cell differentiation *(83,84)* and Th1 immune responses, respectively. This stimulatory milieu produced by activated DCs, combined with the presentation of epitopes of antigens associated with MHC class I and class II determinants and the expression of costimulatory and adhesion molecules, results in the generation of potent antigen-specific CD4+ and CD8+ T-cell responses *(85)*.

In humans there remain difficulties in identifying cells of the DC lineage because no specific marker for these cells has been identified. Human myeloid precursors in peripheral blood express CD2, -4, -13, -16, -32 and -33. With DC maturation, these antigens are gradually lost from the cell surface *(86)*. By contrast, MHC antigens, costimulatory molecules, and adhesins increase with maturation. CD83 is expressed on most activated or mature DCs *(87)*, and antibodies to this molecule label such cells preferentially *(88)*. However, CD83 and other markers of mature DCs are absent or only weakly expressed on DC precursors. Therefore, the identification and isolation of such precursors still requires the exclusion of cells bearing lineage markers such as CD3 (T-cell), CD14 (monocyte), CD19, -20, and -24 (B-cell), CD56 (NK cell), and CD15 (granulocyte), as well as inclusion criteria, typically MHC class II expression *(89)*.

Committed DC precursors as well as activated DCs also typically express adhesins and costimulatory molecules that although not specific for DCs can aid identification *(90,91)*, including CD11a (leukocyte function-associated antigen [LFA-1]), CD11c, CD50 (intercellular adhesion molecule [ICAM-2]), CD54 (ICAM-1), CD58 (LFA-3), and CD102 (ICAM-3). DCs possess nonspecific antigen uptake receptors although at lower levels than macrophages. Some DC express FcγR (CD16, CD32) and complement receptors (CD11b, 11c, CD35). CD11c may also act as a receptor for LPS, as DCs lack the classical LPS receptor, CD14, and yet respond to this stimulus. DCs also can take up antigen through mannose receptors, potentially through the receptor recognized by the DEC-205 antibody *(92)*.

With activation and migration of DCs from peripheral tissues, antigen uptake activity and the associated antigen receptors of DCs are downregulated. As a result, the main function of these cells switches from antigen uptake to antigen presentation *(93)*. DCs are capable of processing antigen via classical pathways, e.g., breakdown of endogenous antigens in the proteosome followed by transfer of peptide fragments into the MHC class I compartment, and transport of exogenous antigens via endocytic lysosomes into the MHC class II compartment *(94)*. DCs also possess alternative pathways of antigen processing and can route soluble antigen into the MHC class I pathway through a mechanism known as crosspriming *(95)*. DCs may also utilize molecular chaperones such as heat shock proteins (e.g., hsp96) to deliver antigens via the class I pathway *(96)*. Finally, as noted earlier, DCs express the CD1 family of antigens, which appear to play important roles in the presentation of nonprotein antigens to T-cells.

As noted above, a number of studies indicate the existence of DC subpopulations. Some controversy remains as to whether these subpopulations represent distinct lineages or cells in different stages of maturation. Regardless of the answer, the possibility that the DC subpopulations differ in their functions has significant implications for DC-based treatment strategies. In humans, the classical "myeloid" DCs, which constitute the majority of circulating DCs and DCs in the periphery, are derived from a committed precursor of granulocyte/monocyte lineage. Myeloid DCs appear in the blood as lymphoid-appearing cells that express high levels of MHC class II antigens and lack most lineage-specific markers. Myeloid DCs can also be derived from several cell types previously thought to be terminally committed. For example, monocytes and committed granulocyte precursors can differentiate into DCs when exposed, in vitro, to appropriate combinations of cytokines including granulocyte/macrophage colony-stimulating factor (GM-CSF) and TNF-α, with or without IL-4 *(97,98)*. In addition to myeloid DC, a human DC subpopulation (plasmacytoid DC) expressing high levels of CD123 (IL-3 receptor) and CD4 and lacking the CD11c myeloid DC marker has been described *(99)*. These CD123+ precursors require IL-3 for their survival and an activation signal, such as CD40L, for maturation. They reportedly bias CD4+ T-cell priming to a Th2 response, in contrast to the classical myeloid CD11c+ DC, which induce a Th1 biased response *(100)*. However, viral infections predominantly induce a Th1 response *(101)*. These CD123^{hi} DC also play an important role in innate immunity by producing type 1 interferons upon viral exposure *(33)*.

Recent reports have appeared describing CD8α+ DCs in the lymph nodes and spleen of mice. These DCs appear to bias CD4+ T-cell priming to a Th1 response, whereas CD8α negative sign DCs appear to bias toward a Th2 response *(102,103)*. Because CD8 is primarily expressed on a subset of T-cells, these CD8+ DC have been postulated to be of lymphoid origin. However, recent studies from our group show clearly that these cells are of myeloid origin and that CD8 is induced on the cells when they migrate from the periphery to lymphoid organs *(104)*. No human CD8+ DCs have been described. Human DCs derived from CD10+ lymphoid precursors have been reported, although their role is not clearly understood *(105,106)*.

METHODS OF DENDRITIC CELL ENRICHMENT

Human DC precursors in blood constitute about 1% of peripheral blood mononuclear cells *(30,107)*. The low frequency of such DCs and the lack of specific DCs markers have been barriers to the isolation of sufficient numbers of DCs for routine study let alone development of DC vaccines. However, DCs can be enriched from the blood using density-based purification *(46)*. Most DC precursors present in peripheral blood are lymphoid-appearing cells that can be separated from monocytes on the basis of their different buoyant densities. Our group currently uses centrifugation through a solution of Percoll for this purpose. After 24–48 hours of culture, the buoyant density of DC precursors decreases, enabling their separation from lymphocytes by centrifugation through solutions of metrizamide, Nycodenz, or Percoll. Our group has made extensive use of this approach to prepare DCs for clinical trials *(46,108)*.

Several other approaches are now being used to generate human DCs. One method utilizes CD34+ precursor cells from bone marrow, cord blood, or G-CSF-mobilized peripheral blood, cultured in the presence of exogenous GM-CSF and IL-4 with or without TNF-α *(109–112)* to generate DCs. DC-like cells can also be generated from CD14+ monocytes after culture of these cells in vitro with GM-CSF, IL-4, and TNF-α for 1–2 weeks. Fifty milliliters of whole blood generates over 10 million such DCs, which are capable of inducing strong immune responses in vivo, in mice and in humans *(113–117)*. However, monocyte-derived DCs (sometimes referred to as dendrophages) are phenotypically unstable and tend to revert back to monocytes if not exposed to additional factors following their culture with GM-CSF and IL-4.

Flt3-ligand, a bone marrow growth factor, can also be used to increase DC yields by inducing the proliferation of DC progenitors, in vivo *(118)*. Flt3-ligand administration in mice results in preferential mobilization or release of DC precursors from the bone marrow to the periphery and into lymphoid organs *(118)*. Flt3-ligand administration in humans can increase the number of circulating blood DCs by 10–30 fold. These DCs can be harvested using a leukapheresis procedure for ex vivo manipulation and potentially used to prime humans to antigen in vivo. Such an approach would avoid the need for prolonged in vitro culture or repeated leukaphereses. Our group is currently using Flt3-L expanded DCs in clinical trials in patients with advanced cancer. The results to date indicate that large numbers of DCs can be obtained from these patients and that following in vitro manipulation, including antigen pulsing, these cells induce strong antigen-specific immunity when reinfused as a vaccine *(119)*.

METHODS OF ANTIGEN DELIVERY TO DENDRITIC CELLS

Several approaches have been used to "educate" DCs with target antigens for use in clinical trials. Microbial or tumor-associated proteins, or HLA-restricted epitopes derived from these proteins, have been used extensively *(53,115,119,120)*. The use of immunogenic epitopes relies on the ability to identify peptides that both bind with high affinity to a particular HLA allele and are recognized by antigen-specific T-cells. For purposes of generating antigen-specific, HLA class I-restricted CTLs, peptides that bind to the HLA*A0201 allele are most frequently used because this allele is very common (33–45%) among most ethnic groups. Peptides that bind HLA class II alleles did induce CD4 T-cell responses and are generally more "promiscuous" than class I binding peptides in that they often bind several alleles rather than just one and may therefore induce an immune response in a higher proportion of the population. Although this approach simplifies the production of target antigens to a limited number of peptides and allows the combined use of both HLA class I and II restricted epitopes, for purposes of generating both CTL and T-helper immune responses, selection of patients is limited. Moreover, since there are practical limits to the number of peptides that can be used (they may compete with each other for binding), a number of biologically important epitopes may be missed.

By introducing whole protein into DCs, immune responses would potentially be available to multiple alleles rather than single alleles as they are with peptides. In general, however, addition of full-length proteins to DCs would be expected to result in antigen processing only through the HLA class II pathway. This will result in the induction of T-helper immune responses but not CTLs. Although exogenous antigens might gain access to the HLA class I processing pathway, which can lead to stimulation of

CD8+ CTLs, this occurs inefficiently. Since CD8+ T-cell mediated immunity is required to control most infections, the use of DC pulsed with full-length proteins is not currently favored.

Several approaches have been developed to solve this problem, including gene transfer, which has been shown to result in antigen processing in the HLA class I pathway of DCs and presentation to CD8+ T-cells. Recombinant viral and bacterial vectors such as adenovirus, vaccinia, fowlpox, salmonella, and listeria expressing the antigen have been used successfully to deliver transgene products into the HLA class I pathway of DCs *(121–125)*. Another approach involves the use of "transporter" peptides to bring proteins into APCs for processing. Conjugating such peptides onto full-length proteins or peptides allows these antigens to translocate across cell membranes and into the HLA class I pathway. One such peptide is obtained from HIV *tat. Tat* is an 86-amino acid protein that has been shown to be rapidly transported from extracellular milieu into the cytosol of most cells. This property presumably plays an important role in viral replication or spread. However, it might also provide the means of delivering antigens into APCs for processing and presentation. When full-length *tat* protein was conjugated to galactosidase, horseradish peroxidase, RNAase, or pseudomonas exotoxin, the conjugated proteins crossed the cellular membrane of fibroblasts with enzymatic activity intact. One problem that must be overcome if *tat* is to be used for antigen delivery is that full-length *tat* protein as well as large (>20 amino acids) peptide fragments of *tat* are highly cytotoxic. We have addressed this issue by identifying the minimal region of *tat* required for transfer into cytosol and have demonstrated that a short, basic sequence corresponding to residues 49–57 enters cells without affecting viability *(126)* and induces both CD8+ and CD4+ T-cell responses. HIV-1 *tat* can increase the efficiency of HLA class I-restricted antigen presentation by more than 100-fold *(126)*.

CLINICAL TRIALS OF DENDRITIC CELL IMMUNOTHERAPY

HIV Trials

Numerous studies in animal models have documented that ex vivo antigen-pulsed DCs are effective inducers of pathogen-specific immunity *(59,63,66,67)*. However, the utility of ex vivo antigen-pulsed DCs for the prophylaxis or therapy of infection has not yet been extensively studied in humans. In the first reported DC clinical trial in HIV-infected patients, the safety and antigen-presenting properties of allogeneic or autologous DCs were investigated in seven HLA-A2+, HIV-infected patients *(46)*. Allogeneic DCs, obtained from the peripheral blood of HLA-identical, HIV-seronegative siblings using the density gradient procedure described earlier, were pulsed with recombinant HIV-1 MN gp160 or synthetic peptides corresponding to HLA-A*0201-restricted cytotoxic epitopes of envelope, Gag and Pol proteins. The antigen-pulsed cells were infused intravenously six to nine times at monthly intervals, and HIV-specific immune responses were monitored.

One allogeneic DC recipient with a CD4+ T-cell count of $460/mm^3$ showed increases in envelope-specific CTLs and lymphocyte proliferative responses, as well as IFN-γ and IL-2 production. Two other allogeneic DC recipients with CD4+ T-cell counts of 434 and $560/mm^3$, respectively, also showed an increase in HIV envelope-specific lymphocyte proliferative responses. A recipient of autologous DC with a CD4+ T-cell count of 723/mm^3 showed an increase in peptide-specific lymphocyte-proliferative responses after three infusions. There was a good correlation between the presence of specific virus sequences obtained by bulk plasma viral RNA sequencing and peptide-specific endogenous CTL responses measured by both direct and indirect CTL assays. Thus, these responses appeared to be recall responses. Three other allogeneic DC recipients with CD4+ T-cell counts <410/mm^3 did not show increases in their HIV-specific immune responses.

No clinically significant adverse effects were noted in this study and CD4+ T-cell numbers and plasma HIV-1 RNA detected by reverse transcriptase polymerase chain reaction of all seven patients were stable during the study period. Thus, both allogeneic and autologous DC infusions were well tolerated, and in patients with normal or near normal CD4+ T-cell counts, administration of these antigen-pulsed cells enhanced the immune response to HIV. Future studies of HIV antigen-pulsed DC infusion in HIV-infected patients will be required to determine whether this approach is clinically beneficial.

Cancer Trials

In contrast to infectious disease, a number of groups are pursuing DC-based immunotherapy trials for cancer. In the first reported DC trial, our group assessed the effect of autologous DCs pulsed ex vivo with tumor-specific antigen in patients with malignant B-cell lymphoma who had failed conventional chemotherapy. Like other B-lymphocytes, the neoplastic cells in these patients express surface immunoglobulin receptors, and because B-cell lymphomas are monoclonal, all the cells of a given tumor express identical surface immunoglobulin. Moreover, this immunoglobulin is potentially immunogenic by virtue of its unique idiotypic determinants, which are formed by the combination of the variable regions of immunoglobulin heavy and light chains *(127–129)*. To prepare idiotype proteins for this clinical study, patients underwent tumor biopsies, and the immunoglobulin (idiotype) produced by each tumor was "rescued" by somatic cell fusion techniques and purified from hybridoma supernatants *(130)*. This protein, together with keyhole limpet hemocyanin, which served as a control antigen, was used to pulse autologous DCs obtained from the patients by leukapheresis, and the antigen-pulsed cells were administered to the patients by intravenous infusion. This procedure was repeated three times at monthly intervals with a booster immunization given 4–6 months later. Throughout the trial the patients were followed for the development of an immune response to the idiotype, and their tumor burden was monitored.

A report of the results obtained in our initial four patients has been published *(108)*. All of these treated patients, as well as six not described in our published report, tolerated their infusions well, and none experienced clinically significant toxicity at any point during the study. In addition, most of the patients developed T-cell-mediated anti-idiotype responses that were not observed prior to treatment initiation. The antiidiotype responses were specific for autologous tumor immunoglobulin compared with irrelevant, isotype-matched immunoglobulins. In addition to these proliferative responses, T-cells from one patient were expanded for several weeks in vitro in the presence of idiotype protein and shown to lyse autologous tumor hybridoma cells but not an isotype-matched, unrelated hybridoma. Most importantly, two of the patients experienced complete tumor regression, including one who entered the trial with bulky disease and remained in complete remission for more than 3 years. A third patient experienced a partial response, whereas three have had stable disease and three have experienced disease progression. Recently, a new cohort of patients has been vaccinated while in remission, and their follow-up is ongoing.

Two vaccine trials for melanoma have also been reported in which the immunogenicity of DCs pulsed with a panel of melanoma-derived HLA-restricted peptides was investigated. Both trials utilized DC derived from monocytes by culture in GM-CSF and IL-4. Nestle et al. limited their clinical trial to patients expressing the HLA*A1 or A2 alleles and reported that 5 of 15 patients developed clinical responses including 2 who developed complete remissions *(115)*. Induction of delayed-type hypersensitivity (as measured by skin testing) to the antigen was seen with this vaccination approach. Lotze et al. also reported the results of their clinical trial in melanoma with one complete response in their cohort of six patients *(116)*.

Recently, we treated a cohort of advanced colorectal cancer patients with recombinant Flt3 ligand, a hematopoietic growth factor, and observed a 20-fold increase in circulating DC *(119)*. Subsequently, these cells were isolated and loaded with a synthetic peptide derived from carcinoembryonic antigen (CEA) and mutated at a single amino acid position to make it a more potent T cell antigen. Following vaccination with these cells, more than half of the patients developed CD8 cytotoxic T cells that recognized tumor cells expressing endogenous CEA. Moreover, two of 12 patients experienced dramatic tumor regression and several other patients had stable disease. Finally, clinical response correlated with the expansion of CEA specific CD8 T cells, confirming the role of such cells in this treatment strategy. Based on these encouraging results, a number of investigators are now pursuing DC-based clinical trials in patients with a variety of malignancies.

FUTURE DIRECTIONS

Although DC-based vaccination trials have yielded promising results, particularly in cancer, the procedures used to date to isolate, load, and activate DCs are cumbersome. As discussed in this review, newer methods for DC mobilization or expression appear to address problems related to cell yield. The potential benefits of coadministration of immunomodulatory cytokines with DCs is another new area being explored. Preliminary results of animal studies in which IL-12 and DC are coadministered have been encouraging. Similarly, synergistic effects of IL-2 with DC vaccination have been demonstrated in an animal model *(131)*. Efforts to genetically engineer DCs to augment their secretion of cytokines and/or chemokines (immune-enhanced DCs) are also advancing. For example, DC precursors transfected with retroviral vectors containing IL-12 and IFN-γ and pulsed with *H. capsulatum, Leishmania donovani,* and *Mycobacterium kansasii* antigens have been used to generate antigen-specific CD8+ T-cell responses in an in vitro system *(132)*. The antiinfective efficacy of Th1 cytokines delivered by genetically modified and microbial antigen-pulsed DCs in animal models of tuberculosis and leishmaniasis is also under investigation *(132)*. Eventually, however, simpler forms of therapy that utilize DCs must be developed before the properties of this cell type can be exploited widely in clinical practice. Identification of agents that induce DC maturation, in vivo, combined with methods of delivering antigens of interest to DC in vivo, would provide an elegant solution.

One such approach using Flt3-ligand and immunostimulatory DNA sequences has recently been described *(133)*.

ACKNOWLEDGMENTS

This work was supported in part by grants from the NIH (CA71725 and HL57443).

REFERENCES

1. Knight S, Stagg AJ. Antigen presenting cell types. Curr Opin Immunol 1993; 5:374–382.
2. Melchers F, Rolink A, Grawunder U, et al. Positive and negative selection events during B lymphopoiesis. Curr Opin Immunol 1995; 7:214–227.
3. Ridge JP, Di Rosa F, Matzinger P. A conditioned dendritic cell can be a temporal bridge between a CD4+ T-helper and a T-killer cell. Nature 1998; 393:474–478.
4. Heufler C, Koch F, Stanzl U, et al. Interleukin-12 is produced by dendritic cells and mediates T helper 1 development as well as interferon-gamma production by T helper 1 cells. Eur J Immunol 1996; 26:659–668
5. Schall TJ, Bacon K, Toy KJ, Goeddel DV. Selective attraction of monocytes and T lymphocytes of the memory phenotype by cytokine RANTES. Nature 1990; 347:669–671.
6. Raychaudhuri S, Jiang W, Farber E, Schall T. Role of fractalkine in cutaneous diseases. J Invest Dermatol 1999; 112:597.
7. Hilkens CMU, Kalinski P, Boer M, Kapsenberg ML. Human dendritic cells require exogenous interleukin-12-inducing factors to direct the development of naïve T-helper cells toward the Th1 phenotype. Blood 1997; 90:1920.
8. Carson DA, Raz E. Oligonucleotide adjuvants for T helper 1 (Th1)-specific vaccination. J Exp Med 1997; 186:1621–1622.
9. Jakob T, Walker PS, Krieg AM, Udey MC, Vogel JC. Activation of cutaneous dendritic cells by CpG-containing oligodeoxynucleotides: a role for dendritic cells in the augmentation of Th1 responses by immunostimulatory DNA. J Immunol 1998; 161:3042–3049.
10. Cella M, Salio M, Sakakibara Y, Langen H, Julkunen I, Lanzavecchia A. Maturation, activation, and protection of dendritic cells induced by double-stranded RNA. J Exp Med 1999; 189:821–829.
11. Carrera L, Gazzinelli RT, Badolateo R, et al. *Leishmania* promastigotes selectively inhibit interleukin 12 induction in bone marrow-derived macrophages from susceptible and resistant mice. J Exp Med 183:515.
12. Reiner SL, Zheng S, Wang ZE, Stowring L, Locksley RM. *Leishmania* promastigotes evade interleukin 12 (IL-12) induction by macrophages and stimulate a broad range of cytokines from CD4+ T cells. J Exp Med 1994; 179:447.
13. Bhardwaj N, Seder RA, Reddy A, Feldman MV. IL-12 in conjunction with dendritic cells enhances antiviral CD8+ CTL responses in vitro. J Clin Invest 1996; 98:715.
14. Seder RA, Grabstein KH, Berzofsky JA, McDyer JF. Cytokine interactions in human immunodeficiency virus-infected individuals: roles of interleukin (IL)-2 IL-12 and IL-15. J Exp Med 1995; 182:1067.
15. Clerici M, Lucey DR, Berzofsky JA, et al. Restoration of HIV-specific cell-mediated immune responses by interleukin-12 in vitro. Science 1993; 262:1721.
16. Chehimi J, Starr SE, Frank I, et al. Impaired interleukin 12 production in human immunodeficiency virus-infected patients. J Exp Med 1994; 179:1361.
17. Trinchieri G. Interleukin-12: a pro-inflammatory cytokine with immunoregulatory functions that bridge innate resistance and antigen specific adaptive immunity. Annu Rev Immunol 1995; 13:251.
18. Guler ML, Gorham JD, Hsieh CS, et al. Genetic susceptibility to *Leishmania:* IL-12 responsiveness in TH1 cell development. Science 1996; 271:984–987.

19. Holland SM, Eisenstein EM, Kuhns DB, Turner ML, Strober WA, Gallin JI. Treatment of refractory disseminated nontuberculous mycobacterial infection with interferon γ: a preliminary report. N Engl J Med 1994; 330:1348.

20. Dupuis M, Peshwa MV, Benike C, et al. Allogeneic dendritic cell induction of HIV specific cytotoxic T lymphocyte responses from T cells of HIV-1 infected and uninfected individuals. AIDS Res Hum Retroviruses 1997; 13:33–39.

21. Macatonia SE, Taylor PM, Knight SC, Askonas BA. Primary stimulation by dendritic cells induces antiviral proliferative and cytotoxic T cell responses in vitro. J Exp Med 1989; 169:1255–1264.

22. Kast WM, Boog CJ, Roep BO, Voorduow AC, Melief CJ. Failure or success in the restoration of virus-specific cytotoxic T lymphocte response defects by dendritic cells. J Immunol 1988; 140:3186–3193.

23. Nonacs R, Humborg C, Tam JP, Steinman RM. Mechanisms of mouse spleen dendritic cell function in the generation of influenza-specific, cytolytic T lymphocytes. J Exp Med 1992; 176:519–529.

24. Mehta-Damani A, Markowicz S, Engleman EG. Generation of antigen-specific CD4+ T cell lines from naïve precursors. Eur J Immunol 1995; 25:1206–1211.

25. Mehta-Damani A, Markowicz S, Engleman EG. Generation of antigen-specific CD8+ CTLs from naïve precursors. J Immunol 1994; 153:996–1003.

26. Huscein LA, Lehner T. Comparative investigation of Langerhans' cells and potential receptors for HIV in oral genitourinary and rectal epithelia. Immunology 1995; 85:474–484.

27. Rowland-Jones SL. HIV: The deadly passenger in dendritic cells. Curr Biol 1999; 9:R248–R250.

28. Patterson S, Gross J, Bedford P, Knight SC. Morphology and phenotype of dendritic cells from peripheral blood and their productive and non-productive infection with human immunodeficiency virus type 1. Immunology 1991; 101:672–680.

29. Weissman D, Li Y, Ananworanich J, et al. Three populations of cells with dendritic morphology exist in peripheral blood, only one of which is infectable with human immunodeficiency virus type 1. Proc Natl Acad Sci USA 1995; 92:826–830.

30. Patterson S, Knight SC. Susceptibility of human peripheral blood dendritic cells to infection by human immunodeficiency virus. J Gen Virol 1987; 68:1177–1181.

31. Cameron PU, Forsum U, Teppler H, Granelli-Piperno A, Steinman RM. During HIV-1 infection most blood dendritic cells are not productively infected and can function normally in clonal expansion of CD4+ T cells. Clin Exp Immunol 1992; 88:226–236.

32. Patterson S, Robinson SP, English NR, Knight SC. Subpopulations of peripheral blood dendritic cells show differential susceptibility to infection with a lymphotropic strain of HIV-1. Immunol Lett 1999; 66:111–116.

33. Kadowaki N, Antonenko S, Ho S, Rissoan MC, Soumelis V, Porcelli SA, Lanier LL, and Liu YJ. Distinct cytokine profiles of neonatal natural killer T cells after expansion with subsets of dendritic cells. J Exp Med 2001; 193(10):1221–1226.

34. Cella M, Jarrossay D, Facchetti F, Alebardi O, Nakajima H, Lanzavecchia A, and Colonna M. Plasmacytoid monocytes migrate to inflamed lymph nodes and produce large amounts of Type I interferon. Nat Med 1999; 5(8):919–923.

35. Knight SC. Infection of dendritic cells with HIV-1. AIDS Res Hum Retroviruses 1994; 10:1591–1595.

36. Vyarkanam A, Matear PM, Cranenburg C, et al. T cell responses to peptides covering the gag p24 region of HIV-1 occur in HIV-1 seronegative individuals. Int Immunol 1991; 3:939–947.

37. Takahashi H, Nakagawa Y, Yokomuro K, Berzofsky JA. Induction of CD8+ cytotoxic T lymphocytes by immunization with syngeneic irradiated HIV-1 envelope derived peptide-pulsed dendritic cells. Int Immunol 1993; 5:849–857.

38. Tschachler R, Groh W, Popovic M, et al. Epidermal Langerhans cells: a target for HTLV-

III/LAV infection. J Invest Dermatol 1987; 88:233–237.

39. Macatonia SE, Gompels M, Pinching AJ, Patterson S, Knight S. Antigen presentation by macrophages but not by dendritic cells in human immunodeficiency virus (HIV) infection. Immunology 1992; 75:576–581.

40. Knight SC, Macatonia SE, Patterson S. HIV-1 infection of dendritic cells. Int Rev Immunol 1990; 6:163–175.

41. Stingl G, Rappersberger K, Tschachler E, et al. Langerhans' cells and HIV-1 infection. J Am Acad Dermatol 1990; 22:1210–1217.

42. Meyaard L, Schnitermaken H, Miedema F. T cell dysfunction in HIV infection: anergy due to defective antigen-presenting cell function? Immunol Today 1993; 14:161–164.

43. Helbert MR, Stehr J-L Mitchison NA. Antigen presentation, loss of immunological memory and AIDS. Immunol Today 1993; 14:340–344.

44. Blauvelt A, Clerici M, Lucey DR, et al. Functional studies of epidermal Langerhans cells and blood monocytes in HIV-infected person. J Immunol 1995; 154:3506–3515.

45. Macatonia SE, Patterson S, Knight SC. Suppression of immune responses by dendritic cells infected with HIV. Immunology 1989; 67:285–289.

46. Kundu SK, Engleman E, Benike C, et al. A pilot clinical trial of HIV antigen-pulsed allogeneic and autologous dendritic cell therapy in HIV-infected patients. AIDS Res Hum Retroviruses 1998; 14:551.

47. Pantaleo G, Graziosi C, Fauci AS. The immunopathogenesis of human immunodeficiency virus infection. N Engl J Med 1993; 328:327–335.

48. Deng H-K, Liu R, Ellmeier W, et al. Identification of a major co-receptor for primary isolates of HIV-1. Nature 1996; 381:661–666.

49. Dragic T, Litwin V, Allaway GP. HIV-1 entry into CD4+ cells is mediated by the chemokine receptor CC-CKR-5. Nature 1996; 381:667–673.

50. Abrahamsohn IA, Coffman RL. *Trypanosoma cruzi:* IL-10, TNF, IFN-γ, and IL-12 regulate innate and acquired immunity to infection. Exp Parasitol 1996; 84:231–244.

51. Van Overtvelt L, Vanderheyde N, Verhasselt V, et al. *Trypanosoma cruzi* infects human dendritic cells and prevents their maturation: inhibition of cytokines, HLA-DR, and costimulatory molecules. Infect Immun 1999; 67:4033–4040.

52. von Stebut E, Belkaid Y, Jakob T, Sacks DL, Udey MC. Uptake of *Leishmania major* amastigotes results in activation and interleukin 12 release from murine skin-derived dendritic cells: implications for the initiation of anti-*Leishmania* immunity. J Exp Med 1998; 188:1547–1552.

53. Seguin R, Kasper LH. Sensitized lymphocytes and CD40 ligation augment interleukin-12 production by human dendritic cells in response to *Toxoplasma gondii.* J Infect Dis 1999; 179:467–474.

54. Klagge IM, Schneider-Schaulies S. Virus interactions with dendritic cells. J Gen Virol 1999; 80:823–833.

55. Redpath S, Angulo A, Gascoigne NRJ, Ghazal P. Murine cytomegalovirus infection down-regulates MHC class II expression on macrophages by induction of IL-10. J Immunol 1999; 162:6701–6707.

56. Frazer IH, Thomas R, Zhou J, et al. Potential strategies utilised by papillomavirus to evade host immunity. Immunol Rev 1999; 168:131–142.

57. West SK, Rapoza P, Munoz B, Katala S, Taylor HR. Epidemiology of ocular chlamydial infection in a trachoma-hyperendemic area. J Infect Dis 1991; 163:752–756.

58. Bavoil PM, Hsia RC, Rank RG. Prospects for a vaccine against chlamydia genital disease. I. Microbiology and pathogenesis. Bull Inst Pasteur 1996; 94:5.

59. Su H, Caldwell HD. CD4+ T cells play a significant role in adoptive immunity to *Chlamydia trachomatis* infection of the mouse genital tract. Infect Immun 1995; 63:3302–3308.

60. Zhang D, Yang X, Lu H, Zhong G, Brunham RC. Immunity to *Chlamydia trachomatis*

mouse pneumonitis induced by vaccination with live organisms correlates with early granulocyte-macrophage colony-stimulating factor and interleukin-12 production and with dendritic cell-like maturation. Infect Immun 1999; 67:1606–1613.

61. Ridge JP, Di Rosa F, Matzinger P. A conditioned dendritic cell can be a temporal bridge between a CD4+ T-helper and a T-killer cell. Nature 1998; 393:474–478.

62. Rehermann B, Fowler P, Sidney J, et al. The cytotoxic T lymphocyte response to multiple hepatitis B virus polymerase epitopes during and after acute viral hepatitis. J Exp Med 1995; 181:1047–1058.

63. Shimizu Y, Guidotti LG, Fowler P, Chisari FV. Dendritic cell immunization breaks cytotoxic T lymphocyte tolerance in hepatitis B virus transgenic mice. J Immunol 1998; 161:4520–4529.

64. Sieling PA, Jullien D, Dahlem M, et al. CD1 expression by dendritic cells in human leprosy lesions: correlation with effective host immunity. J Immunol 1999; 162:1851–1858.

65. Stenger S, Niazi KR, Modlin RL. Down-regulation of CD1 on antigen-presenting cells by infection with *Mycobacterium tuberculosis*. J Immunol 1998; 161:3582–3588.

66. Reis e Sousa C, Sher A, Kaye P. The role of dendritic cells in the induction and regulation of immunity to microbial infection. Curr Opin Immunol 1999; 11:392–399.

67. Barral A, Carvalho JS, Barral-Netto M, et al. Treatment of visceral leishmaniasis with pentavalent antimony and interferon gamma. N Engl J Med 1990; 322:16.

68. Romani L, Puccetti P, Bistoni F. Interleukin-12 in infectious diseases. Clin Microbiol Rev 1997; 10:611.

69. Nathan C. Interferon and inflammation. In: Gallin JI, Goldstein IM, Snyderman R (eds). Inflammation. New York: Raven, 1992, p. 265.

70. Newport MJ, Huxley CM, Huston S. A mutation in the interferon-γ-receptor gene and susceptibility to mycobacterial infection. N Engl J Med 1996; 335:1941.

71. Cocchi F, Devico AL, Garzino-Demo A, Arya SK, Gallo RC, Lusso P. Identification of RANTES, MIP-1α MIP-1β as the major HIV-suppressive factors produced by CD8+ T cells. Science 1995; 270:1811–1815.

72. Papadopoulos EJ, Sassetti C, Saeki H, et al. Fractalkine, a CX3C chemokine, is expressed by dendritic cells and is up-regulated upon dendritic cell maturation. Eur J Immunol 1999; 29:2551–2559.

73. Austyn JM, Larsen CP. Migration patterns of dendritic leukocytes. Implications for transplantation. Transplantation 1990; 49:1–7.

74. Robert C, Fuhlbrigge RC, Kieffer JD, et al. Interaction of dendritic cells with skin endothelium: a new perspective on immunosurveillance. J Exp Med 1999; 189:627–636.

75. Greaves DR, Wang W, Dairaghi DJ, et al. CCR6, a CC chemokine receptor that interacts with macrophage inflammatory protein 3alpha and is highly expressed in human dendritic cells. J Exp Med 1997; 186:837–844.

76. Sozzani S, Allavena P, D'Amico G. Cutting edge: differential regulation of chemokine receptors during dendritic cell maturation: a model for their trafficking properties. J Immunol 1998; 161:1083–1086.

77. Albert ML, Sauter B, Bhardwaj N. Dendritic cells acquire antigen from apoptotic cells and induce class I-restricted CTLs. Nature 1998; 392:86–89.

78. Svensson M, Stockinger B, Wick MJ. Bone marrow-derived dendritic cells can process bacteria for MHC-I and MHC-II presentation to T cells. J Immunol 1997; 158:4229–4236.

79. Pure E, Inaba K, Crowley MT, et al. Antigen processing by epidermal Langerhans cells correlates with the level of biosynthesis of major histocompatibility complex class II molecules and expression of invariant chain. J Exp Med 1990; 172:1459–1469.

80. Dieu MC, Vanbervliet, B, Vicari A, et al. Selective recruitment of immature and mature dendritic cells by distinct chemokines expressed in different anatomic sites. J Exp Med 1998; 188:373–386.

81. Chan VW, Kothakota S, Rohan MC, et al. Secondary lymphoid-tissue chemokine (SLC)

is chemotactic for mature dendritic cells. Blood 1999; 93:3610–3616.

82. Adema GJ, Hartgers F, Verstraten R, et al. A dendritic-cell-derived C-C chemokine that preferentially attracts naïve T cells. Nature 1997; 387:713–717.

83. Armitage RJ, Namen AE, Sassenfeld HM, Grabstein KH. Regulation of human T cell proliferation by IL-7. J Immunol 1990; 144:938–941.

84. Yawalkar N, Brand CU, Braathen LR. IL-12 gene expression in human skin-derived CD1a+ dendritic lymph cells. Arch Dermatol Res 1996; 288:79–84.

85. Steinman RM. The dendritic cell system and its role in immunogenicity. Annu Rev Immunol 1991; 9:271–296.

86. Takamizawa M, Rivas A, Fagnoni F, et al. Dendritic cells that process and present nominal antigens to naïve T lymphocytes are derived from CD2+ precursors. J Immunol 1997; 158:2134–2142.

87. Zhou L-J, Tedder TF. Human blood dendritic cells selectively express CD83, a member of the immunoglobulin superfamily.J Immunol 1995; 154:3821–3835.

88. Knight SC, Fryer PR, Griffiths S, Harding B. Class II histocompatibility antigens on human dendritic cells. Immunology 1987; 61:21–27.

89. Hart DN. Dendritic cells: unique leukocyte populations which control the primary immune response. Blood 1997; 90:3245–3287.

90. Hart DN, Prickett TC. Adhesion molecules in tonsil DC-T cell interactions. Adv Exp Med Biol 1993; 329:65–69.

91. Fagnoni FF, Takamizawa M, Godfrey WR, et al. Role of B70/B7-2 in CD4+ T-cell immune responses induced by dendritic cells. Immunology 1995; 85:467–474.

92. Reis e Sousa C, Stahl PD, Austyn JM. Phagocytosis of antigens by Langerhans cells in vitro. J Exp Med 1993; 178:509–519.

93. Hart DN, McKenzie JL. Isolation and characterization of human tonsil dendritic cells. J Exp Med 1988; 168:157–170.

94. Lanzavecchia A. Mechanisms of antigen uptake for presentation. Curr Opin Immunol 1996; 8:348–354.

95. Norbury CC, Chambers BJ, Prescott AR, Ljunggren HG, Watts C. Constitutive macropinocytosis allows TAP-dependent major histocompatibility complex class I presentation of exogenous soluble antigen by bone marrow-derived dendritic cells. Eur J Immunol 1997; 27:280–288.

96. Arnold-Schild D, Hanau D, Spehner D, et al. Cutting edge: receptor-mediated endocytosis of heat shock proteins by professional antigen-presenting cells. J Immunol 1999; 162:3757–3760.

97. Palucka KA, Taquet N, Sanchez-Chapuis F, Gluckman JC. Dendritic cells as the terminal stage of monocyte differentiation. J Immunol 1998; 160:4587–4595.

98. Oehler L, Majdic O, Pickl WF. Neutrophil granulocyte-committed cells can be driven to acquire dendritic cell characteristics. J Exp Med 1998; 187:1019–1028.

99. Grouard G, Rissoan MC, Filgueira L, Durand I, Banchereau J, Liu YJ. The enigmatic plasmacytoid T cells develop into dendritic cells with interleukin (IL)-3 and CD4-ligand. J Exp Med 1997; 185:1101–1111.

100. Rissoan MC, Soumelis V, Kadowaki N, et al. Reciprocal control of T helper cell and dendritic cell differentiation. Science 1999; 283:1183–1186.

101. Siegal FP, Kadowaki N, Shodell M, et al. The nature of the principal type 1 interferon-producing cells in human blood. Science 1999; 284:1835–1837.

102. Pulendran B, Smith JL, Caspary G, et al. Distinct dendritic cell subsets differentially regulate the class of immune response in vivo. Proc Natl Acad Sci USA 1999; 96:1036–1041.

103. Maldonado-Lopez R, De Smedt R, Michel P, et al. CD8alpha+ and CD8alpha-subclasses of dendritic cells direct the development of distinct T helper cells in vivo. J Exp Med 1999; 189:587–592.

104. Merad M, Fong L, Bogenberger J, and Engleman EG. (2000). Differentiation of myeloid

dendritic cells into CD8alpha-positive dendritic cells in vivo. Blood. 96(5):1865–1872.

105. Galy A, Travis M, Cen D, Chen B. Human T, B, natural killer, and dendritic cells arise from a common bone marrow progenitor cell subset. Immunity 1995; 3:459–473.

106. Olweus J, BitMansour A, Warnke R, et al. Dendritic cell ontogeny: a human dendritic cell lineage of myeloid origin. Proc Natl Acad Sci USA 1997; 94:12551–12556.

107. Markowicz S, Engleman EG. Granulocyte-macrophage colony-stimulating factor promotes differentiation and survival of human peripheral blood dendritic cells in vitro. J Clin Invest 1990; 85:955–961.

108. Hsu FJ, Benike C, Fagnoni F, et al. Vaccination of patients with B-cell lymphoma using autologous antigen-pulsed dendritic cells. Nat Med 1996; 2:52–58.

109. Caux C, Dezutter-Dambuyant C, Schmitt D, Banchereau J. GM-CSF and TNF-alpha cooperate in the generation of dendritic Langerhans cells. Nature 1992; 360:258–261.

110. Romani N, Gruner S, Brang D, et al. Proliferating dendritic cell progenitors in human blood. J Exp Med 1994; 180:83–93.

111. Bernhard H, Disis ML, Heimfeld S, Hand S, Gralow JR, Cheever MA. Generation of immunostimulatory dendritic cells from human CD34+ hematopoietic progenitor cells of the bone marrow and peripheral blood. Cancer Res 1995; 55:1099–1104.

112. Sallusto F, Lanzavecchia A. Efficient presentation of soluble antigen by cultured human dendritic cells is maintained by granulocyte/macrophage colony-stimulating factor plus interleukin 4 and downregulated by tumor necrosis factor alpha. J Exp Med 1994; 179:1109–1118.

113. Zitvogel L, Mayordomo JI, Tjandrawan T, et al. Therapy of murine tumors with tumor peptide-pulsed dendritic cells: dependence on T cells, B7 costimulation and T helper cell 1-associated cytokines. J Exp Med 1996; 183:87–97.

114. Paglia P, Chiodani C, Rodolfo M, Colombo MP. Murine dendritic cells loaded in vitro with soluble protein prime cytotoxic T lymphocytes against tumor antigen in vivo. J Exp Med 1996; 183:317–322.

115. Nestle FO, Alijagic S, Gilliet M, et al. Vaccination of melanoma patients with peptide- or tumor lysate-pulsed dendritic cells. Nat Med 1998; 4:328–332.

116. Lotze MT, Hellerstedt B, Stolinski L, et al. The role of interleukin-2, interleukin-12 and dendritic cells in cancer therapy. Cancer J Sci Am 1997; 3:S109.

117. Rosenzwajg M, Canque B, Gluckman JC. Human dendritic cell differentiation pathway from CD34+ hematopoietic precursor cells. Blood 1996; 87:535–544.

118. Maraskovsky E, Brasel K, Teepe M, et al. Dramatic increase in the numbers of functionally mature dendritic cells in Flt3 ligand-treated mice: multiple dendritic cell subpopulations identified. J Exp Med 1996; 184:1953–1962.

119. Fong L, Hou Y, Rivas A, et al. (2001). Altered peptide ligand vaccination with Flt3 ligand expanded dendritic cells for tumor immunotherapy. Proc Natl Acad Sci USA. 98(15): 8809–8814.

120. Alters SE, Gadea JR, Sorich M, O'Donoghue G, Talib S, Philip R. Dendritic cells pulsed with CEA peptide induce CEA-specific CTL with restricted TCR repertoire. J Immunother 1998; 21:17–26.

121. Dietz AB, Vuk-Pavlovic S. High efficiency adenovirus-mediated gene transfer to human dendritic cells. Blood 1998; 91:392–398.

122. Kim CJ, Cormier J, Roden M, et al. Use of recombinant poxviruses to stimulate antimelanoma T cell reactivity. Ann Surg Oncol 1998; 5:64–76.

123. Matzinger P. Tolerance, danger, and the extended family. Annu Rev Immunol 1994; 12:991.

124. Paglia P, Medina E, Arioli I, Guzman CA, Colombo MP. Gene transfer in dendritic cells induced by oral DNA vaccination with *Salmonella typhimurium,* results in protective immunity against a murine fibrosarcoma. Blood 1998; 92:3172–3176.

125. Pan ZK, Ikonomidis G, Lazenby A, Pardoll D, Paterson Y. A recombinant *Listeria monocytogenes* vaccine expressing a model tumor antigen protects mice against lethal tumor

challenge and causes regression of established tumors. Nat Med 1995; 1:471.

126. Kim DT, Mitchell DJ, Brockstedt DG, et al. Introduction of soluble proteins into the MHC class I pathway by conjugation to an HIV tat peptide. J Immunol 1997; 159:1666–1668.

127. Lynch RG, Rohrer JW, Odermatt B, Gebel HM, Autry JR, Hoover RG. Immunoregulation of murine myeloma cell growth and differentiation: a monoclonal model of B cell differentiation. Immunol Rev 1979; 48:45–80.

128. Hsu FJ, Kwak L, Campbell M, et al. Clinical trials of idiotype-specific vaccine in B-cell lymphomas. Ann NY Acad Sci 1993; 690:385–387.

129. Maloney DG, Kaminski MS, Burowski D, Haimovich J, Levy R. Monoclonal anti-idiotype antibodies against the murine B cell lymphoma 38C13: characterization and use as probes for the biology of the tumor in vivo and in vitro. Hybridoma 1985; 4:191–209.

130. Carroll WL, Lowder JN, Streifer R, Warnke R, Levy S, Levy R. Idiotype variant cell populations in patients with B cell lymphoma. J Exp Med 1986; 164:1566–1580.

131. Shimizu K, Fields RC, Giedlin M, Mule JJ. Systemic administration of interleukin 2 enhances the therapeutic efficacy of dendritic cell-based tumor vaccines. Proc Natl Acad Sci USA 1999; 96:2268–2273.

132. Ahuja SS, Mummidi S, Malech HL, Ahuja SK. Human dendritic cell (DC)-based anti-infective therapy: engineering DCs to secrete functional IFN-γ and IL-12. J Immunol 1998; 161:868–876.

133. Merad M, Sugie T, Engleman EG, and Fong L. (2001). In vivo manipulation of dendritic cells to induce therapeutic immunity. Blood (in press).

6

Cytokines, Cytokine Antagonists, and Growth Factors for Treating Infections

Barbara G. Matthews

INTRODUCTION

Cytokines are proteins involved in all stages of the immune response. The molecular weight of most cytokines ranges between 6 and 60 kD, and these proteins can be glycosylated or myristylated. Although their primary role is in the host-defense response, they can stimulate the growth and differentiation of a number of target cells, e.g., endothelial, neural, and tumor cells. Because of the breadth of their activity, the cytokines have been characterized by investigators in different disciplines, with a resultant variety of names. Colony-stimulating factors (CSFs), tumor necrosis factors (TNFs), interferons (IFNs), interleukins (ILs), growth factors, and chemokines are all considered cytokines.

The intent of this chapter is to provide some background on the biology of cytokines and to describe their role in the earlier stages of the immune response to infectious agents prior to the immune system's commitment to either a cellular or humoral response. Knowledge of their role in infections should help us understand the rationale for use of cytokines or cytokine antagonists as therapy for the specific infections discussed in subsequent chapters. For the sake of simplicity, this chapter discusses chemokines and cytokines separately, with the term cytokines including ILs, CSFs, IRNs, and TNFs. This grouping is based on some gross structural similarities in the receptors for the cytokines within the two groups. The last section provides a sketch of the activity of cytokines in the immune response to infections that are the focus of many of therapeutic interventions intended to modulate cytokine activity.

CYTOKINES

Cytokines are produced by a number of different cells, but most are produced by cells of the immune system. Depending on the type of stimulation, a given cell can produce different cytokines. Induction of cytokine production with measurable tissue or serum concentrations occurs rapidly when cells are stimulated by antigen or bacterial products. Because of the constant surveillance by the immune system, some undetectable to low concentrations of cytokine production is probably ongoing in order to maintain routine maintenance of immunity.

From: *Immunotherapy for Infectious Diseases*
Edited by: J. M. Jacobson © Humana Press Inc., Totowa, NJ

Cytokines can target a number of cells since nearly all cells express one or more cytokine receptors. They can affect both the cells that secrete them (autocrine signals) or cells in the nearby environment (paracrine signals). Cytokines function as a network in which production of one cytokine can affect the production or activity of several other cytokines, either positively or negatively. This cytokine network can become quite complex, not only because of the number of target cells whose function is altered by a given cytokine, but also because of the redundancy in the network, with several cytokines causing a given effect.

The number of cytokines and their roles in different disease processes as identified to date continue to increase. There have been a number of reviews of the clinical role of individual cytokines (*1–4*). To give some idea of the number of cytokines identified,18 interleukins, 20 different growth factors, and 4 types of interferons have been described. Table 1 presents characteristics of the interleukins, and the other cytokines that play a major role in the body's response to infection.

Depending on the type of response to an infectious agent that is being described, cytokines are characterized as either pro-inflammatory or anti-inflammatory or described according to their production by activated T-cell subsets, Th1/Th2. Neither method classifies the cytokines distinctly since some cytokines could be considered either anti-inflammatory or pro-inflammatory in different disease settings. As discussed later, some are produced by both Th1 and Th2 T-cell subsets. Overall, the cytokines considered pro-inflammatory in response to infection include: IFN-γ, granulocyte (G)-CSF, granulocyte/macrophage (GM-CSF), TNF-$\propto$, IL-1, IL-6, IL-8, and IL-12. Those considered anti-inflammatory include IL-4, IL-10, transforming growth factor-β (TGF-β), and IL-1 receptor antagonist (IL-1ra).

Examples of pro-inflammatory cytokines in infections that may have some anti-inflammatory properties in allergic reactions include IFN-γ, and IL-6. For most immune responses, the activities of IFN-γ, are predominantly pro-inflammatory. However, in allergic responses IFN-γ, may play an anti-inflammatory role by lowering IgE concentrations owing to inhibition of the effects of IL-4 (*5*). Although IL-6 activates both T-cells and natural killer (NK) cells and induces preactivated B-cells to synthesize immunoglobulin, it has been shown in a transgenic mouse model to downregulate the production of pro-inflammatory cytokines by monocytes, e.g., TNF and IL-1, and to stimulate the release of IL-1ra. In this model, overproduction of IL-6 was associated with decreased airway inflammation and hyper-reactivity (*6*).

Cytokine Receptors

The effect of a cytokine on the target cell follows the binding of its ligand to high-affinity receptors present on cells throughout the body. This linkage of cytokine ligand to its receptor results in the transduction of a signal, either positive or negative, for transcription of genetic DNA in the nucleus. The type of signal transduced can depend on the type of cell and its state of development, i.e., the cell's state of maturity or activation. The complexity of cytokine activity following receptor linkage is not only caused by the variation in the type of signal sent but also occurs because multiple cytokines can transduce the same biologic response.

In addition to membrane-bound receptors, soluble receptors with similar ligand binding domains have been described for several cytokines, e.g., IL-1, IL-2, and IL-6. These soluble receptors can function as cytokine inhibitors whereby, binding of the cytokine to its soluble receptor prevents the cytokine from effecting target cell function. An analogous approach toward inhibiting cytokine effect by ligand binding may be used by some viruses that code for receptor-like molecules, e.g., IFN-γ *(7)* and TNF-α *(8)*, thereby inhibiting the effects of these cytokines on the host cell.

Receptor Families

Cytokine receptors are membrane glycoproteins with a single transmembrane domain and an external amino terminus. The functional receptor can consist of two or more subunits, and these subunits can be shared among different cytokines. This sharing of the receptor subunits among different cytokines may partially explain some of the functional redundancy and costimulation of their production and activity. The receptors can be grouped into four families according to similarities in their DNA or amino acid sequences: the cytokine receptor superfamily, the TNF superfamily, the immunoglobulin superfamily, and the IFN-R family.

Most cytokine receptors are members of the cytokine receptor superfamily which is characterized by a conserved amino acid motif in the extracellular portion and in a region proximal to the membrane *(9, 10)*. This superfamily can be divided into three subfamilies according to a shared subunit, i.e., those receptors that share the γ chain, the gp 140 β chain, and the gp 130. The receptors in the γ chain subfamily consist of three subunits (α, β, γ): the β, and γ subunits are members of the superfamily and are constitutively expressed on T-cells. Heterodimerization of the βγ chains mediates signal transduction. The receptors for IL-13, IL-4, IL-7, IL-9, and IL-15 are members of this subfamily. An example of the sharing of the subunits of the cytokine receptor is the IL-2 receptor: IL-2Rβ is shared by IL-15, and IL-2Rγ is a subunit of the receptors for IL-4, IL-7, and IL-9. The subfamily of receptors that share the gp 140 β chain includes the receptors for IL-3, IL-5, and GM-CSF. Receptors in this subfamily have two subunits, with the α chain distinct for each receptor. Both the α and β chains are members of the cytokine receptor superfamily, and signaling is mediated through ligand interactions of the cytoplasmic regions on the shared β chain. The subfamily that shares gp 130 includes receptors for IL-6, IL-11, and IL-12. Formation of homodimers and heterodimers with gp 130 mediates signal transduction by these receptors.

The TNF family of receptors includes two distinct receptors that bind TNF, TNFR-I (p75), and TNFR-II (p55). These receptors are homologous and bind both TNF-α and TNF-β with comparable affinity. Interestingly, other receptors in the TNF superfamily do not bind cytokines, e.g., FAS (CD95), which signals apoptosis of thymocytes *(11)* and CD40 ligand, which signals B-cell survival, proliferation, and switch in the Ig isotype *(12)*. The immunoglobulin superfamily of receptors includes the two receptors for IL-1 *(13)*. Although both receptors bind IL-1 well, the type I receptor is the active moiety, and the type II receptor appears to have minimal activity. However, the type II receptor may be the precursor for soluble IL-1 receptor, which can bind IL-1 after being shed from the membrane. A newly described member of the IL-1 receptor family is the receptor for IL-18, which contains a binding and signaling chain that appears to share signal transduction pathways similar to those of IL-1R *(14)*. Members of the IFN-R family include the receptors for IFN-α, IFN-β, and IL-10, which are distant members of the cytokine receptor superfamily. Investigation into the method of gene transcription through signal transduction from the IFN receptors has become a model for signal transduction by several cytokines, i.e., the Jak-Stat paradigm.

Table 1
Source and Activity of Interleukins and Cytokines with a Major Role in Infection

Cytokine	Source	Activity
IL-1α, IL-1β	Macrophages, B-cells	Stimulates macrophages (increases production of IL-6, TNF-α); enhances PMN adhesion; activates lymphocyte increases IL-2); induces acute-phase protein production; enhances production of platelet-activating factor and nitric oxide
IL-2	T-cells	Promotes growth and differentiation of T-cells; enhances cytotoxicity of T-cells and NK cells
IL-3	T-cells, stem cells	Multilineage colony-stimulating factor (stem cells, erythroid, and myeloid)
IL-4	T-cells, B-cells, monocytes, mast cells, endothelial cells	Suppresses production of IL-1, TNF, and IFN-γ (Th1); upregulates IL-1ra production; enhances Th2; promotes B- and cytotoxic T-cells; increases IgG1 and IgE production; enhances MHC class II and IgE receptor function
IL-5	T-lymphocytes	Promotes proliferation and differentiation of B-cells and eosinophils; increases IgA production
IL-6	T- and B-cells, NK cells, monocytes, macrophages, fibroblasts	Activates T- and NK cells; induces immunoglobulin synthesis by B-cells; induces acute-phase protein synthesis by liver
IL-7	Stromal cells of bone marrow	Induces proliferation of T- and B-cells
IL-8	Most cells including leukocyte and myeloid precursors, endothelial cells, fibroblasts	Causes leukocyte chemotaxis, enhances neutrophil adherence and degranulation
IL-9	T-cells	Prolongs T-cell survival; activates mast cells
IL-10	T-cells	Inhibits cytokine production by Th1 (TNF-α and IL-1); upregulates IL-1ra production
IL-11	Stromal cells of bone marrow	Inhibits proinflammatory cytokine production; stimulates osteoclasts and CSF
IL-12	Macrophages, dendritic cells, B-cells, mast cells	Induces production of TH1 cells; enhances IFN-γ production; induces proliferation of NK cells
IL-13	T-cells	Induces proliferation and differentiation of B-cells; enhances IgE and IgG4 production; inhibits production of proinflammatory cytokines
IL-14	T-cells	Induces proliferation of activated B-cells; inhibits secretion of immunoglobulin

Table 1
(continued)

Cytokine	Source	Activity
IL-15	Monocytes, muscle cells, endothelial cells	Induces proliferation of T-cells and activated B-cells
IL-16	Eosinophils, CD8+ T-cells	Chemoattracts CD4+ cells
IL-17	CD4+ T-cells	Stimulates fibroblasts and endothelial cells to release IL-6, IL-8, G-CSF, PGE_2; enhances ICAM-1 production
IL-18	Hepatocytes	Induces IFN-γ production; enhances NK activity
GM-CSF	Fibroblasts, endothelial cells, T-cells	Stimulates proliferation of granulocyte and macrophage precursors; activates mature phagocytes
G-CSF	Macrophages, fibroblasts, endothelial cells	Stimulates proliferation of neutrophil precursors from stem cells
M-CSF	Macrophages, fibroblasts, endothelial cells	Stimulates proliferation of monocytes/macrophage precursors; stimulates monocytes
TNF-α	Macrophages, lymphocytes, mast cells	Increases PMN function; causes PMN degranulation; increases production of GM-CSF; induces acute-phase proteins, cachexia, pyrexia
TNF-β (lymphotoxin)	Lymphyocytes	Similar to TNF-α
IFN-α	Macrophages, lymphocytes, fibroblasts	Increases expression of class I MHC; stimulates Th1 cells and production of IL-12; stimulates NK cells
IFN-β	Fibroblasts, epithelial cells	Similar to IFN-α
IFN-γ	T-cells, NK cells, fibroblasts	Increases PMN and monocyte function; increases MHC class I and II expression; stimulates TH1 (e.g., IL-1, TNF-α)
TGF-β	Lymphyocytes, platelets, activated macrophages	Opposes production of inflammatory cytokines (IL-1 and TNF-α); inhibits T- and B-cell proliferation; mediates extracellular matrix formation (associated with liver and kidney damage)
IL-1ra	T- and B-cells, macrophages	Inhibits synthesis of LPS-stimulated production of IL-1β, TNF. IL-6, and GM-CSF and synthesis of IgE; blocks effect of IL-1

Abbreviations: CSF, colony-stimulating factor; G, granulocyte; GM, granulocyte/macrophage; ICAM, intercellular cell adhesion molecule; IFN, interferon; IL, interleukin; IL-1ra, IL receptor antagonist; NK, natural killer; PGE_2, prostaglandin E_2; PMN, polymorphonuclear neutrophil; TGF, transforming growth factor; TNF, tumor necrosis factor; NAP-2, nucleosome assembly protein-2; GRO, growth related oncogene-α; ENA, epithelial cell-derived neutrophil activating peptide-78; GCP-2, granulocyte chemotactic protein-2.

The Jak-Stat Model of Signal Transduction

Several cytokine receptors lack intrinsic tyrosine kinase activity in their cytoplasmic domains but can activate a family of cytoplasmic protein tyrosine kinases, Jaks *(Janus kinases)*. The model for the signaling mechanism that utilizes Jaks was characterized by activation studies in mutants of the IFN-αβ and IFN-γ receptors *(15)*. In this model, binding of cytokine ligand to the IFN-αβ or IFN-γ receptors results in the dimerization of the receptor subunits. This dimerization (or oligomerization in cytokine receptors with more than two chains) increases the affinity of the dimers' cytoplasmic domain that is proximal to the membrane to bind two Jaks. In the case of IFN-α the two chains bind Jak 1 and Tyk 2; the chains of the IFN-γ receptor bind Jak 1 and Jak 2. Both the Jaks and the cytoplasmic region of the receptor chain become phosphorylated simultaneously. This phosphorylation subsequently becomes a catalyst for the binding and phosphorylation of two latent cytoplasmic transcription factors called Stats, i.e., Signal transducers and activators of transcription. Following the phosphorylation of Stats by Jaks, the Stats dimerize, and this activated Stat-Stat complex enters the nucleus, where it initiates gene transcription by binding to specific promoter sequences in cytokine response genes, resulting in the ultimate step of gene transcription.

Four Jaks have been identified: Jak 1, Jak 2, Jak 3, and Tyk 2. In addition to the IFN-γ receptor, Jak 2 is involved with signaling by granulocyte/macrophage (GM)-CSF, granulocyte (G)-CSF, IL-6, and IL-3. Both Jak 1 and Jak 3 are involved with signaling of the γ chain subfamily of the cytokine receptor superfamily such as IL-2, IL-4, and IL-9. IL-12 activates Jak 2 and Tyk 2. The actual number of Stats is uncertain, but at least six have been characterized. The Stats have structurally conserved binding sites to phosphotyrosine and conserved sequences of their nuclear DNA binding regions. Given the number of Jaks and Stats, it is understandable that different cytokine receptors associate with different Jaks, which then catalyze the binding and phosphorylation of different Stats *(16)*. The network of interaction between the Jaks and Stats can be quite extensive. For example, the Jak 1 and Jak 3 activated by IL-2 receptor binding activates Stat 3 and Stat 5, and the same Jaks activated by IL-4 binding activates Stat 6. To add to the complexity, Stats can be phosphorylated by kinases other than Jaks, e.g., protein tyrosine kinases of the *src* family. Although many receptors related to the cytokine receptor superfamily as well as receptors in some of the other families use the Jak-Stat model of signal transduction, other cytokines such as TNF-α and IL-1-β activate members of the mitogen-activated protein (MAP) kinases, with resultant transcription of nuclear protooncogenes.

CHEMOKINES

Chemokines are low-molecular-weight peptides that have evolved relatively recently. They share a high basic nature and can bind heparin through heparin binding domains. Chemokines are produced by nearly every cell type in response to inflammatory signals, particularly signals that activate interactions between leukocytes and endothelial cells. The first chemokine purified was platelet factor 4 (PF-4) in 1977 *(17),* and IL-8 was purified ten years later *(18)*. Chemokines range between 68 to 100 amino acids in length and are defined by conserved motifs containing either two or four cysteine residues that form disulfide bonds in the protein tertiary structure.

The number and arrangement of these conserved cysteines allow them to be classified into three groups: C, CC, or CXC *(19)*. Both the CXC and CC families of chemokines have four conserved cysteines; the C chemokines have two conserved cysteines. The CXC and CC groups differ by the presence (CC) or absence (CXC) of an intervening amino acid between the first two cysteines. Both the CXC and CC groups have numerous members, whereas the only known members of the C groups include human and mouse lymphotactin and activation-induced, T-cell-derived and chemokine-related molecule (ATAC). Genes encoding members of each group appear to cluster on the same chromosomes, i.e., genes for CXC chemokines are found on chromosome 4, those for CC are on chromosome 17, and those for C are on chromosome 1.

Many CXC chemokines have the tripeptide motif glutamic acid-leucine-arginine (ELR) near the N terminus just prior to the CXC motif, e.g., IL-8, nucleosome assembly protein-2 (NAP-2), growth related oncogene-α (GRO-α), GRO-β, epithelial all-derived neutrophil activating peptide-78 (ENA-78), and granulocyte chemotactic protein-2 (GCP-2). All these chemokines can bind the shared IL-8 receptor type II and are potent mediators of neutrophil chemotaxis *(19, 20)*. The presence of the ELR motif appears to be associated with chemoattractant properties since CXC chemokines that lack the ELR motif, e.g., PF-4, inflammatory protein-10 (IP-10), and monokine inducible by IFN-γ (MIG), do not chemoattract neutrophils nor do they bind the shared IL-8 type II receptor. Although only CC chemokines were initially thought to be able to induce migration of monocytes and macrophages, some CXC chemokines have been found to have monocyte attraction activity. Similarly, only the ERL+ CXC chemokines were thought to induce neutrophil migration. However, several CC chemokines, including macrophage inflammatory protein-1α (MIP-1α) and monocyte chemotactic protein-3 (MCP-3), have been shown to induce migration of neutrophils. In addition to monocytes and macrophages, some CC chemokines have been shown to induce the migration of eosinophils, basophils, and mast cells. The responsiveness to chemokine stimulation depends not only on the specific type of leukocytes but also on the conditions of stimulation, e.g., the migration of mast cells activated by IgE, and specific antigen is enhanced in response to MCP-1 and RANTES compared with nonactivated cells.

In addition to their importance in the recruitment and activation of various leukocytes, chemokines are active on other cell types, including endothelial cells, muscle cells, melanocytes, and hepatocytes. Data suggest that chemokines have a role in several other processes, including angiogenesis, tissue development, and fibrosis.

Chemokine Receptors

Chemokines bind to a distinct class of receptors whose structure is similar to that of rhodopsin. The receptor polypeptide has seven hydrophobic domains passing through the membrane as α-helices with an extracellular aminoterminus and an intracellular carboxy terminus *(21)*. Receptor binding can be restricted to a specific chemokine or shared among several chemokines, e.g., CC CKR1, CC CKR4, and CC CKR5 are selective for MIP-1α and RANTES but also bind a third chemokine that is not shared by the other receptors (MCP-3 for CKR1, MCP-1 for CKR4, and MIP-1β for CKR5).

Humans have one chemokine receptor that is promiscuous since it binds to numerous chemokines. This receptor, the Duffy blood group antigen, was first identified on red blood cells but is also expressed by several nonerythroid cells, e.g., spleen, lung, and heart. Interestingly, the Duffy antigen is a factor in infections with *Plasmodium vivax* in which the parasite utilizes this receptor to invade erythrocytes *(22)*. In people of African descent, this receptor may not be expressed on red blood cells, and they are resistant to infections with *P. vivax*. Chronic exposure to *P. vivax* may have exerted selection pressure for gene expression in different cells since this receptor may be expressed on other tissue cells. In addition to *P. vivax,* some herpes viruses and HIV-1 are also able to use chemokine receptors as factors in their pathogenesis. Human cytomegalovirus (CMV) has genes that encode a functional chemokine receptor that can bind MIP-1α, MIP-1β, RANTES, and MCP-1 *(23, 24)*. The mechanism by which expression of a chemokine receptor is advantageous to the virus is not clear *(21)*.

The signaling of cellular response to chemokines occurs through G proteins (guanine nucleotide binding regulatory proteins) coupling to initiate phosphoinositide hydrolysis. The resultant increase in diacylglycerol and cytosolic Ca^{2+} leads to activation of protein kinase C *(25)*. The ability of some chemokines such as RANTES and MIP-1α to activate Stats suggests that the signaling pathways of Stats and G proteins may act with some communication.

CYTOKINES IN IMMUNE RESPONSE TO INFECTIONS

As discoveries and comprehension of cytokine biology continue to increase, the complexity of the cytokine network has become overwhelming. Despite the complexity of cytokine activity, it is important to appreciate the role of the interplay of the cytokines with their various target cells in the immune response to an inflammatory agent. The immune response during the early stages will either eradicate the infectious agent or set the stage for the type of chronic immune response. When the control mechanism for the type of cytokine response is dysfunctional, the result may be the development of a chronic or progressive infection rather than eradication or containment of the infectious agent, e.g., the development of miliary tuberculosis, lepromatous leprosy, visceral leishmaniasis, and sepsis. The host's genetic background is also a factor in the development of chronic inflammatory response and pathology. Autoimmune diseases result from perturbation of the immune system either intrinsically for unknown reasons, (e.g., systemic lupus, juvenile rheumatoid arthritis) or in response to an infectious agent, (e.g., type I diabetes mellitus).

The purpose of this section is to provide a background sketch of the role of the cytokine network in the responses of the immune system to an infectious agent prior to its commitment to the appropriate immune protective mechanism, i.e., the development of antibody by B-cells, macrophage activation, or cytolysis by T-cells. Two aspects of the immune response that have been the focus of immunomodulators of cytokines to treat infections will be discussed: the initial leukocyte response and the differentiation of the CD4+ T-cells into the Th1 and Th2 subsets.

Initial Inflammatory Response and Leukocyte Migration

The body's innate immune response to an invading organism results in the recruitment of leukocytes and phagocytosis of the organism. Numerous factors, including bacterial components, will stimulate migration of the leukocytes. Bacterial endotoxin or lipopolysaccharide (LPS) stimulates the release of chemokines and cytokines from the surrounding tissue cells and macrophages. Immunotherapies that are intended to interfere with the activity of these cytokines and other inflammatory molecules, e.g., proteins that bind LPS, TNF-α, IL-1, or inhibitors of nitric oxide production, would be expected to diminish the pathologic effects of the acute response to infections. In contrast to the acute increase in serum TNF-α concentrations associated with acute infections, some autoimmune diseases, e.g., rheumatoid arthritis and Crohn's disease, are associated with chronic elevations in tissue TNF-α concentrations. Immunomotherapies that lower levels of TNF-α, such as soluble TNF receptor and monoclonal antibodies to TNF-α, have shown clinical benefit.

The binding of LPS to macrophages stimulates the release of IL-1 and TNF-α. These cytokines in turn stimulate their target cells to produce a number of different molecules. Endothelial cells and macrophages are stimulated by IL-1 and TNF-α (and by bacterial LPS itself) to produce G-CSF and GM-CSF from endothelial cells and macrophages, which further enhances the number of leukocytes and the duration of their recruitment to the site of infection. In response to IL-1, TNF-α, and IFN-γ, endothelial cells will produce prostaglandins, platelet-activating factor, and nitric oxide. One potential effect of these products could be the production of thrombi. These inflammatory cytokines can also stimulate endothelial cells to express molecules involved with leukocyte adhesion and integration through the endothelium including E-selectin, P-selectin, and ICAM-1. These latter molecules are important in the recruitment of leukocytes from the circulation to the infected tissue.

With expression of leukocyte adhesion molecules, the leukocytes loosely attach to the endothelial cells through the oligosaccharides on their membranes. With their movement slowed by this loose attachment, the leukocytes will begin to roll along the endothelial surface. The chemokines released from macrophages, the surrounding tissue cells, and the endothelial cells in response to the bacterial components bind to the endothelium, where they cause the rolling leukocytes to adhere more firmly to the endothelium through binding of the integrins to their ligand. Chemokines involved in this process include MCP-1, RANTES, and MIP-1α. The leukocytes then migrate through the endothelium and move up a gradient of chemokine concentrations to the inflammatory site.

The types of leukocytes recruited to the inflammatory site can differ depending on the source of inflammation, (e.g., bacterial, allergen) and the duration and amount of exposure. The pattern of cytokines produced, i.e., the type and concentration, will depend on these factors as well as the host's genetic background. The predominant cytokines in this pattern (e.g., IL-4, IFN-γ, and (IL-12) will then determine the subsequent T-cell response to chronic infection/inflammation or to immunization *(26)*.

Activation of T-Helper Cells: Th1/Th2 Subsets

When stimulated, T-cells produce different types and amounts of cytokines, which in turn, characterizes the functional response of the T-cells. According to the pattern of cytokines produced, the CD4+ T-cells can be differentiated into the subsets of Th1 or Th2 *(27, 28)*. The cytokines produced by each subset regulates the function and development of the other. IFN-γ produced by Th1 cells inhibits Th2 cell production and function. IL-4 and IL-10 produced by Th2 cells inhibit Th1 cell production and the killing of bacteria by macrophages. Several immunotherapies for infectious diseases have focused on the manipulation of the type or degree of T-cell response, e.g., stimulation of Th1 response by IFN-γ to treat mycobacterial infections or visceral leishmaniasis, and stimulation of CD4+ T-cell production by IL-2.

In humans, Th1 cells produce IFN-γ and TNF-β but not IL-4 or IL-5. Th1 cytokines activate monocytes to generate the cell-mediated immune response. Although this response is intended to eradicate intracellular pathogens, it may also be associated with autoimmune diseases. The primary determinant for Th1 cell differentiation is the predominance of IL-12 in the cytokine response to an inflammatory agent, and full expression of the Th1 response also depends on production of IFN-γ. Macrophages will produce IL-12 in response to bacterial products (e.g., LPS), viral components, intracellular bacteria (e.g., Mycobacteria, *Listeria* organisms), and protozoa (e.g., *Leishmania* organisms). IL-12 was originally described as an NK stimulatory factor, and it induces proliferation and differentiation of NK cells into lymphokine-activated killer (LAK) cells and causes secretion of IFN-γ and TNF-α *(29)*. As a result, IFN-γ will upregulate production IL-12 by the macrophage *(30)* and decrease production of IL-4 by Th2 cells. Because IL-12 potentiates IFN-γ production and promotes a shift toward production of protective antibody isotypes, it may have a potential therapeutic use as a vaccine adjuvant *(31, 32)*. It should be noted that the immunomodulatory activity of other cytokines, e.g., GM-CSF and IL-2, may also increase the activity of vaccines *(33)*.

Human Th2 cells produce IL-4, IL-5, and IL-9 but not IFN-γ or TNF-β. Th2 cytokines activate mast cells, eosinophils, and elevation in IgE levels and are associated with the immune response to allergens and helminths. The major determinant for Th2 cell differentiation is the predominance of IL-4 production early in the immune response. The primary source of IL-4 is uncertain, but it may be other classes of T-cells or mast cells *(28)*.

Both human Th1 and Th2 cells produce GM-CSF, IL-2, IL-3, IL-10, and IL-13. The production of IL-2, IL-10, and IL-13 by both T-cell subsets in humans differs from mice where their production is limited to one subset. T-helper cells that produce IFN-γ, IL-2, IL-6, IL-10, and IL-14 induce proliferation and differentiation of B-cells and function in antibody-dependent immunity. In addition to the Th1/Th2 subsets, there are undifferentiated T-cells, Th0 cells, that produce both Th1 and Th2 cytokines, although the primary cytokine produced is IL-2.

Chemokines have a role in lymphocyte response to infections with the orchestration of the movement of the right lymphocyte, i.e., T-cell, B-cell, or cytotoxic T-cell/NK cell, to the site of infection. The T-helper cell subsets tend to colocalize with different leukocytes (although not always). The Th1 subset of cells tends to colocalize with macrophages and neutrophils, whereas Th2 are more often associated with eosinophils and basophils. The same chemokine receptor can be present on these groups of cells *(34, 35)*. For example, CCR3 (the chemokine for eotaxin, RANTES, and MCP-3), is expressed on Th2 cells as well as on eosinophils and basophils. CCR3 is selectively expressed on Th2 cells that produce high levels of IL-4. Both eosinophils and basophils depend on IL-4 and IL-5, produced by the stimulated Th2 cells to maintain activation. Similarly, the chemokine receptors CCR5 and CCR1 are expressed on Th1 cells and monocytes. Th1 cells have also been shown to express CSCR3, the chemokine receptor for IFN-γ-inducible protein 10 (IP-10) and monokine induced by IFN-γ (MIG). Much of the data on chemokine receptor expression analysis in T-helper subsets are from in vitro experiments, and further studies are needed to improve our comprehension of the role of chemokines in lymphocyte migration.

Since the elucidation of the Th1/Th2 subsets of helper T-cells, their function has probably been oversimplified in the assignment of a Th1 response to intracellular pathogens and a Th2 response to extracellular organisms. However, for many infectious diseases a response by Th1 and Th2 cells at different time points is needed to control or eradicate the infection. In addition, unlike in the mouse, some cytokines are synthesized by both T-cell subsets in humans. This coproduction for some cytokines and the redundancy in the activity of the cytokine network suggest that the immune response to different pathogens represents a weighted response involving both T-cell subsets rather than one limited solely to either Th1 or Th2. Therefore, it is important to recognize that the therapeutic effect of an immunotherapy intended to manipulate the effect of one cytokine will result not only from the modulation of that cytokine but also the effect that that modulation has on other cytokines in the network.

REFERENCES

1. Aggarwal BB, Puri RK (eds). Human Cytokines: Their Role in Disease and Therapy. Cambridge, MA: Blackwell Science, 1995.
2. Kunkel SL, Remick DG (eds). Cytokines in Health and Disease. New York: Marcel Dekker, 1992.
3. Oppenheim JJ, Rossio JL, Gearing, AJ (eds). Clinical Applications of Cytokines. Role in Pathogenesis, Diagnosis, and Therapy. New York: Oxford University Press, 1993.
4. Roilides E, Pizzo PA. Modulation of host defenses by cytokines: evolving adjuncts in prevention and treatment of serious infections in immunocompromised hosts. Clin Infect Dis 1992; 15:508–524.
5. King CL, Gallin JI, Malech HL. Regulation of immunoglobulin production in hyperimmunoglobulin E recurrent-infection syndrome by interferon-gamma. Proc Natl Acad Sci USA 1986; 86:10085–10089.
6. DiCosmo BF, Gebo GP, Picarella D. Airway epithelial cell expression of interleukin-6 in transgenic mice: uncoupling airway inflammation and bronchial hyperreactivity. J Clin Invest 1994; 94:2028–2034.
7. Upton C, Mossman K, McFadden G. Encoding of a homolog of the IFN-gamma receptor by myxoma virus. Science 1992; 258:1369–1372.
8. Smith CA, Davis T, Anderson D, et al. A receptor for tumor necrosis factor defines an unusual family of cellular and viral proteins. Science 1990; 248:1019–1023.
9. Miyajima A, Kitamura T, Haraa N. Cytokine receptors and signal transduction. Annu Rev Immunol 1992; 10:295–331.
10. Bazan JF. Structural design and molecular evolution of a cytokine receptor superfamily. Proc Natl Acad Sci USA 1990; 87:6934–6938.
11. Castro JE, et al. Fas modulation of apoptosis during negative selection of thymocytes. Immunity 1996; 5:617–627.
12. Noelle RJ. CD40 and its ligand in host defense. Immunity 1996; 4:415–419.
13. Dinarello CA, Wolff SM. The role of interleukin-1 in disease. N Engl J Med 1993; 328:106–113.
14. Dinarello CA. Interleukin-18. Methods 1999; 19:121–132.
15. Darnell JE Jr, Kerr IM, Stark GR. Jak-STAT pathways and transcriptional activation in response to IFNs and other extracellular signaling proteins. Science 1994; 264:1415–1421.
16. Fishman S, Hobbs K, Borish L. (1996) Molecular biology of cytokines in allergic diseases and asthma. Immun Allergy Clin North Am 1996; 16:613–642.
17. Walz DA, et al. Primary structure of human platelet factor 4. Thromb Res 1997; 11:893–898.
18. Yoshimura T, et al. Purification of a human monocyte-derived neutrophil chemotactic factor that has peptide sequence similarity to other host defense cytokines. Proc Natl Acad Sci USA 1987; 84:9233–9237.
19. Taub DD. Chemokine-leukocyte interactions—the voodoo that they do so well. Cytokine Growth Factor Rev 1996; 7:355–376.

20. Taub DD, Oppenheim JJ. Chemokines, inflammation and the immune system. Ther Immunol 1994; 1:229–246.

21. Murphy PM. Chemokine receptors: structure, function and role in microbial pathogenesis. Cytokine Growth Factor Rev 1996; 7:47–64.

22. Miller LH, et al. The resistant factor to *Plasmodium vivax* in blacks. The Duffy-blood-group genotype, FyFy. N Engl J Med 1976; 295:302–304.

23. Gao JL, Murphy PM. Human cytomegalovirus open reading frame US28 encodes a functional beta chemokine receptor. J Biol Chem 1994; 269:28539–28542.

24. Price DA, et al. Cytotoxic T lymphocytes, chemokines and anitviral immunity. Immunol Today 1999; 20:212–216

25. Baggiolini M, Walz A, Kunkels SL. Neutrophil activating peptide 1/interleukin 8, a novel cytokine that activates neutrophils. J Clin Invest 1989; 84:1045–1049.

26. Romagnani S. Biology of human Th1 and Th2 cells. J Clin Immunol 1995; 15:121–129.

27. Mosmann TR, Sad S. The expanding universe of T-cell subsets: Th1, Th2 and more. Immunol Today 1996; 17:138–146.

28. O'Garra A. Cytokines induce the development of functionally heterogeneous T helper cell subsets. Immunity 1998; 8:275–283.

29. Brunda MJ. Interleukin-12. Leuk Biol 1994; 55:280–288.

30. Trinchieri G. Interleukin-12: a proinflammatory cytokine with immunoregulatory functions that bridge innate resistance and antigen-specific adaptive immunity. Annu Rev Immun 1995; 13:251–276.

31. Romani L, Puccetti P, Bistoni F. Interleukin-12 in infectious diseases. Clin Microbiol Rev 1997; 10:611–636.

32. Afonso LC, et al. The adjuvant effect of interleukin-12 in a vaccine against *Leishmania major*. Science 1994; 263:235–237.

33. Pasquini S, et al. Cytokines and costimulatory molecules as genetic adjuvants. Immunol Cell Biol 1997; 75:397–401.

34. Syrbe U, Siveke J, Hamann A. Th1/Th2 subsets: distinct differences in homing and chemokine receptor expression?, Springer Semin Immunopathol 1999; 21:263–285.

35. Sallusto F, Lanzavecchia A, Mackay CR. Chemokines and chemokine receptors in T-cell priming and Th1/Th2-mediated responses. Immunol Today 1998; 19:568–574.

7

Principles of Vaccine Development

Constantin A. Bona

INTRODUCTION

Two hundred years ago, Jenner devised the first vaccine able to prevent variola. This vaccine was based on the observation that subsequent to injection of a boy with cowpox, he was protected against two successive inoculations with smallpox virus. After 200 years, global administration of vaccinia has led to almost total eradication of the smallpox virus from the earth. There is no other example in medicine of a new drug or biologic substance leading to eradication of the causative agent and extinction of disease. Vaccinations against other bacteria or viruses prevents the death of millions of people yearly. However, currently vaccines do not cover the entire spectrum of diseases. There is a long list of microbes, among which are HIV and malaria, affecting millions of individuals, for which we do not yet have vaccines. This is why the development of new vaccines is a permanent aim of medical research. This interest grew because scientists have understood that vaccines can be used not only for prevention of infectious diseases but also for therapy, leading to the concept of therapeutic vaccines.

Classical vaccines pioneered by the discoveries of Jenner, Pasteur, and Ramon was based on the principle of inactivation of pathogenicity of a microbe without altering its capacity to induce a protective immune response.

Developments during the past decades in biochemistry, molecular biology, and immunology have provided new tools for the development of a new generation of vaccines. Biochemistry and Immunochemistry contributed to the identification of epitopes endowed with protective capacities. The identification of such antigenic determinants, also called epitopes, on antigens of protein origin allowed for preparation of synthetic peptides or subunit vaccines in the case of antigens of nonprotein origin. Recombinant DNA technology, which revolutionized biomedical research, contributed to the development of genetically engineered antigens used as vaccines, as recombinant protein molecules, microbial vectors, or fusion proteins. Immunology provided the framework for understanding the mechanisms responsible for the activation of lymphocytes following vaccination as well as functional analysis of various epitopes that induce a protective immune response. This is particularly important as antibodies mediate the protection against some bacteria; cellular immune responses are prevalent against obligatory intracellular microbes.

From: *Immunotherapy for Infectious Diseases*
Edited by: J. M. Jacobson © Humana Press Inc., Totowa, NJ

The immune system is composed of two major populations: B-cells, producing antibodies, and T-cells, mediating cellular immunity. T-cells are divided into CD4 and CD8 subsets and the CD4 T-cells are divided, based on the pattern of cytokine secretion, into Th1, Th2 and Th3 cells. The differences between B- and T-cells are not only functional but are also seen in the mechanism of recognition of antigens.

The B-cells, via the Ig receptor, recognize both conformational and linear epitopes directly on the surface of native macromolecules. In certain cases the recognition of epitopes leads to activation and differentiation of B-cells directly, i.e. T-independent antigens. In other cases they need the help of CD4 T-cells, i.e., T-dependent antigens. The isotype of antibodies is dependent on collaboration with T-cells. Whereas Th1 cells polarize the response to IgG2, the collaboration with Th2 leads to IgG1 and IgE *(1)*.

The polarization of isotypes is caused by cytokines secreted by these subsets that represent second signals: interleukin-2 (IL-2), and interferon-γ (INF-γ), in the case of Th1 and IL-4, IL-5, and IL-10 in the case of Th2 cells *(1)*. Antibodies exert their protective capacity by blocking the microbial receptor through which they bind to the cellular receptor of permissive cells, promoting phagocytosis via opsonins and complement-dependent lysis.

In contrast to B-cells, T-cells are unable to recognize the antigens on the surface of native macromolecules. They recognize only fragments of degraded antigens in association with MHC molecules. CD4 T-cells recognize peptides or glycopeptides in association with class II MHC molecules. The peptides are produced from the processing of exogenous proteins in the endosomes of professional antigen-presenting cells (APCs; B-cells, macrophages, and dendritic cells), where they bind to nascent and empty class II molecules. The peptide-class II complex is translocated to the membrane, where interaction with the T-cell receptor (TCR) of T cells occurs.

Figure 1 illustrates cellular events leading to generation of a class II-peptide complex within professional APCs. CD8 T-cells recognize the peptides in association with class I MHC molecules. The peptides are derived from endogenous proteins, including proteins of intracellular microbes. The proteins are fragmented by proteasomes, and the peptides are bound to transporter proteins (TAPs), and taken to the endoplasmic reticulum (ER), where they are released and bind to nascent class I MHC molecules. The peptide-class I complex is transferred via the Golgi apparatus to membranes and is recognized by CD8 T-cells *(2)*.

Figure 2 illustrates the generation of a class I-peptide complex. γ/δ T-cells or natural killer (NK) cells can recognize lipopeptides or glycopeptides in association with CD1 molecules, which are less polymorphic than MHC molecules *(3)*.

Table 1 depicts the major functions of cells involved in host response to vaccines.

Interdisciplinary contributions of accumulated knowledge and new methodologies have led to the development of new vaccines "à la carte," stimulating production of antibodies, cytokines, and cytotoxic responses, contributing to the recovery process from infectious diseases. This also contributed to the development of immunotherapeutic vaccines. Ideally, a vaccine should display the following properties:

1. The antigen should be pure and chemically well defined.
2. It should induce a protective immune response.
3. It should exhibit a constant antigen specificity without being the subject of genetic variation
4. The protection should be lifelong or induced promptly after a booster dose.

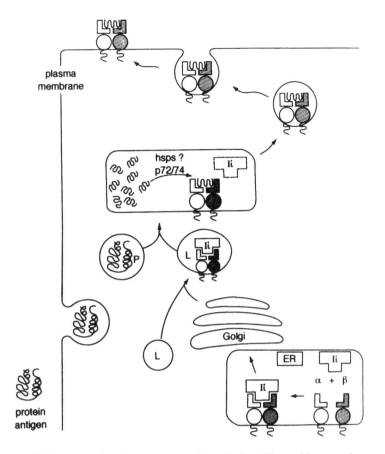

Fig. 1. Intracellular events leading to generation of class II-peptide complex expressed on the surface of professional antigen-presenting cells (APCs). After internalization, a vaccine is digested within endosomes of APCs. Class II molecules are synthesized in the endoplasmic reticulum (ER) as a trimeric complex made up of α, β, and invariant chains. It migrates to endosomes where the invariant chain is partially degraded and a short peptide called CLIP remains attached to class II molecules. After CLIP is released, DM functions as a chaperone that stabilizes the empty class II molecule, allowing the binding of peptides derived from degradation of foreign protein to class II empty molecules. Another molecule called DO stabilizes the class II-peptide complex, which is then pulled to the membrane, where it may be recognized by CD4 T-cells. hsps, heat shock proteins.

5. It should be devoid of side effects.
6. The manufacturing should be inexpensive.

CLASSICAL AND NEWLY DEVELOPED VACCINES

Inactivated Vaccines

The development of inactivated vaccines resulted from the development of methods to grow microbes and to purify the toxins. The preparation of inactivated vaccines is based on a golden rule emerging from Pasteur and Ramon's studies leading to preparation of anti-rabies and toxoid vaccines, respectively: a vaccine should be devoid of pathogenicity but should preserve intact its immunogenicity.

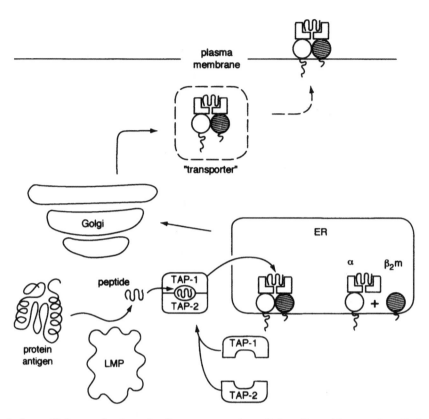

Fig. 2. Intracellular mechanisms leading to generation of class I-peptide complex. Endogenous proteins are degraded by lysosomes and the resulting peptides are translocated to the endoplasmic reticulum (ER) by transporter protein (TAP) molecules. In the ER, the peptides are released from TAP by chaperons such tapasin, calreticulin, and calexin and then bind to the heavy chain of class I molecules, which in turn bind β_2-microglobulin (β_2m). The class I-peptide complex is then transferred via a Golgi secretory pathway to the membrane, where it is recognized by CD 8 T-cells.

The killing of bacteria can be achieved by physical means (heat) or by chemical agents. For example, currently used influenza and Salk polio vaccines are produced by inactivation with formalin. Similarly, the conversion of toxins to toxoids was obtained by treatment with formalin. Table 2 lists currently used inactivated vaccines.

Immunity

Inactivated vaccines can induce only a humoral response. Functional antibodies are produced subsequent to recognition by the Ig receptor of B-cells of a protective epitope on the bacterial membrane or secreted toxins. Activation and differentiation of resting B-cells into antibody-forming cells requires a second signal by cytokines produced by activated CD4 T-cells. The activation of CD4 T-cells is achieved by APCs, which take up the microbes, process them in endosomes, and present the peptide-class II complex to CD4 T-cells.

Advantages

Inactivated vaccines display several advantages:

1. Simple manufacturing methodology.
2. Inability of reverse mutations that might lead to pathogen microbes.

Table 1
Function of Immunocytes in Immune Responses Elicited by Vaccines

Cell type	Function
Dendritic and B-cells	Presentation of epitopes
Macrophages	Phagocytosis of opsonized microbes
B-cells	Synthesis of antibodies against T-independent antigens
B+CD4 T-cells	Synthesis of antibodies against T-dependent antigens
CD4 T-cells	Secretion of antiinflammatory cytokines
CD8 T-cells	Lysis of infected cells

Table 2
Inactivated Vaccines

Vaccine	Licensed	In trials
Rabies	Yes	
Influenzavirus	Yes	
Salk polio	Yes	
Hepatitis B	Yes	
Japanese encephalitis	Yes	Yes
Bordetella pertussis	Yes	
Mycobacterium leprae		Yes
Vibrio cholerae	Yes	
Salmonella typhi	Yes	
Tetanus toxin	Yes	
Diphtheria toxin	Yes	

3. Stability.
4. Good induction of antibody synthesis.
5. Can be administered as combined vaccines such as trivalent or quatrivalent vaccines, e.g., influenza vaccine composed of H1N1, H3N3, and a subtype B-strain, or diphtheria, tetanus, and pertussis trivalent or quatrivalent when polio vaccine is added to trivalent vaccine. Combined vaccines induce similar responses, as do monovalent vaccines, indicating that is no antigen competition.

Disadvantages

The inactivated vaccines exhibit some drawbacks:

1. Poor antibody response is seen owing to weak generation of memory B-cells; several boosts are often required.
2. The antibody-mediated response against the protective epitope can be diluted by production of antibodies against the multitude of bacterial macromolecules bearing nonprotective epitopes.
3. There is an inability to stimulate the cell-mediated immune responses that contribute to recovery from disease or alter the course of disease in the case of therapeutic vaccines.
4. Some inactivated vaccines exhibit side effects (e.g., pertussis vaccine [4]).

Subunit Vaccines

Subunit vaccines represent a variant of inactivated vaccines. These vaccines can easily be developed when the disease is caused by a single or a few serotypes of infectious agents (e.g., *Neisseria meningitidis, Streptococcus pneumoniae,* and *Hemophilus influenzae* b serotype). They cannot be generated when multiple serotypes are involved in pathogenicity, as in the case of the nosocomial infection caused by *Klebsiella pneumoniae.*

Subunit vaccines are produced by purification from bacteria of antigens bearing protective epitopes or by molecular methods of expression and purification of recombinant proteins. With the exception of the hepatitis B subunit vaccine (which is of a protein nature), these are bacterial polysaccharides

Immunity

Polysaccharide vaccines are generally poor immunogens and induce T-independent responses dominated by IgM. The immune response results from direct activation of a subset of B-cells subsequent to the crosslinking of B-cell receptor (BCR) by antigens exibiting repetitive epitopes. This subset is under the control of an X-linked gene. Mutation of this gene, as in Wiscott-Aldrich syndrome, makes such patients unresponsive to subunit polysaccharide vaccines.

Advantages

Subunit vaccines are very stable and safe. Antibody response is more restricted than that induced by inactivated vaccines.

Disadvantages

Antibody response is generally weak, requires several boosts, and is dominated by low-affinity IgM antibodies. Generally, the vaccines are inefficient in newborns and infants because of the ontogenic delay of expression of a B-cell subset responding to polysaccharide antigens. Induction of high-affinity IgG antibodies can be obtained by coupling the polysaccharide to a protein bearing strong T-cell epitopes. This procedure was successfully used in the case of *H. influenzae* b serotype vaccine, in which the polysaccharide was coupled to tetanus toxoid. This vaccine is efficient not only in adults but also in infants. Finally, subunit vaccines cannot induce cytotoxic T-lymphocyte (CTL) responses. Table 3 lists licensed subunit vaccines.

Live Attenuated Vaccines

The possibility of preparation of live attenuated vaccines is based on Enders *(5)* discovery of a method of culturing viruses in vitro in permissive cells. Live attenuated vaccines are produced by culturing the microbe in special conditions, leading to loss of pathogenicity without altering immunogenicity. To achieve this goal, several methods were and are currently used:

1. Passage of virus many times in tissue culture or chicken embryonated eggs.
2. Selection of temperature-sensitive mutants that do not grow above 37°C.
3. Selection of naturally occurring mutants (e.g., Sabin vaccine).
4. Deletion of pathogenic genes.

Immunity

Live attenuated vaccines induce humoral and cellular responses. The humoral response results from the interaction of CD4 T-cells recognizing a peptide generated by APCs,

Table 3
Licensed Subunit Vaccines

Hemophilus influenzae
Streptococcus pneumoniae
Neisseria meningitidis
Bordetella pertussis (acellular)
Hepatitis B (recombinant protein)

which have taken up the microbe with B-cells able to recognize an epitope on the surface of virus. The CD4 T-cells secrete cytokines, which represent the second signal required for the activation of B-cells responding to T-dependent antigens. The infected cells can produce peptides subsequent to fragmentation of endogenous viral or microbial proteins. The peptide associated with class I molecules is expressed on the membrane. The CD8 T-cells are activated subsequent to recognition of the class I-peptide complex.

Advantages

1. Live attenuated vaccines elicit a long-lasting immunity comparable to that induced during natural infection. Therefore, immunity can be induced by a single or several injections.
2. These vaccines induce both humoral and cellular immunity.

Disadvantages

The preparation of live attenuated vaccines requires a tedious procedure to select the microbes that are devoid of pathogenicity, and manufacturing is costly. A possible drawback is the occurrence of reverse mutations. Table 4 lists currently used live attenuated vaccines.

Internal Image Idiotype Vaccines

Idiotypes are phenotypic markers of antigen receptors of lymphocytes. The diversity of antigen receptors is reflected in the diversity of idiotypes. Idiotype are immunogenic and able to induce antiidiotypic antibodies (Ab2s), which in turn express their own idiotypes. As a statistical necessity, Jerne *(6)* introduced the concept that the idiotypes of antiidiotype antibodies could mimic the antigen recognized by antibody-Ab1. This concept is not a simple consequence of the "lock and key" rule of complementary of antigen-antibody interaction but can be owing to molecular mimicry or sharing of similar sequences between antigen and Ab2.

This hypothesis is strongly supported by crystallographic studies. Fields et al. *(7)* had determined the crystal structure of an antibody specific for lysozyme and of its corresponding antiidiotype antibody. Of the 18 residues that contact Ab1 with Ab2, and the 17 that interact with lysozyme, 13 were in contact with both lysozyme and Ab2. This important information clearly demonstrated that some antiidiotypic antibodies are internal images of antigens and therefore they may function as antigen surrogates because they represent the positive imprint of antigen.

An Ab1 antibody specific for a protective epitope is prepared, and then Ab2 antiidiotype antibodies are generated. Antigen-inhibitable Ab2, which then can be used as internal image idiotype vaccines, is then selected *(8)*.

Table 4
Live Attenuated Vaccines

Vaccine	Licensed	In trials
Vaccinia	Yes	
Sabin polio	Yes	
Measles	Yes	
Mumps	Yes	
Rubella	Yes	
Adenovirus	Yes	
Varicella-zoster	Yes	
Cytomegalovirus		Yes
Dengue		Yes
Rotavirus		Yes
Parainfluenza		Yes
Japanese encephalitis		Yes
Hepatitis A	Yes	
Influenza (cold attenuated)		Yes
Salmonella typhi (aromutant)		Yes
Bacille Calmette-Guérin	Yes	

In various animal models it has been shown (Table 5) that antibodies produced subsequent to injection of internal image idiotype elicited a protective response. However, this type of vaccine was not introduced in human trials.

Immunity

The immune response elicited by idiotype vaccines results either from activation of B-cells subsequent to the binding of Ab2 to BCR of Ab1 or by interaction of B-cells with CD4 T-cells that recognize idiopeptides produced by digestion of antiidiotype by APC.

Advantages

The internal image idiotype vaccines are safe, induce humoral immunity, and are able to circumvent the ontogenic delay responsible for unresponsiveness of infants to some vaccines *(8)*.

Disadvantages

Internal image vaccines are poor immunogens and require coupling with carrier protein, which increases their immunogenicity. Generally they do not induce memory cells, an intrinsic property of a good vaccine. In addition, they are unable to induce mucosal immunity or CTL activity *(9)*.

Recombinant Protein Vaccines

The preparation of this type of vaccine is limited to microbial proteins bearing protective epitopes. The generation of recombinant proteins is based on cloning a gene encoding a protein, which is then aligned with a promoter and inserted into a suitable plasmid replicon. The plasmid is used to transform bacteria such as *E. coli* or to stably transfect mammalian, insect or yeast cells. Recombinant proteins can also be obtained from genetically engineered viruses. In this case, the flanking region of the

Table 5
Idiotype Vaccines

Microbe	Antigen mimicked by internal image	Property of antibodies
E. coli	Capsular polysaccharide	Protective
Streptococcus pneumoniae	Phosphocholine	Protective
Streptococcus pyogenis	Group A carbohydrate	Protective
Pseudomonas aeruginosa	Capsular antigen	Protective
Corynebacterium diphtheriae	Toxin	Protective
Legionela pneumoniae	Cytolysin	Nonprotective
Reovirus type 3	Hemagglutinin	Neutralizing
Poliovirus type II	?	Neutralizing
Influenzavirus	Hemagglutinin	Neutralizing
Rabies virus	Glycoprotein	Neutralizing
SV40 virus	T-antigen	Suppressive
Coxsackievirus B4	Binding receptor	Nonneutralizing
Coronavirus	A59 epitope	?
Blue tongue virus	?	Neutralizing
Foot and mouth disease virus	Surface antigen	Nonneutralizing
Hepatitis B virus	S antigen	?
Schisostoma mansoni	Glycoprotein	Protective
Trypanosoma organisms	Variable antigen type (VAT)	Protective
Trichothecene	Mycotoxin T2	Protective

Adapted from ref. 9.

foreign gene permits homologous recombination between plasmid and the viral genome, and double reciprocal recombination results in transfer of plasmid DNA into the viral genome. Permissive cells infected with virus will drive the synthesis of recombinant protein. The production of recombinant protein in mammalian cells has a lower yield, but such proteins are correctly glycosylated. Whatever the system, the production of recombinant protein requires purification procedures from the culture medium.

Immunity

By virtue of their protein nature, recombinant proteins require a B-CD4 T-cell collaboration.

Advantages

Recombinant protein vaccines are safe and can induce a strong humoral response. They can be immunogenic in adults as well as in infants.

Disadvantages

The stability of recombinant protein is high but costly procedures are required to prevent alteration of proteins. They cannot induce mucosal immunity except when they are administered intranasally or orally. They are unable to stimulate CTL activity. There are only a few recombinant proteins licensed with proven efficacy: recombinant hepatitis B protein produced in yeast, Osp A protein produced in yeast (recently approved as vaccine to prevent Lyme disease), and a protein used as a vaccine against Japanese encephalitis virus.

Recombinant Vectors Vaccines

Recombinant viruses or bacteria may act as vectors of a foreign gene, bearing protective epitopes that would be transcribed, translated, and capable of inducing an immune response. The preparation of recombinant microbial vaccines is carried out in two steps: first, the selection or engineering of a live attenuated virus or bacterium and second, expression of foreign gene in the vector. It is possible to express several genes in a single vector and therefore to prepare polyvalent vaccines. In recent years, poxvirus, adenovirus, Bacille Calmette-Guérin (BCG), *Salmonella* and recently *B. anthracis* have been used as vectors in attempts to develop recombinant vectors.

Vaccinia vectors

Since vaccinia displays reactogenicity, sometimes causing postvaccinal encephalitis or even generalized and fatal infection in immunodeficient subjects, new poxviruses were developed. One new vector called NYVAC has 18 complete open reading frames (ORFs) deleted, including two genes contributing to the ability of virus to replicate in vitro in various cells. It can replicate in Vero cells only in the presence of wild-type virus *(10)*. The second is ALVAC, which is an avipox virus that can infect mammalian cells but does not replicate *(11)*.

There are two methods to insert the foreign DNA in poxviruses:

Homologous recombination. Recombinant vaccinia vectors are prepared by infection of permissive cells with vaccinia virus and transfection with a plasmid expressing an antigen gene. Since the rate of homologous recombination is high, about 0.1% of virions incorporate the foreign gene. The recombinants are easily selected by common techniques. The genes of more than 20 RNA and more than 10 DNA viruses, bacteria, or parasites have been expressed in vaccinia *(12)*.

Genetic engineering. A foreign gene can also be introduced into the vaccinia genome by cutting the DNA at a unique endonuclease site, after which the foreign gene can be ligated at compatible ends in vitro.

Recombinant Adenovirus Vector

Adenovirus vectors express antigen genes that are translated in replicas of native protein. The proteins do not exhibit posttranslational modifications and are capable of inducing neutralizing antibodies in both permissive and abortive animal models *(13)*. Several viral genes have been expressed in adenovirus vectors: hepatitis B, VSV, *env* and *gag* genes of HIV-1, HSV, CMV glycoprotein, rabies glycoprotein, F and HN of parainfluenza virus, and F and G of RSV viruses. The recombinant adenovirus vectors are able to elicit mucosal immunity.

Recombinant Salmonella *Vectors*

Attenuated *Salmonella* strains were obtained by deletion of genes encoding for virulence as toxins or invasin. The attenuated strains were then used to insert a foreign gene into a bacterial chromosome *(14)*. Since it was observed that synthesis of protein encoded by the foreign gene is low, an effort was made to increase the number of copies of foreign gene in the *Salmonella* genome. Several properties are required for an ideal *Salmonella* vector vaccine:

1. It should be complete avirulent and highly immunogenic.
2. It should be genotypically stable, with two or more deletions that do not revert and are not influenced by environmental factors. This is an important requirement since it was shown

that attenuated *Salmonella* organisms recovered from immunized animals lose the plasmid of avirulence or the foreign gene.

3. Finally, it should colonize to allow for a continuous synthesis of foreign protein.

Recombinant *Salmonella* vectors can be administered orally and therefore are able to induce mucosal immunity.

Recombinant BCG Vectors

Recombinant BCG vector vaccines were obtained by transfer of replicative or integrative plasmids by electroporation, gene replacement, plasmid conjugation, and phage lysogeny *(15)*. These vectors are able to induce a long-lasting humoral and cellular immunity conferred by the expression of foreign gene and by the nature of the BCG vector, respectively.

Bacillus anthracis (Stern strain)

B. anthracis (non-pathogenic Stern strain) was used to express foreign genes. This strain contains a pX01 gene coding for toxin but lacks pX02 plasmid coding for capsular polysaccharide, which is responsible for virulence. A vector expressing the *listeriolysine* gene was able to deliver Listeria protein to the cytoplasm and to induce a CTL response mediated by CD8 T-cells *(16)*.

DNA Vaccines

The utilization of DNA as a vaccine is based on the fact that the injection of a plasmid bearing a reporter gene leads to in vivo transfection of cells as well as to transcription of the foreign gene inserted into plasmid *(17)*. There has been an explosion of research in this area, leading to human trials of DNA vaccines.

DNA vaccines are constructed by insertion into plasmid of a foreign gene and a strong promoter, which ensures a high level of expression of the antigen gene, bearing protective epitopes. Recent studies have established the best conditions for constructing the plasmids used for vaccination. The spacing required between the regulatory and inserted genes, the stability of RNA transcripts, and the minimum number of copies required for a significant synthesis of foreign antigen able to induce immune responses have also been studied. Table 6 lists the systems in which DNA vaccination against viruses, bacteria, and parasites were assessed.

Immunity

The induction of a humoral immune response depends on the type of protein encoded by the foreign gene. Whereas a protein bearing epitopes recognized by a B-cell will induce the synthesis of antibodies, a protein expressing CD8 T-cell epitopes induces a CTL response.

In the case of the humoral immune response, the B-cells can recognize the conformational or linear epitopes on the surface of antigens secreted by transfected cells. In contrast, in the case of CD8 T-cells, the peptides required for activation of CTL precursors are generated via endogenous pathways, and the class I-peptide complexes translocated on the membrane are recognized by T-cells.

The CD4 T-cells are stimulated by in vivo transfected APCs, which synthesize the protein, process it, and present the peptides in association with class II molecules to CD4 T-cells. Recent reports showed that both macrophages *(18)* and dendritic cells *(19)* are transfected in vivo and are able to activate the CD4 T-cells

Table 6
DNA Vaccines Used in Experimental Models

Microbe	Virus
Negative-strand RNA viruses	Influenza
	Measles
	Newcastle
	Sendai
	Bovine respiratory syncytial
	Rabies
	Lymphocytic choriomeningitis
	Ebola
Positive, single-strand RNA viruses	Hepatitis C
	St. Louis encephalitis
	Tick-borne encephalitis
	Japanese encephalitis
	Russian-spring encephalitis
	Bovine viral diarrhea
	Infectious bronchitis
	Foot and mouth disease
Double-strand RNA	Rotavirus
Retroviruses	Human, simian, and feline immunodeficiency
	Human T-cell leukemia/lymphoma
	Cas murine leukemia
DNA viruses	Hepatitis B
	Bovine herpes
	Herpes simplex
	Cytomegalovirus
	Pseudorabies
	Papilloma

Advantages

Several advantages have made genetic immunization appealing for vaccination:

1. The DNA vaccine is very stable and easy to manufacture; it is easy to construct new plasmids in the case of vaccines against microbes exhibiting natural genetic variation.
2. Long-lasting persistence of plasmid and sustained synthesis of low doses of antigen preclude induction of high-dose tolerance and favor the generation of memory cells.
3. Lack of contaminant proteins in plasmid preparation prevents side effects such as allergic reactions.
4. DNA immunization does not require adjuvants since the plasmids rich in CpG motifs are endowed with intrinsic adjuvanticity.
5. It can induce humoral and cellular immune responses.
6. It can prime neonates, which may lead to development of vaccines for neonates or infants otherwise unresponsive to inactivated or live attenuated vaccines.

Disadvantages

Various studies have demonstrated the safety of DNA vaccines. However, DNA vaccination has two possible drawbacks: first, the induction of anti-DNA antibodies and second, the possibility of integration of plasmid into the host genome by non-homologous recombination. Such phenomena can lead to the occurrence of mutated structural genes, inhibition of expression of suppressor genes, or mutation of protooncogenes favoring the development of cancers.

Peptide-Based Vaccines

In contrast to B-cells able to recognize the epitopes on the surface of native antigen, T-cells recognize peptides derived from the processing of proteins in association with MHC molecules. Thus, the peptide-based vaccines can be efficient only against protein antigens and can be used only against infectious agents for which the cellular immunity is the major arm of the immune responses

The peptide-based vaccines can be divided into two categories: CD4 T-cell vaccines having potential usage against obligatory intracellular microbes (*Mycobacterium, Salmonella, Brucella, Francisella, Listeria, Rickettsia, Candida, Nocardia, Histoplasma, Leishmania, Babesia, Trypanosoma,* and *Schistosma* organisms) and CD8 vaccines against all viruses *(20)*.

Synthetic peptides corresponding to epitopes recognized by CD4 or CD8 T-cells represent ideal safe vaccines. However, the peptides themselves cannot be used as efficient vaccines because of a short half-life and poor immunogenicity. Because of these drawbacks, several approaches have been taken to present the peptides loaded in liposomes and adjuvants or on platforms in which oligonucleotide sequences coding for peptides are inserted by genetic engineering.

Synthetic Peptide as a Vaccine

Because of drawbacks of induction of an immune response by peptides, several artificial systems have been used to increase immunogenicity such as immunization with liposomes containing peptides, synthetic lipopeptides, or coadministration with immunostimulating complex (ISCOM). Whereas injected peptides can bind directly to surface MHC molecules on the surface of APCs, the peptides delivered within liposomes or trapped in ISCOM are released subsequent to processing by APCs. Figure 3 illustrates the mechanisms of activation of CD8 T-cells by peptides.

Viruses Expressing Foreign Peptide Epitopes

DNA or RNA viruses expressing foreign peptides are constructed by genetic engineering. Briefly, a minigene encoding a given peptide is inserted in a viral gene by PCR mutagenesis. These viruses produce chimeric protein made up of viral protein expressing the foreign epitope. This chimeric protein elicits an immune response against viral protein as well as against foreign peptide.

This approach may contribute to the preparation of polyvaccines, an example being an influenza HK strain expressing a CD8 epitope on its nucleoprotein and a different CD8 epitope inserted in hemagglutinin. This virus was able to induce a strong CTL response against nucleoprotein peptides recognized in association with class I K^d and D^b molecules *(21)*. Similarly, a chimeric Sindbis virus expressing a minigene encoding two distance epitopes was able to prime CD8 cytotoxic T-cells *(22)*.

The advantage of these vaccines lie in their ability to induce immune responses not only against proteins of host virus but also against foreign peptides. These vaccines induce immune responses subsequent to penetration and eventual replication of virus in APCs, followed by processing of protein in endogenous pathways and presentation

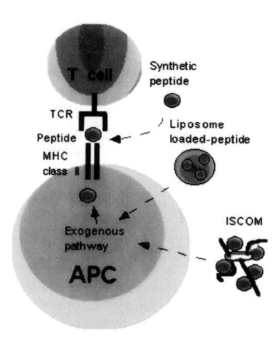

Fig. 3. Mechanisms of activation of CD4 T-cells by peptides. Soluble peptides can bind directly to MHC molecules by displaying the endogenous peptides. Once the complex is formed, it can activate the T-cells. The peptides trapped in liposomes or adjuvants are internalized and released in endosomes. APC, antigen-presenting cell; ISCOM, immunostimulating complex; TCR, T-cell receptor.

of peptide in association with class I and eventually class II molecules. Figure 4 illustrates the mechanism of activation of T-cells by chimeric viruses expressing foreign epitopes.

The disadvantages of this approach consist in the induction responses against viral proteins devoid of protective epitopes as well as fast clearing owing to the presence of antiviral antibodies, which precludes efficient boosting.

Delivery of T-Cell Peptides by Recombinant Proteins

Molecular engineering methods allowed for the in-frame insertion of oligonucleotides encoding a given peptide within coding regions of genes coding for otherwise unrelated proteins. The translation of this chimeric gene led to synthesis of a chimeric protein expressing the epitopes recognized by T-cells. In constructing such molecules several factors should be taken into consideration:

1. The insertion of foreign peptide should not alter the correct folding of carrier molecule nor preclude its secretion.
2. The carrier molecule should have permissive sites where the peptide is inserted.
3. The flanking sequences of carrier molecules at the site of insertion should be accessible to processing by APC proteolytic enzymes.

Various T-cell epitopes were expressed in bacterial organelles or in secreted proteins *(23,24)*.

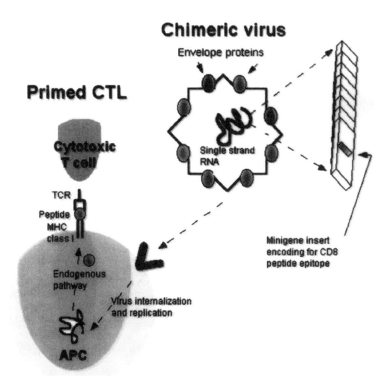

Fig. 4. Mechanism of activation of CD8 T-cells by chimeric viruses expressing T-cell epitopes. APC, antigen-presenting cell; CTL, cytotoxic T-lymphocyte; TCR, T-cell receptor.

The immune response elicited by recombinant proteins follows the uptake by APCs and their processing in the endosomal compartment. Figure 5 illustrates the mechanisms of induction of immune response by recombinant protein expressing T-cell epitopes, which are contained in various bacterial organelles.

Although the recombinant molecules are safe, they can induce strong responses against multiple antigenic determinants of carrier, and therefore the protective response might be diluted.

Receptor-Mediated Delivery of Peptides

The principle of this procedure is to artificially conjugate a peptide to a ligand interacting with a receptor or to a molecule expressed on the surface of APCs. Among the receptors able to internalize the conjugates are transferrin, ferritin, and α_2-macroglobulin receptors

The internalization of peptides can be achieved by conjugation of peptides with antibodies specific for a molecule expressed on APCs such as class I, class II, or Ig *(20)*.

The T-cells are activated subsequent to internalization of conjugates and their processing within APCs (Fig. 6). Until now this approach has had only academic interest because it is difficult to optimize coupling conditions as well as to preclude the formation of aggregates.

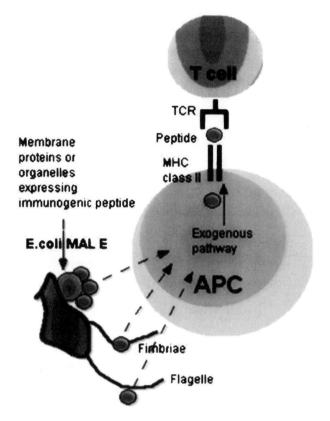

Fig. 5. Mechanism of generation of peptides by proteins expressing foreign epitopes. Chimeric viruses are internalized within the cell subsequent to binding to cellular receptors. Subsequent to replication, viral proteins are produced and processed in endogenous pathways leading to the release of foreign peptide from the viral protein in which it was inserted. APC, antigen-presenting cell; TCR, T-cell receptor.

Delivery of Peptides by Self Molecules

Self protein molecules are an ideal tool to deliver peptides since they are safe and do not elicit immune responses against carrier protein. Three major approaches have been undertaken to construct such molecules:

1. Genetically engineered replacement of a segment of the V_H gene (i.e., *CDR3*) with an oligonucleotide encoding a peptide recognized by T-cells. The resulting "antigenized" immunoglobulin molecules are taken up by APCs, which process chimeric Ig molecules and generate the peptide.
2. The peptide is attached to the sugar moiety of the Ig molecule by enzymatic engineering. This type of molecules can activate T-cells without the need for antigen processing since the molecule, by its Fc fragment, binds to the Fc receptor of APCs as well as to class II via the peptide attached to the sugar moiety *(25)*.
3. Generation by genetic engineering of soluble class I or class II molecules in which the peptide is covalently linked to the heavy chain of class I or to the β chain of class II molecules respectively *(26)*.

Depending on the dose used, these molecules can stimulate or anergize the T-cells. Figure 7 illustrates the structure of such molecules. In the future new approaches will develop toward safe and efficient delivery of peptides using various self molecules.

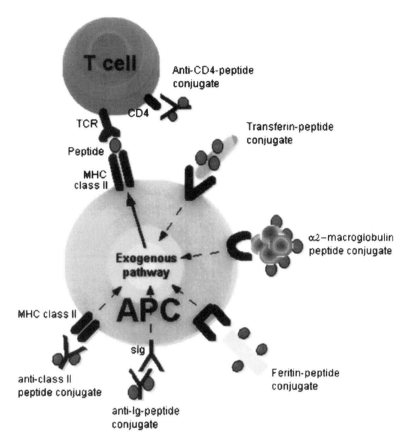

Fig. 6. Receptor delivery systems of peptides. Peptides chemically conjugated to ligands of cellular receptor or antibodies specific for membrane antigens are internalized by antigen-presenting cells (APC). After processing within the endosomal compartment, the peptides are released and then bind to MHC molecules. TCR, T-cell receptor.

IMMUNOTHERAPEUTIC VACCINES

Vaccines were initially conceived to prevent the infectious diseases associated with morbidity and mortality. The vaccine concept was extended to therapeutic reagents to cure chronic infection caused by persistent viruses or bacteria, autoimmune diseases, or cancers. The concept of therapeutic vaccines derives from the understanding of T-cell biology and pathophysiology: T-cells are not simply good soldiers fighting microbes or tumor cells but also vicious mercenaries contributing to the destruction of tissues that leads to autoimmune diseases.

Therapeutic vaccines against chronic infectious diseases (*Mycobacterium leprae*, HSV virus hepatitis B virus) are aimed at harnessing the immune response in carriers or cancer patients who are otherwise tolerant or unresponsive to microbial or tumor-associated antigens. In the case of autoimmune disease, therapeutic vaccines are used to eliminate autoreactive lymphocytes.

Most of the approaches used to develop the vaccines discussed in this chapter have been undertaken to prepare therapeutic vaccines.

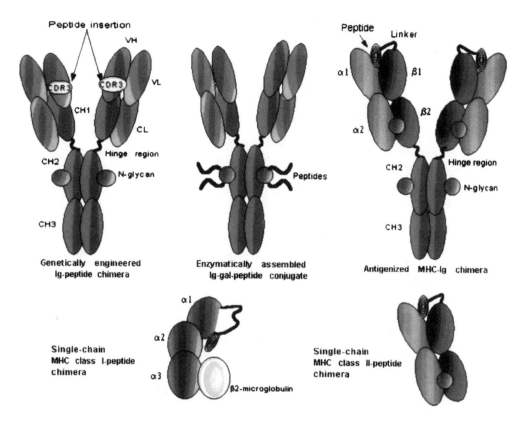

Fig. 7. Structure of self molecules expressing peptides recognized by CD4 or CD8 T-cells.

REFERENCES

1. Revillard JP (ed). Cytokine series. Int Rev Immunol 1998; 17:1–53.
2. Braciale TL, Braciale VL. Antigen presentation: structural theme variation. Immunol Today 1992; 12:124–129.
3. Moody DB, Reinhold BB, Guy MR, et al. Structural requirements for glycolipid recognition by CD1b-restricted T-cells. Science 1997; 278:283–286.
4. Institute of Medicine. Vaccine Supply and Innovation. Washington: National Academy Press, 1985.
5. Enders JF, Weller TH, Robbins FC. Cultivation of the Lansing strain of poliomyelitis virus in culture of various human embryonic tissues. Science 1949; 109:85–87.
6. Jerne NK. Towards a network theory of the immune system. Ann Inst Pasteur Immunol 1974; 125C:373–389.
7. Fields B, Goldbaum FA, Ysern X, Poljak RJ, and Mariuzza RA. Molecular basis of antigen mimicry by an anti-idiotype. Nature 1995; 374:739–742.
8. Bona CA. Idiotype vaccines: forgotten but not gone. Nat Med 1998; 4:668–669.
9. Bona CA. Internal image concept revisited. PSEBM 1996; 213:32–42.
10. Tartaglia J, Percus ME, Taylor J, et al. NYVAC: a highly attenuated strain of vaccinia virus. Virology 1992; 188:217–232.
11. Taylor J, Weinberg W, Kaawaoka Y, Webster R, Paoletti E. (1988) Protective immunity against avian influenza induced by fowlpox recombinant virus. Vaccine 1988; 6:497–503.
12. Moss B. Vaccinia virus vectors. In: Elis RW (ed). Vaccines: New Approaches to Immunological Problems. Boston, Butterworth-Heineman, pp. 345–357.

13. Natuk AR, Davis PK, Chanda MD, et al. Adenovirus vectored vaccines. In: Brown F (ed). Recombinant Vectors in Vaccine Development. Dev Biol Stand 1994; 82:71–78
14. Curtis R, Kelly SM, Tinge SM, et al. Recombinant *Salmonella* vactors in vaccine development. In: Brown F (ed). Recombinant Vectors in Vaccine Development. Dev Biol Stand 1994; 82:23–33
15. Giquel B. Towards new mycobacterial vaccines. In: Brown F. (ed). Recombinant Vectors in Vaccine Development. Dev Biol Stand 1994; 82:171–178.
16. Sirard J-C, Fayolle C, Chastellier C, Mock M, Leclerc C, Berche P. Intracytoplasmic delivery of liseriolysine O by a vaccinal strain of *Bacillus anthracis* induces CD8-mediated protection. J Immunol 1997; 159:4453–4443.
17. Wolff JA, Ludtke JJ, Acsadi G, Williams P, Jani A. Long-time persistence of plasmid DNA and foreign gene expression in mouse cells. Hum Mol Genet 1992; 1:363–369.
18. Chattergoon MA, Robinson TM, Boyer LD, Weiner DB. (1998) Specific immune induction following DNA-based immunization through in vivo transfection and activation of macrophages/antigen presenting cells, J Immunol 1998; 160:5705–5718.
19. Casares S, Inaba K, Brumeanu T-D, Steinaman RM, Bona C. Antigen presentation by dendritic cells after immunization with DNA encoding a major histocompatibility complex class II-restricted viral epitope. J Exp Med 1997; 186:1481–1486.
20. Bona CA, Casares S, Brumeanu T-D. Towards development of T-cell vaccines. Immunol Today 1998; 19:126–133.
21. Isobe H, Moran T, Li S, et al. Presentation by a major histocompatibility class I molecule of nucleoprotein peptide expressed in two different genes of an influenza virus transfectant. J Exp Med 1995; 181:202–213.
22. Hahn CS, Hahn YS, Braciale TJ, Rice CM. Infectious Sindbis virus transient expression vector for studying antigen processing and presentation. Proc Natl Acad Sci USA 1992; 89:2679–2683.
23. Leclerc C (ed). Immunogenicity of foreign epitopes expressed in chimeric molecules. Int Rev Immunol 1994; 11:103–178.
24. Russman H, Shams H, Poblete F, Fu Y, Galan JE, Donis RO. Delivery of epitopes by the *Salmonella* type III secretion systen for vaccine development. Science 1998; 281: 565–567
25. Bona CA, Bot A, Brumeanu T-D Immunogenicity of viral epitopes expressed on genetically and enzymatically engineered immunoglobulins. Chem Immunol 1997; 65:179–206.
26. Casares S, Bot A, Brumeanu T-D, Bona C. Foreign peptides expressed in engineered chimeric molecules. Biotech Gen Eng Rev 1998; 15:159–198.

III
Immunotherapy for HIV Infection

8

Immunopathogenesis of HIV Infection

Lawrence M. Fox

INTRODUCTION

AIDS was recognized in the United States in 1981, when scientists at the Centers for Disease Control and Prevention (CDC) noted a cluster of cases of *Pneumocystis carinii* pneumonia and Kaposi's sarcoma in homosexual men in New York City and Los Angeles. HIV was isolated in 1983 and was demonstrated to be the agent of AIDS in 1984. HIV is a retrovirus of the lentivirus family, which includes the human lymphotropic viruses (human T-cell lymphoma virus [HTLV]-I and II) and HIV-1 and -2. HIV-2 infection is largely confined to West Africa. HIV-1 is responsible for the world AIDS pandemic, which is now the number one cause of death owing to infectious disease in the world. Currently, 34 million people are estimated to be infected with HIV-1, and 14 million have died from AIDS *(1)*.

HIV DISEASE

Etiology

HIV-1 is divided into subtypes or clades. The major clades, group M, are designated A–I; the less common group O has been largely confined to West and Central Africa. Based on maps of genetic diversity between clades and compared with the simian immunodeficiency viruses (SIVs) that are endemic in African monkeys, HIV-1 is believed to have derived from mutation of an SIV, whose original host was probably a chimpanzee *(2)*. HIV-1 is thought to have then infected human groups that lived in close proximity to infected chimpanzees, and possibly kept them as pets or hunted them. Most likely, HIV remained for decades a disease largely confined to rural African villages, until urbanization of Africa eventually permitted worldwide spread.

The disease is spread through contact of infected body fluids, usually blood, semen or breast milk, by the mucous membranes or directly into the recipient's blood or an open wound. The vast majority of cases of HIV-1 infection in the world are the result of heterosexual intercourse. In the United States, the disease was originally largely confined to homosexual men and then spread into intravenous drug users through the sharing of needles. HIV infection is now rapidly increasing among women, both through intravenous drug use and via sexual intercourse with infected men. Pediatric HIV infection usually occurs during labor and delivery from an infected mother but may also occur earlier in gestation or later, as a result of breast feeding.

From: *Immunotherapy for Infectious Diseases*
Edited by: J. M. Jacobson © Humana Press Inc., Totowa, NJ

Scope of the Epidemic

Worldwide, approximately 1 in every 100 adults aged 15–49 years is HIV-1-infected. At least 1.2 million children under the age of 15 years are also infected. In 1998, approximately 16,000 new HIV infections occurred each day, more than 95% in developing countries *(1)*. The greatest risk factor for HIV infection is heterosexual intercourse, which has been responsible for 75% of the infections in the world *(1,3)*. The epidemic is especially concentrated in sub-Saharan Africa, where approximately 80% of the infections have occurred. The disease is increasing most rapidly in South Africa. The epidemic spread along truck routes from West to East Africa and from there to India and the Orient. India has the largest number of HIV-infected people in any one country in the world. The disease has spread through Southeast Asia and into China and Indonesia. In Europe, especially since the end of the Soviet Union, the disease has become particularly concentrated in some of the former Eastern Block nations, where economic collapse has fostered the drug trade and prostitution.

In the United States, up to 900,000 people are currently living with HIV infection and 688,200 cases of AIDS were reported to the CDC as of December, 1998 *(3,4)*. The proportion of new AIDS cases diagnosed in women increased from 7% in 1985, to 23% in 1998. Of the U.S. AIDS cases reported in 1998, 45% were among blacks, 33% among whites, and 20% among Hispanics *(3)*. Heterosexual transmission accounts for an increasing proportion of AIDS cases in the United States. From 1994 to 1997, the estimated proportion of adult U.S. AIDS cases attributed to heterosexual contact grew from 8.5% to 22.1% *(4)*.

Throughout the world, HIV infection is particularly a scourge of the most impoverished and disenfranchised nations and members of society. It has greatly reduced life expectancy in many developing countries, created millions of orphans, reduced the healthy labor force, and placed huge burdens on businesses and health care structures. It is fed by and contributes to social, political, and economic instability. Throughout most of the world, the worst consequences of the HIV epidemic will not be felt for at least another decade.

Typical Disease Course

HIV-1 disease typically follows a course of acute HIV syndrome, which occurs in the weeks immediately after primary infection, and then years of clinical latency, with AIDS usually manifesting 6–10 years later.

Plasma viremia is greatest during the period of acute infection and at end-stage disease, and most transmission probably occurs during the acute and early infection phase. HIV-1 replication occurs primarily in activated CD4+ T-lymphocytes. During acute infection, the CD4+ T-cell count falls from the normal level of about 1000 cells/mL to about half that level, accompanied by wide dissemination of virus and the seeding of lymphoid organs; it then usually rises again to about 75% of baseline as the plasma viremia falls. The virus becomes largely sequestered in lymphoid tissue, with the plasma viral burden reflecting only a small fraction of total body viral burden. A small fraction of the activated CD4+ T-cells that have been infected with HIV revert to an inactive state, continuing to harbor the HIV provirus in their chromosomes. This "latent pool" of HIV infected CD4+ memory T-cells is extremely long lived and can release HIV at any time the cells become reactivated *(5)*.

Viral replication continues within lymphoid tissue during the years of clinical latency *(6)*, and the CD4+ T-cell count gradually falls. As the lymphoid architecture becomes disrupted and the host immune defenses become exhausted, the virus reemerges. The patient experiences constitutional symptoms when the CD4+ T-cell count falls to about 300 cells/mL. Opportunistic infections, wasting disease, and rare cancers occur when the CD4+ T-cell count drops below 200 cells/mL. If this pattern is not reversed by potent antiretroviral therapy, death typically follows within 2 years.

Variant Disease Courses

Although progression from time of HIV infection to end-stage disease typically takes 8–10 years in the absence of potent antiretroviral therapy, there are also cases of either very rapid or slow disease progression. This variation has sometimes been linked to the characteristics of the infecting virus but more often seems to be a function of host immune response. Rapid progressors have sometimes been infected with an overwhelmingly large burden of virus, for instance, in the case of transfusion with heavily contaminated blood products. Other cases of rapid progression have been associated with primary HIV infection with strains that usually only arise late in disease course and that are able to bind to the β-chemokine receptor CXCR4 and induce syncytium formation. Failure to mount a broad enough host immunologic defense is a risk factor for rapid progression *(7)*.

At the other end of the spectrum are those rare individuals who exhibit long-term non-progression, maintaining low levels of plasma viremia and elevated CD4+ T-cell counts in the absence of antiretroviral therapy, despite 10 or more years of infection. In a few cases, this has been associated with infection with a virus strain defective in essential viral genes *(8–10)*. More often, these individuals are found to have competent viruses, but also a more preserved immune response, particularly characterized by retention of HIV-specific T-helper lymphocyte activity. Relative resistance to HIV infection or disease progression has been associated with different HLA groups *(11)* and with expression of mutant cell surface receptors for HIV, particularly the β-chemokine receptors *(12)*. Pediatric HIV infection is also characterized by variation in rate of disease progression, with rapid progression to AIDS occurring about one-third of the time in the absence of potent therapy.

Biology and Life Cycle of the Virus

HIV-1 is icosahedral in structure, with an inner (p18) and outer membrane, a protein core (p24) containing two strands of genomic RNA bound to reverse transcriptase, and glycoprotein spikes extending from the outer membrane. The glycoprotein spikes are the two major viral envelope proteins, gp120 and gp41. Most of the outer envelope consists of host cell-derived proteins, including major histocompatibility complex antigens, acquired as the virus particle buds from the cell. The genome of HIV-1 is similar to that of other retroviruses, with *gag* encoding virion core proteins, *env* encoding envelope glycoproteins, and *pol* encoding the reverse transcriptase and integrase enzymes. In addition, the HIV-1 genome contains the regulatory genes *nef, rev, tat, vif, vpr,* and *vpu*. Regulatory elements are located in the long terminal repeats that flank the other genes.

HIV infection begins with the binding of the gp120 V1 region to the cellular CD4+ molecule, found predominantly on T-helper lymphocytes and monocytes/macrophages. This then results in a conformational change that exposes the gp120 V3 loop. Second receptor binding by the V3 loop is the next key step, which confers infectious tropism depending on the host receptor that the virus is able to utilize. Early in HIV infection, the infecting strains are typically best able to bind to the receptor CCR5 and are macrophage-tropic *(13–17)*. With disease progression, more pathogenic strains arise that are able to bind to CXCR4 *(18)*. These strains are able to replicate in transformed T-cell lines that express CXCR4, but not CCR5, and they induce syncytium formation. Other chemokine receptors have also been identified that HIV strains are able to utilize.

Resistance to HIV infection has been linked to production of high levels of the natural ligands for these receptors, competing for binding with HIV *(19,20)*, and with mutations in the genes coding for the receptors, yielding a poor match for HIV binding *(21–23)*. Following binding by gp120 to both primary and secondary receptors, gp41 binding leads to fusion of viral and host cell membranes, uncoating of the HIV genomic RNA and its associated proteins, and its entry into the cell. HIV reverse transcriptase then makes a double-stranded DNA copy of the viral RNA, which is transported to the nucleus and integrated into the host cell chromosome by the viral integrase enzyme. The relative infidelity of the reverse transcriptase enzyme to the RNA template leads to a high mutation rate. Transcription of the integrated provirus is dependent on host cell activation and DNA-dependent RNA-polymerase activity. Initially, double-spliced viral mRNA is produced, coding for viral proteins. Later, as a result of the action of the HIV *rev* gene product, single-spliced and full-length HIV genomic RNA is produced and transported to the cytoplasm, where it is encapsulated in viral proteins. The virion buds from the host cell membrane and then matures into an infectious virus particle after cleavage of immature viral proteins by HIV protease. Each step of this complex life cycle presents opportunities for intervention with antiviral agents.

PATHOLOGIC MANIFESTATIONS

Host Response

HIV disease is characterized by immune activation, which becomes chronic owing to its failure to clear the infection. This eventually leads to exhaustion of immunologic resistance and vulnerability to opportunistic disease. The unremitting inflammatory immune response also results in tissue damage, contributing to wasting, renal disease, cardiac disease, dementia, and neuropathy. Proinflammatory cytokines have been shown to stimulate HIV replication; therefore this response, which is elicited by HIV antigens, contributes to persistence of infection *(24)*. The viremia during acute HIV infection falls as HIV is sequestered in lymphoid tissue, largely bound to follicular dendritic cells (FDCs), and as cytotoxic lymphocyte (CTL) response to HIV arises. Both infected and uninfected T-lymphocytes are also sequestered in the lymphoid tissues, in response to cytokine signaling and adhesion molecule expression. A significant amount of neutralizing antibody to HIV is usually detectable in the peripheral blood weeks after the plasma viral burden has fallen, suggesting that cell-mediated immunity is the more important initial host immune response *(25)*.

Studies of the breadth of CTL receptor V-β repertoire demonstrated more rapid disease progression when the repertoire was most limited *(26)*. In contrast to the fall in CD4+ T-cell numbers and function, CD8+ T-cells are increased in both number and activation state throughout most of the course of HIV disease. This produces the characteristic reversal of CD4+/CD8+ cell ratio. CD8+ T-cells suppress HIV replication through CTL activity and through noncytolytic suppressor action. Much of the latter activity is thought to be due to production of the β-chemokines that are the natural ligands for the second receptors utilized by HIV during binding to target cells, although additional suppressor factors also seem to be involved *(27)*.

Late in the course of HIV disease, the numbers of circulating CD8+ T-cells fall, heralding much more rapid disease progression. Although clinical manifestations of HIV disease may not occur for a decade after infection, HIV replication in lymphoid tissues continues throughout this time. The high mutation rate of the virus leads to steady escape from immunologic containment, as well as development of resistance to antiretroviral drugs. With progression to AIDS, the architecture of the lymphoid tissue collapses, as both T- and B-cell regions involute and the FDC network is disrupted. HIV previously contained in lymphoid tissue is then released, with a sharp increase in plasma viremia.

In the absence of potent antiretroviral therapy, any condition that causes an inflammatory immune response is likely to induce increased HIV replication in the infected host. This has been observed with a relatively mild stimulus, such as vaccination, as well as with the more potent stimulus of intercurrent illness, such as influenza. As the disease progresses to AIDS, the opportunistic infections that follow may do the added damage of driving HIV expression by the inflammatory response they provoke, in addition to the harm the infection itself causes. Globally, infection with both HIV and tuberculosis continues to be the most difficult public health problem complicating the HIV epidemic *(28)*. HIV disease progresses much more rapidly in persons infected with tuberculosis, who are also at greater risk of harboring multidrug-resistant tuberculosis. Chronic parasitic infections also frequently accompany HIV infection, particularly in Africa. Successful treatment of the parasite disease has been shown to ameliorate the course of the HIV coinfection. Coinfection at the cellular level with herpesviruses and HIV may also directly drive HIV replication, through promotor stimulation.

Immune Dysfunctions in HIV Disease

AIDS is characterized by the progressive loss of reaction to antigenic stimulation and vulnerability to infection. Response is first lost to recall antigen, next to alloantigen, and finally to mitogen. In pediatric AIDS, failure to resist common bacterial infections is frequently seen, whereas in adults, this is less common, reflecting the adult's more mature humoral immunity. In both populations, loss of resistance to intracellular parasites, viruses, protozoa, fungi, and mycobacteria demonstrates impaired cell-mediated immunity. Polyclonal B-cell activation contributes to inappropriate antibody production, autoimmune disease, and B-cell lymphomas.

The primary target for HIV infection is the activated CD4+ T-cell. The central role of this cell type in coordinating both the humoral and cell-mediated immune response means that physical or functional loss of these cells leads to a broad array of immune dysfunctions. B-cells that encounter a matching antigen engulf it, digest it, and display antigen fragments on their surface in complex with MHC molecules. A mature CD4+ T-cell with a matching receptor for the antigen and MHC display must next supply lymphokines to allow the B-cell to multiply and mature into antibody-producing plasma cells. Failure of this T-helper cell function leads to loss of humoral response to the antigen against which the T-cell was primed. Similarly, cell-mediated immunity depends on antigen display by an antigen-presenting cell (APC) such as a B-cell, macrophage, or circulating dendritic cell, encounter with a matching receptor on a mobilized T-cell, stimulation of the T-cell by second receptor binding and lymphokines from the APC, and appropriate activation of the T-cell. The activated cell then secretes lymphokines that may attract immune cells (including macrophages, granulocytes, and other lymphocytes), stimulate the growth of T-cells, and induce killer cell activity. Defects in any of these steps leads to failure of all the subsequent responses.

Both the number and function of CD4+ T-cells is compromised by HIV infection. Many factors seem to contribute to the fall in CD4+ T-cell number, including lysis by HIV itself, lysis by HIV-specific CTL, syncytia formation, apoptosis, and reduced rate of T-cell synthesis *(29)*. Sequestration in lymphoid tissue also reduces the number of CD4+ T-cells in the peripheral blood. The rate of CD4+ T-cell infection is inadequate to account for most of the cell loss, particularly early in HIV disease. Apoptosis seems to contribute significantly to this cell loss, which affects uninfected as well as infected cells. Many auxiliary HIV proteins, such as Nef, Tat, and Vpr, which have regulatory functions in HIV maturation, also appear to contribute to this immune dysfunction *(30)*. Linking of gp120, which is shed by HIV, with CD4 can program cells for apoptosis upon receipt of a second stimulatory signal delivered via the T-cell receptor. Thus cells exposed to soluble HIV proteins, but uninfected by HIV, may undergo apoptosis. This may lead to deletion of clones of memory cells at the moment they are activated by the antigen to which they are programmed to respond.

It is not surprising, then, in the constant presence of HIV antigen, that HIV-specific CD4+ T-helper cells are rapidly depleted *(31)*. The same mechanism may underlie the loss of response to recall antigens, with accompanying vulnerability to other infectious agents. Binding of HIV-induced proinflammatory cytokines with the apoptosis-inducing CD95 or tumor necrosis factor receptor 1 (TNFR-1) receptors may also contribute to cell death. The rate of synthesis of T-cells has been shown to be reduced by HIV infection and to increase when HIV replication is suppressed by antiviral drugs *(32)*. The reason for this inhibition of T-cell synthesis is unclear, but it may involve more than one mechanism. The maturation of thymus-derived naive T-cells is probably inhibited by effects of HIV on both thymic epithelial cells and immature thymic precursor cells *(33)*. The extrathymic expansion of T-cells is inhibited by the disruption of cytokine signaling, in particular by the reduced expression of interleukin-2 (IL-2) and the IL-2 receptor *(34)*.

The failure of CD4+ T-cell function seems to be due to disruption of the normal cellular and intercellular signaling mechanisms. CD4+ T-cell anergy can result from inappropriate signaling after gp120 binding to CD4. Stimulation by superantigen binding nonspecifically to the T-cell receptor may cause the massive overexpansion of T-cell subsets and may also cause deletion of these subsets if they are already primed for apoptosis *(35)*. APC interaction with T-cells may fail, if the proper cytokine signal does not accompany antigen presentation. HIV-infected monocytes/macrophages express decreased MHC class II, CD80/86 costimulatory molecule, and IL-12 and increased IL-10, Fas (CD-95), and Fas ligand (CD-95L). Interaction of such APCs with CD4+ T-cells predisposes to T-cell death, either through apoptosis or HIV infection

(36). In the absence of appropriate APC signaling, CD4+ T-helper function will not be induced, leading to poor development of HIV-specific CD8+ T-cell CTLs and noncytolytic suppressor activity.

In addition to defective APC activity, HIV-infected monocytes/macrophages are also impaired in migration, phagocytosis, oxidative burst, and tumor surveillance. This contributes to the vulnerability to opportunistic infections and cancer seen in AIDS. These cells also seem to play a key role in HIV spread across tissue barriers, especially during primary infection and in infection of the central nervous system. Microglial cells in central nervous system are of monocytic lineage and can be infected by HIV. Expression of proinflammatory cytokines by HIV-infected microglia, as well as from invading macrophages, seems to contribute to neurotoxicity.

In summary, the failure of the immune system to clear HIV, although it may successfully contain the infection for many years, coupled with the central importance of the primary target cells in regulating the immune response, leads to chronic immune activation and immune dysregulation. Initially, the lesions in the immune repertoire are those directed at HIV itself, especially the loss of HIV-specific CD4+ T-helper cell function. Chronic immune activation and apoptosis eventually lead to loss of cell-mediated immunity directed against ubiquitous opportunistic agents. The chronic inflammation causes bystander damage, leading to complications such as dementia and wasting. Successful therapy with antiviral drugs leads to rapid clearance of HIV from the peripheral blood and from most tissue sites. This is followed by reduced immune activation and partial restoration of immune function *(37)*. Although resistance to many opportunistic infections are frequently restored by successful potent antiretroviral therapy, resistance to HIV itself remains an illusive goal.

THERAPY

Range of Possible Therapeutic Modalities

As will be discussed in detail in the chapters that follow, a variety of strategies are being explored in attempts to halt and reverse the immune dysfunction caused by HIV disease. Foremost has been the use of antiviral agents to suppress HIV replication and the use of antibiotic prophylaxis to prevent the emergence of opportunistic infections. With the recent advent of potent antiretroviral therapy, the ability of the immune system to recover spontaneously has been demonstrated, and the limits of this recovery have also been seen *(38–40)*. Other strategies being tested involve modulation of the immune response, to reduce the excessive activation. Supplementation of cytokines depressed by HIV disease, to restore the number and function of T-cells and monocytic cells, may yield improved resistance to opportunistic disease, and conceivably to HIV itself. Therapeutic vaccines and strategies of treatment interruption to deliberately permit reexposure of the immune system to HIV antigen, in an effort to boost host immune response to HIV, are being tried. Attempts are being made to reduce the size of the pool of cells latently infected with HIV, or to make it more difficult for these cells to become activated and to express HIV. Gene-based therapies are being developed to confer resistance to HIV infection at the cellular level. As these and other therapeutic interventions are developed, they present great challenges in clinical trial design.

Challenges of Therapeutic Trial Design

The limitations of the available animal models of HIV infection have forced researchers to go to human trials with more limited data than we would prefer to have. Only chimpanzees can be infected with HIV, and the development of immunodeficiency following their infection is as slow as in human disease, if in fact it occurs at all. They are therefore used primarily in testing vaccines, since the prevention of infection can be measured, but the impact of a therapy on disease course cannot. Their use is further complicated by the fact that they are an intelligent, endangered species, whose use as a laboratory animal is tightly restricted and very expensive. The macaque model is the next best choice.

Strains of simian immunodeficiency virus (SIV) have been developed that produce a predictable range of immunodeficiency disease course, from months to years. Recently, the simian/human immunodeficiency virus, engineered to express antigens of both SIV and HIV (SHIV), has been used in the macaque model to test vaccines. Unfortunately, there are sufficient differences between some of the SIV and HIV proteins that are the targets of antiviral drugs to make it impossible to use the potent antiretroviral cocktails that have been developed against HIV in the macaque model. The expense of caring for macaques restricts the size of experiments using this model.

There are no good small animal models for HIV. The use of genetically immunodeficient mice, in which human tissues have been implanted (the SCID-hu mouse model) has limited application and is very labor intensive. The feline immunodeficiency (FIV) model is likewise too far removed from HIV for much data to be gleaned about therapy. Human clinical trials are therefore the setting in which therapeutic interventions for HIV disease are generally first tested.

Clinical trials of therapies to reverse or prevent the immunopathology of HIV disease must be carefully designed to account for practical and ethical considerations. Once trials have grown beyond the pilot stage, in which interventions in small numbers of subjects yield data that help to guide the planning of larger trials, sufficient numbers of participants must be enrolled so that the outcome can be reliably attributed to something other than chance.

The choice of end points is critically important to make sure that meaningful results are eventually obtained. In the past, disease progression and survival were the outcomes most frequently used to judge effectiveness of therapeutic interventions for HIV disease. However, the slow rate of progression of the disease required very large trials with long-term follow-up before sufficient numbers of events could display a significant difference between arms in a protocol. The correlation of fall in CD4+ T-cell count with disease progression led to that measure being viewed as the first surrogate marker in therapeutic trials. With the development of reliable techniques for quantitatively measuring HIV in the peripheral blood, and the demonstration of the correlation between viral load and risk of disease progression, HIV plasma viral load has become accepted as a partial surrogate for clinical progression. However, CD4+ T-cell count and HIV plasma viral load taken together still do not account for the full risk of disease progression. Markers of immune activation, especially CD8+ CD38+ phenotype, seem to be at least as powerful predictors *(41)*.

With the development of immune-based therapies given with a background of potent antiviral therapy, and the ensuing rate of disease progression being as low as 1% per year or less, surrogate marker end points are essential. At the same time, although interventions that may result in change in viral load can be tested against that measure, it is quite conceivable that an intervention could confer significant immunologic benefit with little impact on viral load. Interventions that reverse immune dysregulation, increase CD4+ T-cell levels, modulate excessive immune activation, or decrease apoptosis all might fall into this category. Validation of appropriate surrogate markers for immune-based therapies is the next hurdle in the advancement of this field.

The choice of the population in which to test interventions is also an important consideration in clinical trial design. Patients with advanced disease, who have failed potent antiretroviral therapy, are eager to find alternate therapies, and their outcome might be relatively quickly learned. Unfortunately, many of the interventions being tried are the least effective and most toxic in subjects with advanced disease. Populations with a more intact immune response are therefore currently favored for trials of immune-based therapies. At the same time, if surrogate markers are being relied on for end points, there must be something to measure in the population chosen. For example, if change in viral load is chosen, then either the subjects must not have their viral load suppressed below the level of detection to begin with, or must have a likelihood of sufficient numbers of participants to experience viral breakthrough to be able to measure benefit from the intervention. An alternate model being explored is to withdraw therapy at some time and measure the rate or the magnitude of viral load resurgence as an end point. The possible risks to participants of this study design are being carefully examined.

Further complicating the design of clinical trials is the rapid evolution of the standard of care of HIV disease. In trials that may take years to develop, enroll, and then follow to end points, care must be devoted to considering incorporation of the use of new antiviral drugs, new measures of efficacy of therapy, and new techniques for determining suitable antiviral regimens. (Examples are the routine use of potent antiretroviral cocktails, plasma viral load for assessing efficacy of therapy, and screening for antiviral resistance.) Otherwise, the outcome of the trial may not be relevant in the context of the current standard of care at the trial's conclusion.

Ethical considerations are extremely important in clinical trial design. Consideration must be given not only to the risk to the individual participant but also to the benefit to the community from which participants are recruited. In the United States, for instance, consideration must be given to including women and minorities in the participants in clinical trials and to not unnecessarily barring participation by pregnant women. The greatest challenge is in designing trials suitable for developing countries. The data gathered from such trials must be relevant to the population of that country and the prospect must exist for the therapy being tested to be available there if found to be effective. An exquisite tension exists between the dire need for therapies in developing nations and the barriers of cost that may be insurmountable. The unavailability of potent antiretroviral therapy in developing nations and the rapid rate of HIV disease progression still seen there makes this setting suitable for therapeutic trials with clinical end points. However, the lack of therapeutic options outside the clinical trials mechanism makes this group especially vulnerable to exploitation, and careful ethical review of clinical trials planned for developing nations is extremely important.

REFERENCES

1. UNAIDS. Report on the Global HIV/AIDS Epidemic, December, 1998. UNAIDS, 1998.
2. Gao F, Baile E, Robertson DL, et al. Origin of HIV-1 in the chimpanzee *Pan troglodytes*. Nature 1999; 397:436–441.
3. Quinn T. Global burden of the HIV pandemic. Lancet 1996; 348:99–106.
4. Centers for Disease Control and Prevention, unpublished data.
5. Perelson AS, Neumann AU, Markowitz M, et al. HIV dynamics in vivo: virion clearance rate, infected cell life-span, and viral generation time. Science 1996; 271:1582–1586.
6. Panteleo G, Fauci AS. New concepts in the immunopathogenesis of HIV infection. Annu Rev Microbiol 1996; 50:825–845.
7. Panteleo G, Demarest JF, Schacker T, et al. The quantitative nature of the primary immune response is a prognosticator of disease progression independent of the initial level of plasma viremia. Proc Natl Acad Sci USA 1997; 94:254–258.
8. Kirchoff F, Greenough TC, Brettler DB, et al. Brief report of the absence of intact *nef* sequences in a long-term noprogressing survivor of HIV-1 infection. N Engl J Med 1995; 332:228–232.
9. Deacon NJ, Tsykin A, Slomon A, et al. Genomic structure of an attenuated quasi species of HIV-1 from a blood transfusion donor and recipients. Science 1995; 270:988–991.
10. Salvi R, Garbuglia AR, Di Caro A, et al. Grossly defective *nef* gene sequences in a human immunodeficiency virus type-1-seropositive long-term nonprogressor. J Virol 1998; 72:3646–3657.
11. Houria H, Caillat-Zucman S, Lebuanec H, et al. New class I and II HLA alleles strongly associated with opposite patterns of progression to AIDS. J Immunol 1999; 162:6942–6946.
12. D'Souza MP, Harden VA. Chemokines and HIV second receptors. Confluence of two fields generates optimism in AIDS research. Nat Med 1996; 2:1293–1300.
13. Dragic T, Litwin V, Allaway GP, et al. HIV-1 entry inot CD4+ cells is mediated by the chemokine receptor CC-CKR-5. Nature 1996; 381:667–673.
14. Doranz BJ, Rucker J, Yi Y, et al. A dual-tropic primary HIV-1 isolate that uses fusin and the beta-chemokine receptors CKR-5. CKR-3, CKR-2b as fusion co-factors. Cell 1996; 85:1149–1158.
15. Choe H, Farzan M, Sun Y, et al. The beta-chemokine receptors CCR3 and CCR5 facilitate infection by primary HIV-1 isolates. Cell 1996; 85:1135–1148.
16. Alkhatib G, Combardiere C, Broder CC, et al. CC CKR5: a RANTES, MIP1alpha, MIP-1beta receptor as a fusion cofactor for macrophage-tropic HIV-1. Science 1996; 272:1955–1958.
17. Deng H, Liu R, Ellmeier W, et al. Identification of a major co-receptor for primary isolates of HIV-1. Nature 1996; 381:661–666.
18. Feng Y, Broder CC, Kennedy PE, Berger EA. HIV-1 entry cofactor: functional cDNA cloning of a seven-transmembrane, G protein-coupled receptor. Science 1996; 272:872–877.
19. Bleul CC, Farzan M, Choe H, et al. The lymphocyte chomeattractant SDF-1 is a ligand for LESTR/fusin and blocks HIV-1 entry. Nature 1996; 382:829–833.
20. Oberlin E, Amara A, Bachelerie F, et al. The CXC chemokine SDF-1 is the ligand for LESTR/fusin and prevents infection by T cell line-adapted HIV-1. Nature 1996; 382:833–835.
21. Liu R, Paxto WA, Choe S, et al. Homozygous defect in HIV-1 coreceptor accounts for resistance of some multiply-exposed individuals to HIV-1 infection. Cell 1996; 86:367–377.
22. Samson M, Libert F, Doranz BJ, et al. Resistance to HIV-1 infection in Caucasian individuals bearing mutant alleles of the CCR-5 chemokine receptor gene. Nature 1996; 382:722–725.
23. Dean M, Carrington M, Winkler C, et al. Genetic restriction of HIV-1 infection and progression to AIDS by a deletion allele of the CKR5 structural gene. Hemophilia Growth and

Development Study, Multicenter AIDS Cohort Study, Multicenter Hemophilia Cohort Study, San Francisco City Cohort, ALIVE Study. Science 1996; 273:1856–1862.

24. Fauci AS. Multifactorial nature of human immunodeficiency virus disease: implications for therapy. Science 1993; 262:1011–1018.

25. Moore JP, Cao Y, Ho DD, Koup RA. Development of the anti-gp120 antibody response during seroconversion to human immunodeficiency virus type 1. J Virol 1994; 68:5142–5155.

26. Panteleo G, Demarest JF, Soudeys H, et al. Major expansion of CD8 T cells with a predominant V beta usage during the primary immune response to HIV. Nature 1994; 370:463–467.

27. Mackewicz CE, Yang LC, Lifson JD, Levy JA. Non-cytolytic CD8 T-cell anti-HIV responses in primary HIV-1 infection. Lancet 1994; 344:1671–1673.

28. Dye C, Scheele S, Dolin P, et al. Global burden of tuberculosis: estimated incidence, prevalence, and mortality by country. JAMA 1999; 282:677–686.

29. Pantaleo G, Fauci AS. New concepts in the immunopathogenesis of HIV infection. Annu Rev Immunol 1995; 13:487–512.

30. Cullen BR. HIV-1 auxilliary proteins: making connections in a dying cell. Cell 1998; 93:685–692.

31. Rosenberg ES, Walker BD. Characterization of HIV-1 specific T helper cells in acute and chronic infection. Immunol Lett 1999; 66:89–93.

32. Hellerstein M, Hanley MB, Ktzin BL, et al. Directly measured kinetics of circulating T lymphocytes in normal and HIV-1 infected humans. Nat Ned 1999; 5:83–89.

33. Douek DC, McFarland RD, Keisre PH, et al. Changes in thymic function with age and during the treatment of HIV infection. Nature 1998; 396:690–695.

34. Fan J, Bass HZ, Fahey JL. Elevated IFN-gamma and decreased IL-2 gene expression are associated with HIV infection. J Immunol 1993; 151:5031–5040.

35. Laurence J, Hodtsev A, Posnett DN. Suprantigen implicated in dependence of HIV-1 replication in T cells on TCR V beta expression. Nature 1992; 58:255–259.

36. Shearer GM. HIV-Induced Immunopathogenesis (review). Immunity 1998; 9:587–593.

37. Andersson J, Fehniger TE, Patterson BK, et al. Early reduction of immune activation in lymphoid tissue following highly active HIV therapy. AIDS 1998; 12:F123–F129.

38. Li TS, Tubiana R, Katlama C, et al. Long-lasting recovery in CD4 T-cell function and viral-load reduction after highly active antiretroviral therapy in advanced HIV disease. Lancet 1998; 351:1682–1686.

39. Lederman MM, Conick E, Landay A, et al. Immunologic reponses associated with 12 weeks of antiretroviral therapy consisting of zidovudine, lamivudine, and ritonavir: results of AIDS clinical trials group protocol 315. J Infect Dis 1998; 178:70–79.

40. Connick E, Lederman MM, Kotzin BL, et al. Immune reconstitution in the first year of potent antiretroviral therapy and its relationship to virologic resonse. J Infect Dis 2000; 181:358–363.

41. Giorgi JV, Liu Z, Huitlin LE, et al. Elevated levels of CD38+CD8+ T cells in HIV infection add to the prognostic value of low CD4+ T cell levels: results of 6 years of follow-up. J Acquir Imm Defic Syndr 1993; 6:904–912.

9

Immune Reconstitution
with Antiretroviral Chemotherapy

Elizabeth Connick

INTRODUCTION

Infection with HIV-1 results in the progressive loss of CD4+ T-lymphocytes and a variety of immune functions, leading ultimately to premature death in most untreated individuals. The introduction of potent combination antiretroviral chemotherapy for HIV-1 infection in the mid-1990s resulted in unprecedented decreases in HIV-1 replication and increases in CD4+ T-cell counts in many treated individuals. Simultaneous to the introduction of potent combination antiviral drug therapy, substantial declines in morbidity and mortality from HIV-1-associated illnesses have been observed. The study of immune reconstitution in the context of viral suppression has already provided some important insights into the immune pathogenesis of HIV-1. Many questions remain, however, concerning the extent and clinical significance of the immune reconstitution that occurs in the setting of antiretroviral drug therapy.

IMPACT OF ANTIRETROVIRAL CHEMOTHERAPY
ON HIV-1-RELATED MORBIDITY AND MORTALITY

Before the introduction of potent antiretroviral therapy for HIV-1 infection, the standard of care for treatment consisted of monotherapy and dual therapy with HIV-1 nucleoside analog reverse transcriptase inhibitors. These therapies were shown to produce modest increases in CD4+ T-cell counts and some improvements in survival (1–4). With the introduction of protease inhibitors in the mid-1990s and their use in combination with other antiviral drugs, much more profound and sustained viral suppression and larger increases in CD4+ T-cell counts were observed than ever before.

The first widely used potent combination antiretroviral therapies for HIV-1 infection consisted of an HIV-1 protease inhibitor and two nucleoside analog reverse transcriptase inhibitors (5–7). After 6 months of therapy with the HIV-1 protease inhibitor indinavir and two reverse transcriptase inhibitors, the plasma HIV-1 RNA copy number was diminished by a median of over 2 $\log_{10}$ in subjects treated with potent antiretroviral therapy compared with less than 1 $\log_{10}$ in subjects receiving only two nucleoside analog reverse transcriptase inhibitors (6,7). Increases in CD4+ T-lymphocyte

From: *Immunotherapy for Infectious Diseases*
Edited by: J. M. Jacobson © Humana Press Inc., Totowa, NJ

counts ranged from 73 to 86 cells/mm^3 in the combination therapy groups after 6 months of therapy, almost double that of the subjects receiving only two nucleoside analog drugs. Over the past 4 years, a variety of combinations of antiviral drugs have been shown to be equally if not more potent in suppressing HIV-1 replication and inducing increases in CD4+ T-cell counts (8–12). These various combinations of potent antiviral medications, frequently referred to as highly active antiretroviral therapy (HAART), have become the standard of care for HIV-1 infection (13).

Commensurate with the introduction of HAART, there has been a dramatic decline in mortality and morbidity from HIV-1 infection in the United States and other industrialized countries. In the United States, AIDS-related deaths in adults declined from a peak of 50,610 in 1995 to 16,273 in 1999 (14). The Adult/Adolescent Spectrum of HIV Disease (ASD) sentinel surveillance project, which prospectively reviews medical records of HIV-1-infected individuals in 11 U.S. cities, reported a significant decline in the incidence of 15 of the 26 AIDS-defining illnesses between 1992 and 1997 (15). A study of 1255 subjects in eight different U.S. cities with a history of at least one CD4+ T-cell count under 100 cells/mm^3 found significant declines in the incidence of *Pneumocystis carinii* pneumonia (PCP), *Mycobacterium avium* complex (MAC), and cytomegalovirus (CMV) retinitis between 1994 and 1997 (Fig. 1) (16).

These declines in opportunistic infections (OIs) cannot be explained by increases in prophylactic measures to prevent them (15,16). Similar declines in the incidence of OIs have been reported by other studies in the United States as well as Europe and Australia (17–24). Randomized trials of potent combination antiretroviral therapy compared with less potent regimens have demonstrated that it is the superior control of HIV-1 replication and the increase in CD4+ T-lymphocyte counts induced by potent regimens that are associated with the reduced incidence of OIs (6,25,26).

Further evidence to suggest that HAART results in immune reconstitution comes from numerous case reports of the resolution of OIs after initiation of therapy. Progressive multifocal leukoencephalopathy (PML) (27–33) diarrhea owing to cryptosporidia and microsporidia (34,35), treatment-refractory oral candidiasis (36,37), molluscum contagiosum (38,39), and Kaposi's sarcoma (40–42) have been reported to regress after the initiation of potent combination antiretroviral therapy. Individuals with a history of CMV retinitis, which in the absence of CMV-specific therapy usually progresses within a few weeks, have had primary anti-CMV therapy withdrawn without disease recurrence after receiving HAART (43–45). Similarly, disseminated MAC infection, which previously required lifelong therapy for containment, has failed to recur in several individuals despite cessation of primary therapy after a good response to HAART (46). Primary prophylaxis for both PCP (47–51) and MAC (52–54) have been safely withdrawn in subjects previously at risk after they had achieved sustained increases in CD4+ T-cell counts on HAART. These data suggest that the decrease in OIs seen with potent antiretroviral therapy is owing not only to a halt in the progression of HIV-1-induced immune deficiency but also to reconstituted immunity, which allows individuals to contain infections immunologically that they were unable to control previously. As a result of these data, guidelines regarding prophylaxis of OIs have been modified to allow for the discontinuation of primary PCP and MAC prophylaxis in individuals with sustained elevations in CD4+ T-cell counts above threshold levels in the setting of HAART (55).

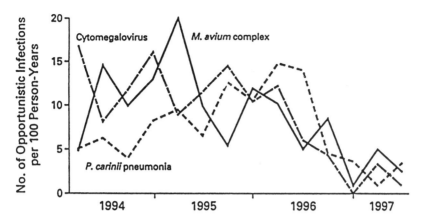

Fig. 1. Rates of cytomegalovirus infection, *Pneumocystis carinii* pneumonia, and *Mycobacterium avium* complex disease among 1255 HIV-infected patients in eight U.S. cities with fewer than 100 CD4+ T-cells/mm^3 on at least one occasion, according to calendar quarter, from January 1994 through June 1997. (From ref. *16.*)

The immune reconstitution associated with HAART may be deleterious to the host in some instances. Several distinct immune inflammatory syndromes have been reported in the setting of initiation of HAART. These syndromes, which consist of severe and sometimes unusual clinical manifestations of OIs shortly after the introduction of HAART, are believed to be caused by reconstitution of immunity to preexisting, but clinically occult OIs. Severe CMV retinitis, including the unusual presentation of vitritis associated with retinitis, has been reported in patients recently initiated on HAART *(56–58).* PML *(59,60),* including one atypical case in which contrast-enhancing lesions developed 2 months after presentation, has been observed to develop shortly after initiation of HAART as well. Focal lymphadenitis, as well as other unusual clinical manifestations of MAC, other atypical mycobacteria, and *Mycobacterium tuberculosis* (MTB) *(61–63),* have been reported in individuals who had recently started HAART. Similar immunopathology has been suggested as the cause for elevations in liver function tests in patients with chronic hepatitis B or C infection following initiation of HAART *(64,65).* An association has been described between initiation of HAART and serious and sometimes fatal cases of Castleman's disease, which is believed to be caused by human herpesvirus-8 (HHV-8) infection *(66).* In general, with the continuation of potent antiretroviral therapy and, in some instances, treatment with steroids, these immune inflammatory syndromes have resolved.

Although many lines of evidence suggest that substantial immune reconstitution occurs in individuals treated with HAART, clinical data suggest that this immune reconstitution is not necessarily uniform or complete in every treated individual. Despite evidence that prophylaxis against CMV and PCP can be safely discontinued when CD4+ T-cell counts rise above the traditional threshold values for prophylaxis, several studies have reported the presentation of these and other OIs at higher CD4+ T-cell counts than was usually seen in the past *(23,67).* The CD4+ T-cell nadir has been shown to be a significant risk factor for AIDS-defining illnesses or death even after CD4+ T-cell increases on HAART have occurred *(68,69).* A few case reports, such as recurrent CMV retinitis in an individual treated with HAART for over 1 year and with a CD4+ T-cell count over 400 cells/mm^3 *(70)*, suggest that some individuals may have persistent immunologic lacunae despite sustained increases in CD4+ T-cell numbers.

Further evidence that immune reconstitution in the setting of HAART may not be complete comes from the observation that not all HIV-1-associated illnesses have been found to decline. HIV-1-associated malignancies in particular have had quite variable responses to HAART. Declines in the incidence of Kaposi's sarcoma *(71–74)*, as well as primary brain lymphoma *(71)*, have been reported since the introduction of HAART. However, the incidence of other HIV-1-associated malignancies, including immunoblastic lymphoma, invasive cervical cancer, Hodgkin's lymphoma, and Burkitt's lymphoma, have not declined or have declined more slowly than Kaposi's sarcoma over the same time interval *(71,73–75)*. It may be that it takes longer for HAART to reverse the oncogenic diathesis induced by HIV-1 infection than the susceptibility to OIs. Alternatively, or in addition, there may be a persistent oncogenic risk induced by HIV-1 infection that cannot be eliminated by the immune restoration induced by HAART. Studies examining the clinical outcomes of individuals treated with HAART over the long term are needed to assess the immune reconstitution induced by HAART more fully.

NUMERICAL CHANGES
IN CD4+ T-LYMPHOCYTES IN THE SETTING OF HAART

Progressive loss of CD4+ T-cells is the hallmark of HIV-1 infection. During the course of untreated disease, CD4+ T-cell counts drop from normal values, which are usually over 800 cells/mm^3, to less than 200 CD4+ T-cells/mm^3, which in and of itself constitutes a diagnosis of AIDS. Historically, CD4+ T-cell counts have been used to guide clinical decisions as to when to start antiretroviral therapy or prophylaxis for OIs because they are highly predictive of the risk of OIs and death *(76)*. An average increase of 150 CD4+ T-cells/mm^3 in the first year of therapy has been seen in individuals with moderately advanced disease *(5–7,77)*. The magnitude of CD4+ T-cell increases in the first year of therapy has been shown to be directly correlated with the magnitude of virus suppression *(5–7,77,78)*.

Peripheral blood CD4+ T-cell increases in the first year of potent antiretroviral therapy have been described as biphasic *(77–84)*, although there is substantial variability in CD4+ T-cell changes among treated individuals *(85)*. The first phase increase, which occurs over the first 8–12 weeks of therapy, is usually more precipitous than the second and consists primarily of CD4+ T-cells with a memory phenotype. The second phase increase, which occurs after the first 8–12 weeks of therapy, is usually less rapid and consists primarily of CD4+ T-cells with a naive phenotype. The magnitude of the two different phases of CD4+ T-cell increases is highly variable and appears to be related to a number of factors. Both phases are inversely correlated with the magnitude of viral suppression *(71,86–88)* and the rate of CD4+ T-cell decline prior to initiation of therapy *(86)*. Thus, subjects with higher plasma virus concentrations or more rapid loss of CD4+ T-cells experience greater CD4+ T-lymphocyte increases than others on HAART. The first phase increase is positively correlated with the baseline CD4+ T-cell count *(86,88)* and inversely correlated with the age of the host *(86)*. The second phase increase has been found to correlate with age in some *(89)*, but not all, studies *(71,86)*.

Significant controversy exists over the origins of the increases in CD4+ T-cell counts that occur in the setting of HAART. Multiple mechanisms for reconstitution of peripheral blood CD4+ T-cell numbers have been proposed, including preservation of cells from HIV-1 infection and death, diminished activation-induced death of uninfected cells, increased thymic output, peripheral expansion of preexisting cells, and redistribution of CD4+ T-cells to the periphery from lymphoid tissues. When the remarkable peripheral blood first phase increases induced by protease inhibitor therapies were initially observed, it was assumed that they reflected preservation of CD4+ T-cells that previously would have been infected by HIV-1 and destroyed either by viral lysis or immune clearance *(90–92)*. However, studies of lymphoid tissues, which contain more than 95% of the body's T-lymphocytes, as well as the vast majority of HIV-1 replication, revealed that 10-fold fewer lymphoid cells were productively infected than would have been predicted by this model *(93)*. Although HAART was demonstrated to result in significant declines in measures of immune activation *(82,83,87,94,95)* and apoptosis *(96)* in both lymphoid tissues and peripheral blood, the fact that the peripheral blood first-phase increases were not observed in lymphoid tissues *(97)* argued against this mechanism as the major source of peripheral blood CD4+ T-cell reconstitution. Studies of peripheral blood CD4+ T-cell turnover during the first 12 weeks of HAART (using a novel method of measuring lymphocyte half-life through incorporation of deuterated glucose) indicated that T-cell half-life is reduced, not increased by HAART *(98)*, arguing against either diminished apoptosis or decreased viral infection and death as the major causes of increased CD4+ T-cell counts.

The observation that levels of expression of lymphocyte adhesion molecules in lymphoid tissues of untreated HIV-1-infected individuals were high, and diminished substantially in the setting of HAART, led to the interpretation that most of the first-phase increase may be caused by redistribution of cells from the lymphoid tissues to the peripheral blood, rather than a true increase in total body CD4+ T-cells *(95)*. The fact that the T-cell receptor (TCR) repertoire after the first phase resembles that of the pretreatment repertoire, which is often aberrant *(87,99–101)*, further supports this interpretation. In addition, the observation that CD8+ lymphocytes as well as B-lymphocytes also increase during the first 12 weeks of HAART *(77–83)* suggests that other lymphocyte populations may be redistributed from lymphoid tissues during the first 12 weeks of HAART as well. Thus, although there is not complete consensus, multiple lines of evidence suggest that the major source of the first-phase increases in peripheral blood CD4+ T-cells is redistribution of these cells from lymphoid tissues.

The origins of the second-phase increase in peripheral blood CD4+ T-cell counts are also unclear, but most likely these increases do not represent redistribution from lymphoid tissues. The second-phase increase, which primarily consists of cells with a naive phenotype, is similar in tempo to what has been observed in cancer patients treated with chemotherapy *(102)*. Phenotypically naive cells are not necessarily newly synthesized, as reversion of cells from a memory to a naive phenotype has been reported *(103,104)*. Studies of lymphoid tissues, however, have demonstrated CD4+ T-cell increases during the second phase, suggesting that these represent true increases in total body CD4+ T-cells *(97)*. The TCR repertoires of the second phase increases have been less extensively studied, but several studies suggest that they may be trending toward a more normal repertoire than that prior to HAART *(100,101)*, further bolstering the theory that HAART results in new CD4+ T-cell synthesis.

A novel method of identifying thymically derived cells using TCR excision circles (TRECs) that are a byproduct of TCR rearrangement in the thymus as a marker, has demonstrated increases in TRECs in the naive pool of peripheral blood cells in HIV-1-infected individuals following initiation of HAART *(105),* suggesting that new CD4+ T-cells are being generated by the thymus. The number of phenotypically naive cells in HAART-treated individuals has been correlated with the abundance of thymic tissue determined by computed tomography scan, further suggesting that the thymus may be an important source of newly synthesized cells in patients on HAART *(106).* However, it has been argued that the increase in TREC-containing cells observed in the setting of HAART may be the result of diminished proliferation in the naive CD4+ T-cell pool and not necessarily because of synthesis of naive cells in the thymus *(107).* Thus, the origin of the second-phase increases in CD4+ T-cells, whether from thymically or peripherally derived T-cells, remains unclear.

Increasing evidence suggests that there may be a third (or plateau) phase, when CD4+ T-cell reconstitution stops. Although some treated individuals achieve and maintain normal CD4+ T-cell counts, many others, particularly those with moderately advanced HIV-1 infection, do not fully reconstitute their CD4+ T-cells to normal numbers *(108,109).* The determinants of the long-term ability to reconstitute CD4+ T-cell numbers have not been defined. Whether this could represent an HIV-1-induced defect in the generation of CD34+ bone marrow precursors or in thymic regeneration is unclear. The clinical consequences of incomplete CD4+ T-cell regeneration are also unknown. The failure to reconstitute any CD4+ T-cells has been shown to be associated with a worse outcome among individuals with moderately advanced HIV-1 infection *(110),* but it is unknown what the implications of partial CD4+ T-cell reconstitution are.

IMPACT OF HAART ON RECONSTITUTION OF IMMUNE RESPONSES

Prior to the inception of HAART, an individual's immune status and clinical prognosis was inferred from the CD4+ T-cell count, which provided the basis for recommendations for prophylaxis against OIs. This was based not only on clinical observations, but on laboratory data demonstrating that CD4+ T-cell declines paralleled the loss of a variety of immune functional responses *(111,112).* An important clinical question since the advent of HAART is whether the CD4+ T-cell count remains an accurate indicator of immune function and consequently clinical prognosis.

The sequential loss of T-lymphocyte proliferative responses to antigens, alloantigens, and mitogens in HIV-1 infection is well described and has been found to be prognostic of disease progression independently of CD4+ T-cell counts *(111,112).* The recovery of T-lymphocyte proliferative responses to antigens such as CMV, MAC, *Candida,* and MTB following initiation of HAART has been reported by several groups *(77,78,113–115).* The development of new mycobacteria-specific T-cell lymphoproliferative responses has been correlated with immune inflammatory reactions in patients with unusual clinical manifestations of mycobacterial infections following the initiation of HAART *(63).* In general, the restoration of these responses has occurred rapidly, within the first 3 months of therapy.

T-lymphocyte proliferative responses do not appear to be unilaterally reconstituted in the setting of HAART, however. Despite some reports of recovery of tetanus-specific lymphocyte proliferative responses in small numbers of patients, particularly in relatively early stages of disease *(113,115,116),* a larger study of individuals with moderately advanced HIV-1 infection did not reveal reconstitution of tetanus-specific lymphocyte proliferative responses after 1 year of HAART therapy *(77)*. The selective failure of tetanus responses to increase is probably owing to the infrequency of exposure to tetanus compared with *Candida,* CMV, MAC, and MTB, to which individuals are probably reexposed endogenously. Indeed, a tetanus booster vaccination given to subjects after 1 year of HAART therapy resulted in reconstitution of tetanus-specific lymphocyte proliferative responses *(117),* suggesting that antigen-specific precursors had not been completely eliminated in these subjects, but only depleted. These findings suggest that HAART improves the immune system's ability to respond to antigen on exposure but that HAART does not reconstitute preexisting responses in the absence of reexposure. Thus, the rejuvenated immune system on HAART is not identical to the one prior to HIV-1 infection.

Delayed-type hypersensitivity (DTH) skin test responses are lost in chronic HIV-1 infection and are prognostic of disease progression independently of CD4+ T-cell count and lymphocyte proliferative responses *(112,118).* DTH responses to *Candida* and mumps were found to be recovered in adults with moderately advanced HIV-1 disease after 1 year of treatment with HAART *(77).* However, the recovery of responses was asynchronous; *Candida* responses were restored within 12 weeks of therapy, whereas mumps responses only increased after 12 weeks of therapy. One interpretation of these findings is that HAART reconstituted the booster phenomenon *(119)* such that the mumps skin test at week 12 boosted preexisting mumps-specific memory cells, resulting in subsequent positive DTH responses. These findings support the hypothesis that reexposure to antigen is necessary to reconstitute functional immune responses.

Although improvements in functional immunity in individuals treated with HAART have been demonstrated by numerous studies, few studies have actually compared these reconstituted responses with those in HIV-1-seronegative individuals. Lymphoproliferative responses to *Candida* normalized relative to HIV-1-seronegative individuals in one study *(77).* However, although lymphoproliferative responses to tetanus toxoid as well as keyhole limpet hemocyanin increased in HAART-treated HIV-1-infected individuals after vaccination, they were still significantly lower than those in HIV-1-seronegative controls who received the same vaccines *(117).*

A study of pneumococcal vaccination in HIV-1 infected individuals receiving HAART found that antibody responses were poor, regardless of the degree of virus suppression on HAART *(120).* In contrast, antibody responses to pneumococcal vaccination in recent HIV-1 seroconverters have been reported to be equivalent to those in HIV-1-seronegative individuals *(121),* suggesting that chronic untreated HIV-1 infection may induce a long-term deficit in immune responsiveness that cannot be completely reversed by HAART. HAART regimens themselves may impair immune responsiveness. Protease inhibitors have been shown to exhibit an antiproliferative effect on human cells in vitro *(122)* and also to impair antigen presentation and CTL activity in mice *(123).* Thus, functional immune reconstitution is substantial, but not necessarily complete, in individuals treated with HAART, although the reasons why this immune reconstitution is incomplete remain to be determined.

IMPACT OF HAART ON HIV-1-SPECIFIC IMMUNE RESPONSES

It is not fully understood why most HIV-1-infected individuals are unable to mount an immune response that is capable of controlling and eradicating HIV-1 replication. Loss of HIV-1-specific CD4+ T-lymphocyte proliferative responses, which usually occurs quite early in infection *(124–126)*, has been hypothesized to be critical to the immunopathogenesis of HIV-1 infection. The finding that these responses are preserved in long-term nonprogressors *(127,128)*, who have low levels of virus replication, has been interpreted as evidence that HIV-1-specific CD4+ T-cell functions are essential for immunologic control of the virus. A critical question is whether HAART may reverse defects in HIV-1-specific immune responses and thereby enhance immunologic control in infected individuals.

Studies of HAART in chronically infected individuals have shown that HIV-1-specific CD4+ lymphocyte proliferative responses are usually not reconstituted *(77,78,115,129)*. There are exceptions, however, as reconstitution of HIV-1-specific lymphocyte proliferative responses have been reported in some individuals in early stages of disease *(116)*, as well as after 2 years of antiretroviral therapy *(122)*. Virus-specific lymphoproliferative responses have been reported to develop in individuals with transient interruptions of HAART as well *(130,131)*, suggesting that reexposure to HIV-1 antigens may reconstitute these responses. HIV-1-specific CD4+ T-cells have been detected in untreated individuals using flow cytometric studies of antigen-induced interferon-γ production *(132)*. Long-term administration of HAART to chronically infected individuals results in a decrease in HIV-1-specific CD4+ lymphocytes detected by these flow cytometric assays *(132)*.

Other HIV-1-specific immune responses appear to decline in the setting of HAART as well, presumably owing to decreased antigen concentration. HIV-1-specific CD8+ cytotoxic T-lymphocyte (CTL) memory and effector responses decline in chronically infected individuals treated with HAART *(133–136)*. Humoral immune responses to HIV-1 decline in chronically infected individuals treated with HAART as well. HIV-1 gp120-specific antibody-secreting cells rapidly decline in number with the institution of HAART, and anti-gp120 titers fall more gradually *(137)*.

Treatment of acute seroconverters with HAART appears to have different immune consequences than treatment of chronically infected individuals. Institution of HAART during or shortly after seroconversion has been reported to result in preservation of HIV-1-specific lymphocyte proliferative responses *(138)*. In addition, treatment of acute seroconverters has been reported to result in strong HIV-1-specific neutralizing antibodies *(139)*, which are distinctly unusual in chronic HIV-1 infection *(140)*. HIV-1-specific CTL responses in seroconverters who receive HAART appear to be affected in the same way as those in chronically infected individuals treated with HAART in that they decline in subjects with maximal virus suppression but are maintained or increase in those in whom viral suppression is incomplete *(141,142)*.

Because virus-specific responses could potentially synergize with HAART and enhance control of viral replication *(143)*, a number of strategies are currently under investigation to bolster HIV-1-specific CD4+ and CD8+ T-cell responses. Based on the observations that interruption of HAART can result in augmentation of both CD4+ and CD8+ HIV-1-specific responses, studies of the immunologic and virologic effects of intermittent withdrawal of antiretroviral therapy have been undertaken. Preliminary results suggest that interruption of treatment in subjects treated during acute HIV-1 seroconversion may result in enhanced virologic control *(138)*, perhaps through preservation of HIV-1-specific CD4+ T-cell responses. Multiple interruptions in therapy have been suggested to be important in augmenting virologic control, perhaps through additional stimulation of HIV-1-specific cellular responses *(138)*. Interruption of therapy in chronically infected individuals, on the other hand, has not yielded much evidence of enhanced virologic control thus far *(130,144,145)*. Further studies are needed to determine whether these strategies are safe or successful in inducing HIV-1-specific immune responses and whether these immune responses are associated with more effective elimination of virus or more sustained viral suppression.

Therapeutic vaccination is another approach currently under investigation to augment HIV-1-specific immunity in HAART-treated individuals. SIV-infected macaques who were treated with HAART 15 days after experimental infection and then subsequently vaccinated have demonstrated enhanced virologic control upon discontinuation of antiretroviral therapy compared with animals who received antiretroviral therapy alone *(146)*. Similar studies in humans are ongoing, but there are no definitive results to date.

CONCLUSIONS

Immune reconstitution in the setting of potent combination antiretroviral chemotherapy has resulted in remarkable decreases in morbidity and mortality from HIV-1 infection over the past 5 years. Both clinical and laboratory data suggest that HAART restores the ability of the immune system to respond to antigens upon reexposure. Nevertheless, immune reconstitution is neither uniform nor complete in all treated individuals. Some HIV-1-associated malignancies have not declined in frequency, and the long-term impact of HAART on these and other HIV-1-associated illnesses remains to be determined. CD4+ T-cell counts do not normalize in all treated individuals, and CD4+ T-cell functional studies suggest that many HIV-1-infected individuals treated with HAART continue to have selected defects. The clinical implications of subnormal CD4+ T-cell numbers and incomplete immune restoration are unknown.

Although HAART has revolutionized the treatment of HIV-1 infection, it is not the solution for this disease. A small fraction of individuals are absolutely intolerant of the medications and therefore unable to take them. Many others suffer side effects but continue to use them with substantial impairments in their quality of life *(147)*. As many as two-thirds of treated individuals do not achieve or maintain complete virologic suppression *(147)*. Although partial suppression of virus has been shown to result in clinical benefits, ultimately individuals with incomplete virologic suppression will develop resistant viruses and then lose the immune benefits that they have achieved with HAART. Transmission of resistant virus is increasing *(148)*, which limits the medications that individuals infected with resistant strains may receive. Lastly, most of the HIV-1-infected people in the world currently do not have access to HAART and therefore do not benefit from it at all. A better understanding of the immunopathogenesis of HIV-1 infection that has been brought about by HAART may ultimately lead to better therapies for this infection and possibly decrease or eliminate the need for antiretroviral drug therapy in the future.

REFERENCES

1. Hammer SM, Katzenstein DA, Hughes MD, et al. A trial comparing nucleoside monotherapy with combination therapy in HIV-infected adults with CD4 cell counts from 200 to 500 per cubic millimeter. AIDS Clinical Trials Group Study 175 Study Team. N Engl J Med 1996; 335:1081–1090.

2. Delta Coordinating Committee. Delta: a randomized double-blind controlled trial comparing combinations of zidovudine plus didanosine or zalcitabine with zidovudine alone in HIV-infected individuals. Lancet 1996; 348:283–291.

3. Marschner IC, Collier AC, Coombs RW, et al. Use of changes in plasma levels of human immunodeficiency virus type 1 RNA to assess the clinical benefit of antiretroviral therapy. J Infect Dis 1998; 177:40–47.

4. Katzenstein DA, Hammer SM, Hughes MD, et al. The relation of virologic and immunologic markers to clinical outcomes after nucleoside therapy in HIV infected adults with 200 to 500 CD4 cells per cubic millimeter. AIDS Clinical Trials Group Study 175 Virology Study Team. N Engl J Med 1996; 335:1091–1098.

5. Collier AC, Coombs RW, Schoenfeld DA, et al. Treatment of human immunodeficiency virus infection with saquinavir, zidovudine, and zalcitabine. AIDS Clinical Trials Group. N Engl J Med 1996; 334:1011–1017.

6. Hammer SM, Squires KE, Hughes MD, et al. A controlled trial of two nucleoside analogues plus indinavir in persons with human immunodeficiency virus infection and CD4 cell counts of 200 per cubic millimeter or less. AIDS Clinical Trials Group 320 Study Team. N Engl J Med 1997; 337:725–733.

7. Gulick RM, Mellors JW, Havlir D, et al. Treatment with indinavir, zidovudine, and lamivudine in adults with human immunodeficiency virus infection and prior antiretroviral therapy. N Engl J Med 1997; 337:734–739.

8. D'Aquila RT, Hughes MD, Johnson VA, et al. Nevirapine, zidovudine, and didanosine compared with zidovudine and didanosine in patients with HIV-1 infection. A randomized, double-blind, placebo-controlled trial. Ann Intern Med 1996; 124:1019–1030.

9. Riddler S, Stein D, Mayers D, et al. Durable clinical anti-HIV-1 activity (48 weeks) and tolerability (24 weeks) for DMP 266 in combination with indinavir (IDV): DMP 266–003, Cohort IV. In: Abstracts of the 35th Annual Meeting of the Infectious Diseases Society of America, San Francisco, CA, 1997 [Abstract 770].

10. Albrecht M, Katzenstein D, Bosch RJ, et al. ACTG 364: virologic efficacy of nelfinavir (NFV) and/or efavirenz (EFV) in combination with new nucleoside analogs in nucleoside experienced subjects. In: Proceedings of the XII World AIDS Conference, Geneva, Switzerland, 1998 [Abstract 12203].

11. Murphy RL, Gulick R, Smeaton L, et al. Treatment with indinavir, nevirapine, stavudine, and 3TC following therapy with an amprenavir-containing regimen [Abstract OP2.4]. AIDS 1998; 12(suppl 4):S9.

12. Murphy RL, Gulick RM, DeGruttola V, et al. Treatment with amprenavir alone or amprenavir with zidovudine and lamivudine in adults with human immunodeficiency virus infection. AIDS Clinical Trials Group 347 Study Team. J Infect Dis 1999; 179:808–816.

13. Carpenter CC, Cooper DA, Fischl MA, et al. Antiretroviral therapy in adults. Updated recommendations of the international AIDS society-USA panel. JAMA 2000; 283:381–390.

14. Centers for Disease Control and Prevention. HIV/AIDS Surveillance Report, no. 10. Atlanta, GA: CDC, 1999, p. 38.

15. Jones JL, Hanson DL, Dworkin MS, et al. Surveillance for AIDS-defining opportunistic illnesses, 1992-1997. MMWR 1999; 48:1–22.

16. Palella FJ, Delaney KM, Moorman AC, et al. Declining morbidity and mortality among patients with advanced human immunodeficiency virus infection. HIV Outpatient Study Investigators. N Engl J Med 1998; 338:853–860.

17. Brodt HR, Kamps BS, Gute P, et al. Changing incidence of AIDS-defining illnesses in the era of antiretroviral combination therapy. AIDS 1997; 11:1731–1738.

18. Egger M, Hirschel B, Francioli P, et al. Impact of new antiretroviral combination therapies in HIV infected people in Switzerland: prospective multicentre study. BMJ 1997; 315:1194–1199.

19. Holtzer CD, Jacobson MA, Hadley WK, et al. Decline in the rate of specific opportunistic infections at San Francisco General Hospital (SFGH): 1994–1997 [Letter]. AIDS 1998; 12:1931–1933.

20. Mocroft A, Vella S, Benfield TL, et al. Changing patterns of mortality across Europe in patients infected with HIV-1. EuroSIDA Study Group. Lancet 1998; 352:1725–1730.

21. Correll PK, Law MG, McDonald AM, et al. HIV disease progression in Australia in the time of combination antiretroviral therapies. Med J Aust 1998; 169:469–472.

22. Hogg RS, Heath KV, Yip B, et al. Improved survival among HIV-infected individuals following initiation of antiretroviral therapy. JAMA 1998; 279:450–454.

23. Pezzotti P, Dal Maso L, Serraino D, et al. Has the spectrum of AIDS-defining illnesses been changing since the introduction of new treatments and combination of treatments? [Letter]. J Acquir Immun Defic Syndr Hum Retroviruses 1999; 20:515–516.

24. Paul S, Gilbert HM, Ziecheck W, et al. The impact of potent antiretroviral therapy on the characteristics of hospitalized patients with HIV infection. AIDS 1999; 13:415–418.

25. Cameron DW, Heath-Chiozzi M, Danner S, et al. Randomized, placebo-controlled trial of ritonavir in advanced HIV-1 disease. The Advanced HIV Disease Ritonavir Study Group. Lancet 1998; 351:543–549.

26. Hirsh M for Protocol 039 (Indinavir) Study Group, Meibohm A, Rawlins S, et al. Indinavir (IDV) in combination with zidovudine (ZDV) and lamivudine (3TC) in ZDV-experienced patients with CD4 cell counts $<$ 50 cells/mm^3. In: Abstracts of the 4th Conference on Retroviruses and Opportunistic Infections, Washington, DC, 1997 [Abstract #LB7].

27. Baqi M, Kucharczyk W, Walmsley SL. Regression of progressive multifocal leukoencephalopathy with highly active antiretroviral therapy [Letter]. AIDS 1997; 11:1526–1527.

28. Baldeweg T, Catalan J. Remission of progressive multifocal leukoencephalopathy after antiretroviral therapy. Lancet 1997; 349:1554–1555.

29. Domingo P, Guardiola JM, Iranzo A, et al. Remission of progressive multifocal leukoencephalopathy after antiretroviral therapy. Lancet 1997; 349:1554–1555.

30. Elliot B, Aromin I, Gold R, et al. 2.5 year remission of AIDS-associated progressive multifocal leukoencephalopathy with combined antiretroviral therapy [Letter]. Lancet 1997; 349:850.

31. Power C, Nath A, Aoki FY, Bigio MD. Remission of progressive multifocal leukoencephalopathy following splenectromy and antiretroviral therapy in a patient with HIV infection. N Engl J Med 1997; 336:661–662.

32. Cinque P, Casari S, Bertelli D. Progressive multifocal leukoencephalopathy, HIV, and highly active antiretroviral therapy. N Engl J Med 1998; 339:848–849.

33. Albrecht H, Hoffmann C, Degen O, et al. Highly active antiretroviral therapy significantly improves the prognosis of patients with HIV-associated progressive multifocal leukoencephalopathy. AIDS 1998; 12:1149–1154.

34. Carr A, Marriott D, Field A, Vasak E, et al. Treatment of HIV-1-associated microsporidiosis and cryptosporidiosis with combination antiretroviral therapy. Lancet 1998; 351:256–261.

35. Goguel J, Katlama C, Sarfati C, et al. Remission of AIDS-associated intestinal microsporidiosis with combined antiretroviral therapy. In: Abstracts of the 37th Interscience Conference on Antimicrobial Agents and Chemotherapy. Toronto, Canada, 1997 [Abstr. #I-32].

36. Zingman BS. Resolution of refractory AIDS-related mucosal candidiasis after initiation of didanosine plus saquinavir. N Engl J Med 1996; 334:1674–1675.

37. Valdez H, Gripshover BM, Salata RA, et al. Resolution of azole-resistant oropharyngeal candidiasis after initiation of potent combination antiretroviral therapy [Letter]. AIDS 1998; 12:538.

38. Hicks CB, Myers SA, Giner J. Resolution of intractable molluscum contagiosum in a human immunodeficiency virus infected patient after institution of antiretroviral therapy with ritonavir. Clin Infect Dis 1997; 24:1023–1025.

39. Hurni MA, Bohlen L, Furrer H, et al. Complete regression of giant molluscum contagiosum lesions in an HIV-infected patient following combined antiretroviral therapy with saquinavir, zidovudine and lamivudine. AIDS 1997; 11:1784–1785.

40. Murphy M, Armstrong D, Sepkowitz KA, et al. Regression of AIDS related Kaposi's sarcoma following treatment with an HIV-1 protease inhibitor. AIDS 1997; 11:261–262.

41. Conant MA, Opp KM, Poretz D, et al. Reduction of Kaposi's sarcoma lesions following treatment of AIDS with ritonavir. AIDS 1997; 11:1300–1301.

42. Parra R, Leal M, Delgado J, et al. Regression of invasive AIDS-related Kaposi's sarcoma following antiretorviral therapy. Clin Infect Dis 1998; 26:218–219.

43. Uthayakumar S, Birthistle K, Dalton R, Hay PE. Cytomegalovirus retinitis after initiation of highly active antiretroviral therapy. Lancet 1997; 350:588–589.

44. Jabs DA, Bolton SG, Dunn JP, et al. Discontinuing anticytomegalovirus therapy in patients with immune reconstitution after combination antiretroviral therapy. Am J Ophthalmol 1998; 126:817–822.

45. Whitcup S, Fortin E, Lindblad A, et al. Discontinuation of anticytomegalovirus therapy in patients with HIV infection and cytomegalovirus retinitis. JAMA 1999; 282:1633–1637.

46. Aberg JA, Yajko DM, Jacobson MA. Eradication of AIDS-related disseminated *mycobacterium avium* complex infection after 12 months of antimycobacterial therapy combined with highly active antiretroviral therapy. J Infect Dis 1998; 178:1446–1449.

47. Weverling GJ, Mocroft A, Ledergerber B, et al. Discontinuation of *Pneumocystis carinii* pneumonia prophylaxis after start of highly active antiretroviral therapy in HIV-1 infection. EuroSIDA Study Group. Lancet 1999; 353:1293–1298.

48. Schneider MME, Borleffs JCC, Stolk RP, et al. Discontinuation of *Pneumocystis carinii* pneumonia prophylaxis in HIV-1 infected patients treated with highly active antiretroviral therapy. Lancet 1999; 353:201–203.

49. Dworkin M, Hanson D, Jones J, et al. The risk for *Pneumocystis carinii* pneumonia (PCP) and disseminated nontuberculous mycobacteriosis (dMb) after an antiretroviral therapy (ART) associated increase in the CD4+ T lymphocyte count. In: Abstracts of the 6th Conference on Retroviruses and Opportunistic Infections, Chicago, IL, 1999 [Abstract No. 692].

50. Lopez JC, Pena JM, Miro JM, et al. Discontinuation of PCP prophylaxis (PRO) is safe in HIV-infected patients (PTS) with immunological recovery with HAART. Preliminary results of an open randomized and multicenter clinical trial (GESIDA 04/98). In: Abstracts of the 5th Conference on Retroviruses and Opportunistic Infections, Chicago, IL, 1999 [Abstract No. LB7].

51. Furrer H, Egger M, Opravil M, et al. Discontinuation of primary prophylaxis against *Pneumocystis carinii* pneumonia in HIV-1-infected adults treated with combination antiretroviral therapy. Swiss Cohort Study. N Engl J Med 1999; 340:1301–1306.

52. Currier JS, Williams PL, Koletar SL, et al. Discontinuation of *Mycobacterium avium* complex prophylaxis in patients with antiretroviral therapy-induced increases in CD4+ cell count. A randomized, double-blind, placebo-controlled trial. Ann Intern Med 2000; 133:493–503.

53. El-Sadr WM, Burman WJ, Grant LB, et al. Discontinuation of prophylaxis for *Mycobacterium avium* complex disease in HIV-infected patients who have a response to antiretroviral therapy. Terry Beirn Community Programs for Clinical Research on AIDS. N Engl J Med 2000; 243:1085–1092.

54. Furrer H, Telenti A, Rossi M, Ledergerber B. Discontinuing or withholding primary prophylaxis against *Mycobacterium avium* in patients on successful antiretroviral combination therapy. The Swiss HIV Cohort Study. AIDS 2000; 14:1409–1412.

55. Anonymous. 1999 USPHS/IDSA guidelines for the prevention of opportunistic infections in persons infected with human immunodeficiency virus. MMWR 1999; 48:1–59.

56. Jacobson MA, Zegans M, Pavan PR, et al. Cytomegalovirus retinitis after highly active antiretroviral therapy. Lancet 1997; 349:1443–1445.

57. Gilquin J, Piketty C, Thomas V, et al. Acute cytomegalovirus infection in AIDS patients with CD4 counts above $100 \times 10(6)$ cells/l following combination antiretroviral therapy including protease inhibitors [Letter]. AIDS 1997; 11:1659–1660.

58. Karavellas MP, Lowder CY, Macdonald JC, Avila CP, Freeman WR. Immune recovery vitritis associated with inactive cytomegalovirus retinitis: a new syndrome. Arch Ophthalmol 1998; 116:169–175.

59. Mayo J, Collazos J, Martinez E. Progressive multifocal leukoencephalopathy following initiation of highly active antiretroviral therapy. AIDS 1998; 12:1720–1722.

60. Kotecha N, George MJ, Smithe TW, et al. Enhancing progressive multifocal leukoencephalopathy: an indicator of improved immune status? Am J Med 1998; 105:541–543.

61. Race EM, Adelson-Mitty JA, Kriegel GR, et al. Focal mycobacterial lymphadenitis following initiation of protease-inhibitor therapy in patients with advanced HIV-1 disease. Lancet 1998; 351:252–255.

62. Chien JW, Johnson JL. Paradoxical reactions in HIV and pulmonary TB. Chest 1998; 114:933–936.

63. Foudraine NA, Hovenkamp E, Notermans DW, et al. Immunopathology as a result of highly active antiretroviral therapy in HIV-1-infected patients. AIDS 1999; 13:177–184.

64. Carr A, Cooper DA. Restoration of immunity to chronic hepatitis B infection in HIV-infected patient on protease inhibitor. Lancet 1997; 349:995–996.

65. Vento S, Garofano T, Renzini C, et al. Enhancement of hepatitis C virus replication and liver damage in HIV-coinfected patients on antiretroviral combination therapy [Letter]. AIDS 1998; 12:116–117.

66. Zietz C, Bogner JR, Goebel FD, et al. An unusual cluster of cases of Castleman's disease during highly active antiretroviral therapy for AIDS (letter). N Engl J Med 1999; 340:1923–1924.

67. Law MG, de Winter L, McDonald A, et al. AIDS diagnoses at higher CD4 counts in Australia following the introduction of highly active antiretroviral treatment. AIDS 1999; 13:263–269.

68. Miller V, Mocroft A, Reiss P, et al. Relations among CD4 lymphocyte count nadir, antiretroviral therapy, and HIV-1 disease progression: results from the EuroSIDA study. Ann Intern Med 1999; 130:570–577.

69. Ledergerber B, Egger M, Erard V, et al. AIDS-related opportunistic illnesses occurring after initiation of potent antiretroviral therapy: the Swiss HIV cohort study. JAMA 1999; 282:2220–2226.

70. Johnson SC, Benson CA, Johnson DW, Weinberg A. Recurrence of cytomegalovirus retinitis in a human immunodeficiency virus-infected patient, despite potent antiretroviral therapy and apparent immune reconstitution. Clin Infect Dis 2001; 32:815–819.

71. Jones JL, Hanson DL, Dworkin MS, et al. Effect of antiretroviral therapy on recent trends in selected cancers among HIV-infected persons. Adult/Adolescent Spectrum of HIV Disease Project. J Acquir Immun Defic Syndr 1999; 21:Suppl 1:11–17.

72. Sparano JA, Anand K, Desai J, et al. Effect of highly active antiretroviral therapy on the incidence of HIV-associated malignancies at an urban medical center. J Acquir Immun Defic Syndr 1999; 21:Suppl 1:S18–S22.

73. Rabkin CS, Testa MA, Huang J, Von Roenn JH. Kaposi's sarcoma and non-Hodgkin's lymphoma incidence trends in AIDS clinical trial group study participants. J Acquir Immun Defic Syndr 1999; 21:S31–S33.

74. Jacobson LP, Yamashita TE, Detels R, et al. Impact of potent antiretroviral therapy on the incidence of Kaposi's sarcoma and non-Hodgkin's lymphomas among HIV-1-infected individuals. Multicenter AIDS Cohort Study. J Acquir Immun Defic Syndr 1999; 21:Suppl 1:S34–S41.

75. Grulich AE. AIDS-associated non-Hodgkin's lymphoma in the era of highly active antiretroviral therapy. J Acquir Immun Defic Syndr 1999; 21:Suppl 1:S27–S30.

76. Dolan M.J., Clerici M., Blatt S.P., et al. In vitro T cell function, delayed type hypersensitivity skin testing, and CD4+ T cell subset phenotyping independently predict survival time in patients infected with human immunodeficiency virus. J Infect Dis 1995; 172:79–87.

77. Connick E, Lederman MM, Kotzin BL, et al. Immune reconstitution in the first year of potent antiretroviral therapy and its relationship to virologic response. J Infect Dis 2000; 181:358–363.

78. Autran B, Carcelain G, Li TS, et al. Positive effects of combined antiretroviral therapy on CD4+ T cell homeostasis and function in advanced HIV disease. Science 1997; 277:112–116.

79. Pakker NG, Roos M, Leeuwen R, et al. Patterns of T-cell repopulation, virus load reduction, and restoration of T-cell function in HIV-infected persons during therapy with different antiretroviral agents. J Acquir Immun Defic Syndr Hum Retroviruses 1997; 16:318–326.

80. Li TS, Tubiana R, Katlama C, et al. Long-lasting recovery in CD4 T-cell function and viral-load reduction after highly active antiretroviral therapy in advanced HIV-1 disease. Lancet 1998; 351:1682–1686.

81. Pakker NG, Notermans DW, de Boer RJ, et al. Biphasic kinetics of peripheral blood T cells after triple combination therapy in HIV-1 infection: a composite of redistribution and proliferation. Nat Med 1998; 4:208–214.

82. Gray CM, Schapiro JM, Winters MA, et al. Changes in CD4+ and CD8+ T cell subsets in response to highly active antiretroviral therapy in HIV type 1-infected patients with prior protease inhibitor experience. AIDS Res Hum Retroviruses 1998; 14:561–569.

83. Giorgi JV, Majchrowicz MA, Johnson TD, et al. Immunologic effects of combined protease inhibitor and reverse transcriptase inhibitor therapy in previously treated chronic HIV-1 infection. AIDS 1998; 12:1833–1844.

84. Bisset LR, Cone RW, Huber W, et al. Highly active antiretroviral therapy during early HIV infection reverses T-cell activation and maturation abnormalities. AIDS 1998; 12:2115–2123.

85. Wu H, Connick E, Kuritzkes DR, et al. Multiple CD4+ cell kinetic patterns and their relationships with baseline factors and virologic responses in HIV-1 patients receiving HAART. AIDS Res Human Retroviruses 2001; 13:1231–1240.

86. Renaud M, Katlama C, Mallet A, et al. Determinants of paradoxical CD4 cell reconstitution after protease inhibitor-containing antiretroviral regimen. AIDS 1999; 13:669–676.

87. Lederman MM, Connick E, Landay A, et al. Immunologic responses associated with 12 weeks of combination antiretroviral therapy consisting of zidovudine, lamivudine, and ritonavir: results of AIDS clinical trials group protocol 315. J Infect Dis 1998; 178:70–79.

88. Drusano GL, Stein DS. Mathematical modeling of the interrelationship of CD4 lymphocyte count and viral load changes induced by the protease inhibitor indinavir. Antimicrob Agents Chemother 1998; 42:358–361.

89. Lederman MM, McKinnis R, Kelleher D, et al. Cellular restoration in HIV infected persons treated with abacavir and a protease inhibitor: age inversely predicts naïve CD4 cell count increase. AIDS 2000; 14:2635–2642.

90. Wei X, Ghosh SK, Taylor ME, et al. Viral dynamics in human immunodeficiency virus type 1 infection. Nature 1995; 373:117–122.

91. Ho DD, Neumann AU, Perelson AS. Rapid turnover of plasma virions and CD4 lymphocytes in HIV-1 infection. Nature 1995; 373:123–126.

92. Perelson AS, Neumann AU, Markowitz M, et al. HIV-1 dynamics in vivo: virion clearance rate, infected cell life-span, and viral generation time. Science 1996; 271:1582–1586.

93. Haase AT, Nehry K, Zupancic M, et al. Quantitative image analysis of HIV-1 infection in lymphoid tissue. Science 1996; 274:985–989.

94. Andersson J, Fehniger TE, Patterson BK, et al. Early reduction of immune activation in lymphoid tissue following highly active HIV therapy. AIDS 1998; 12:F123–F129.

95. Bucy RP, Hockett RD, Derdeyn CA, et al. Initial increase in blood CD4+ lymphocytes after HIV antiretroviral therapy reflects redistribution from lymphoid tissues. J Clin Invest 1999; 103:1391–1398.

96. Badley AD, Dockrell DH, Algeciras A, et al. In vivo analysis of Fas/FasL interactions in HIV-infected patients. J Clin Invest 1998; 102:79–87.

97. Zhang Z, Notermans DW, Sedgewick G, et al. Kinetics of CD4+ T cell repopulation of lymphoid tissues after treatment of HIV-1 infection. Proc Natl Acad Sci 1998; 95:1154–1159.

98. Hellerstein M, Hanley MB, Cesar D, et al. Directly measured kinetics of circulating T lymphocytes in normal and HIV-1-infected humans. Nat Med 1999; 5:83–89.

99. Connors M, Kovacs JA, Krevat S, et al. HIV infection induces changes in CD4+ T-cell phenotype and depletions within the CD4+ T-cell repertoire that are not immediately restored by antiviral or immune-based therapies. Nat Med 1997; 3:533–540.

100. Gorochov G, Neumann AU, Kereveur A, et al. Perturbation of CD4+ and CD8+ T-cell repertoires during progression to AIDS and regulation of the CD4+ repertoire during antiviral therapy. Nat Med 1998; 4:215–221.

101. Kostense S, Raaphorst FM, Notermans DW, et al. Diversity of the T-cell receptor BV repertoire in HIV-1-infected patients reflects the biphasic CD4+ T-cell repopulation kinetics during highly active antiretroviral therapy. AIDS 1998; 12:F235–F240.

102. Hakim FT, Cepeda R, Kaimei S, et al. Constraints on CD4 recovery postchemotherapy in adults: thymic insufficiency and apoptotic decline of expanded peripheral CD4 cells. Blood 1997; 90:3789–3798.

103. Bell EB, Sparshott SM. Interconversion of CD45R subsets of CD4 T cells in vivo. Nature 1990; 348:163–166.

104. Walker RE, Carter CS, Muul L, et al. Peripheral expansion of pre-existing T cells is an important means of CD4+ T-cell regeneration in HIV-infected adults. Nat Med 1998; 4:852–856.

105. Douek DC, McFarland RD, Keiser PH, et al. Changes in thymic function with age and during the treatment of HIV infection. Nature 1998; 396:690–695.

106. McCune JM, Hanley MB, Cesar D, et al. Factors influencing T-cell turnover in HIV-1-seropositive patients. J Clin Invest 2000; 105:565–616.

107. Hazenberg MD, Otto SA, Cohen Stuart JW, et al. Increased cell division but not thymic dysfunction rapidly affects the T-cell receptor excision circle content of the naive T cell population in HIV-1 infection. Nature Med 2000; 6:1036–1042.

108. Notermans DW, Pakker NG, Hamann D, et al. Immune reconstitution after 2 years of successful potent antiretroviral therapy in previously untreated human immunodeficiency virus type 1-infected adults. J Infect Dis 1999; 180:1050–1056.

109. Valdez H, Connick E, Lederman M, et al. T-lymphocyte changes after 3 years of controlled viral replication. In: 8th Conference on Retroviruses and Opportunistic Infections, Chicago, IL, 2001 [Abstract 372].

110. Grabar S, Le Moing V, Goujard C, et al. Clinical outcome of patients with HIV-1 infection according to immunologic and virologic response after 6 months of highly active antiretroviral therapy. Ann Intern Med 2000; 133:401–410.

111. Clerici M, Stocks NI, Zajac RA, et al. Detection of three distinct patterns of T helper cell dysfunction in asymptomatic human immunodeficiency virus-seropositive patients: independence of CD4+ cell numbers and clinical staging. J Clin Invest 1989; 84:1892–1899.

112. Dolan MJ, Clerici M, Blatt SP, et al. In vitro T cell function, delayed type hypersensitivity skin testing, and CD4+ T cell subset phenotyping independently predict survival time in patients infected with human immunodeficiency virus. J Infect Dis 1995; 172:79–87.

113. Rinaldo CR Jr, Liebmann JM, Huang XL, et al. Prolonged suppression of human immunodeficiency virus type 1 (HIV-1) viremia in persons with advanced disease results in enhancement of CD4 T cell reactivity to microbial antigens but not to HIV-1 antigens. J Infect Dis 1999; 179:329–336.

114. Komanduri KV, Viswanathan MN, Wieder ED, et al. Restoration of cytomegalovirus-specific CD4+ T-lymphocyte responses after ganciclovir and highly active antiretroviral therapy in individuals infected with HIV-1. Nat Med 1998; 4:953–956.

115. Pontesilli O, Kerkhof-Garde S, Notermans DW, et al. Functional T cell reconstitution and human immunodeficiency virus-1-specific cell-mediated immunity during highly active antiretroviral therapy. J Infect Dis 1999; 180:76–86.

116. Al-Harthi L, Siegel J, Spritzler J, Pottage J, Agnoli M, Landay A. Maximum suppression of HIV replication leads to the restoration of HIV-specific responses in early HIV disease. AIDS 2000; 14:761–770.

117. Valdez H, Smith K, Landay A, et al. Response to immunization with recall and neoantigens after prolonged administration of an HIV-1 protease inhibitor-containing regimen. AIDS 2000; 14:11–21.

118. Blatt SP, Hendrix CW, Butzin CA, et al. Delayed-type hypersensitivity skin testing predicts progression to AIDS in HIV-infected patients. Ann Intern Med 1993; 119:177–184.

119. Thompson NJ, Glasroth J, Sinder D, et al. The booster phenomenon in serial tuberculin testing. Am Rev Respir Dis 1979; 119:587–597.

120. Fleming C, Cilento J, Steger K, McNamara E, Pelton S, Craven D. Immunogenicity of revaccination with penumococcal vaccine in HIV-infected patients on combination antiretroviral therapy. In: 7th Conference on Retroviruses and Opportunistic Infections. San Francisco, 2000 [Abstract 249].

121. Weiss PJ, Wallace MR, Oldfield EC, O'Brien J, Janoff EN. Response of recent human immunodeficiency virus seroconverters to the penumococcal polysaccharide vaccine and *Haemophilus influenzae* type b conjugate vaccine. J Infect Dis 1995; 171:1217–1222.

122. Angel JB, Parato KG, Kumar A, et al. Progressive human immunodeficiency virus-specific immune recovery with prolonged viral suppression. J Infect Dis 2001; 183:546–554.

123. Andre P, Klenerman P, Groettrup M, et al. An inhibitor of HIV-1 protease blocks proteasome activity, antigen presentation and CD8 T cell responses. Proc Natl Acad Sci USA 1998; 95:13120–13125.

124. Wahren B, Morfeldt-Mansson L, Biberfeld G, et al. Characteristics of the cell-mediated immune response in human immunodeficiency virus infection. J Virol 1987; 61:2017–2023.

125. Berzofsky JA, Bensussan A, Cease KB, et al. Antigenic peptides recognized by T lymphocytes from AIDS viral envelope-immune human. Nature 1988; 334:706–708.

126. Krowka JF, Stites DP, Jain S, et al. Lymphocyte proliferative responses to human immunodeficiency virus antigens in vitro. J Clin Invest 1989; 83:1198–1203.

127. Schwartz D, Sharma U, Busch M, et al. Absence of recoverable infectious virus and unique immune responses in an asymptomatic HIV+ long term survivor. AIDS Res Hum Retroviruses 1994; 10:1703–1711.

128. Rosenberg ES, Billingsley JM, Caliendo AM, et al. Vigorous HIV-1-specific CD4+ T cell responses associated with control of viremia. Science 1997; 278:1447–1450.

129. Plana M, Garcia F, Gallart T, et al. Lack of T-cell proliferate response to HIV-1 antigens after 1 year of highly active antiretroviral treatment in early HIV-1 disease. Immunology Study Group of Spanish EARTH-1 Study. Lancet 1998; 352:1194–1195.

130. Ruiz L, Martinez-Picado J, Romeu J, et al. Structured treatment interruption in chronically HIV-1 infected patients after long-term viral suppression. AIDS 2000; 14:397–403.

131. Haslett PA, Nixon DF, Shen Z, et al. Strong human immunodeficiency virus (HIV)-specific CD4+ T cell responses in a cohort of chronically infected patients are associated with interruptions in anti-HIV chemotherapy. J Infect Dis 2000; 181:1264–1272.

132. Pitcher CJ, Quittner C, Peterson DM, et al. HIV-1-specific CD4+ T cells are detectable in most individuals with active HIV-1 infection, but decline with prolonged viral suppression. Nat Med 1999; 5:518–525.

133. Ogg GS, Jin X, Bonhoeffer S, et al. Decay kinetics of human immunodeficiency virus-specific effector cytotoxic T lymphocytes after combination antiretroviral therapy. J Virol 1999; 73:797–800.

134. Gray CM, Lawrence J, Schapiro JM, et al. Frequency of class I HLA-restricted anti-HIV CD8+ T cells in individuals receiving highly active antiretroviral therapy (HAART). J Immunol 1999; 162:1780–1788.

135. Kalams SA, Goulder PJ, Shea AK, et al. Levels of human immunodeficiency virus type 1-specific cytotoxic T-lymphocyte effector and memory responses decline after suppression of viremia with highly active antiretroviral therapy. J Virol 1999; 73:6721–6728.

136. Moilet L, Li T-S, Samri A, et al. Dynamics of HIV-specific CD8+ T lymphocytes with changes in viral load. J Immunol 2000; 165:1692–1704.

137. Morris L, Binley JM, Clas BA, et al. HIV-1 antigen-specific and -nonspecific B cell responses are sensitive to combination antiretroviral therapy. J Exp Med 1998; 188:233–245.

138. Rosenberg ES, Altfeld M, Poon SH, et al. Immune control of HIV-1 after early treatment of acute infection. Nature 2000; 407:523–526.

139. Barassi C, De Santis C, Pastori C, et al. Early production of HIV-1 neutralising antibodies in patients following highly active antiretroviral treatment (HAART) during primary HIV infection. J Biol Regul Homeostatic Agents 2000; 14:68–74.

140. Wrin T, Crawford L, Sawyer L, et al. Neutralizing antibody responses to autologous and heterologous isolates of human immunodeficiency virus. J Acquir Immun Defic Syndr Hum Retrovirol 1994; 7:211–219.

141. Dalod M, Harzic M, Pellegrin I, et al. Evolution of cytotoxic T lymphocyte responses to human immunodeficiency virus type 1 in patients with symptomatic primary infection receiving antiretroviral triple therapy. J Infect Dis 1998; 178:61–69.

142. Markowitz M, Vesanen M, Tenner-Racz K, et al. The effect of commencing combination antiretroviral therapy soon after human immunodeficiency virus type 1 infection on viral replication and antiviral immune responses. J Infect Dis 1999; 179:527–537.

143. Rosenberg ES, Walker BD. HIV type 1-specific helper T cells: a critical host defense. AIDS Res Hum Retroviruses 1998; 14:Suppl 2:S143–S147.

144. Ortiz GM, Nixon DF, Trkola A, et al. HIV-1-specific immune responses in subjects who temporarily contain virus replication after discontinuation of highly active antiretroviral therapy. J Clin Invest 1999; 104:677–678.

145. Neuman AU, Tubiana R, Calvez V, et al. HIV-1 rebound during interruption of highly active antiretroviral therapy has no deleterious effect on reinitiated treatment. Comet Study Group. AIDS 1999; 13:677–683.

146. Hel Z, Venzon D, Poudyal M, et al. Viremia control following antiretroviral treatment and therapeutic immunization during primary SIV251 infection of macaques. Nat Med 2000; 6:1140–1146.

147. Lucas GM, Chaisson RE, Moore RD. Highly active antiretroviral therapy in a large urban clinic: risk factors for virologic failure and adverse drug reactions. Ann Intern Med 1999; 131:81–87, 1999.

148. Little SK, Daar ES, D'Aquila RT, et al. Reduced antiretroviral drug susceptibility among patients with primary HIV infection. JAMA 1999; 282:1142–1149.

10

Active Immunization as Therapy for HIV Infection

Spyros A. Kalams

INTRODUCTION

Emerging data over the past several years have confirmed the role of the HIV-specific immune response in determining viral setpoint and delaying HIV disease progression. Despite advances in the control of HIV-1 viremia with highly active antiretroviral therapy (HAART), these therapies carry the risk of toxicities with long-term use. This has led to accelerated efforts designed to augment HIV-1-specific immune responses in infected subjects with the hope that the use of antiretroviral medications can be reduced or eliminated. This chapter reviews the current state of knowledge regarding the immune responses directed against HIV and summarizes efforts that are in progress or that will be under way to augment these responses in infected individuals.

IMMUNE RESPONSES
IN CONTROLLED CHRONIC VIRAL INFECTIONS

Although there are examples of acute infections with viruses that are subsequently cleared by the immune system (e.g., influenza), for several viral infections recovery from illness is the result of immune-based containment of viremia. Patients with acute Epstein-Barr virus (EBV) infection contain the initial infection with a vigorous immune response, yet despite almost uniform resolution of symptoms, the virus remains present for the life of the infected individual. In the presence of an intact immune response, viremia is contained, and disease does not recur. Evidence for the continued need for immune surveillance is provided by the well-documented occurrence of EBV-associated malignancies in patients on immunosuppressive agents, as well as the regression of tumors when immunosuppression is decreased *(1,2)*.

The lymphocytic choriomeningitis virus (LCMV) infection model in mice has been a useful tool for dissecting the roles of the humoral and cellular immune system in viral containment. After acute infection there are large expansions of CD8+ T-cells (CTLs) and up to 70% of total CD8 T-cells are LCMV-specific 8 days after infection *(3,4)*. Another important component of immune control is the virus-specific T-helper cell response. If CD4 T-cells are either absent by genetic knockout of CD4, or depleted by anti-CD4 antibodies CTL are still generated, but they decline during the chronic phase of infection. In this instance viremia is not controlled. These studies suggest that in this

From: *Immunotherapy for Infectious Diseases*
Edited by: J. M. Jacobson © Humana Press Inc., Totowa, NJ

model, immune control is mediated through CTL, but the ability of these cells to persist and maintain normal function is dependent on the presence of an intact CD4 T-helper cell response *(5,6)*.

IMMUNE CONTROL OF HIV-1 INFECTION

HIV infection is almost invariably associated with progressive destruction of the immune system, but some patients are able to contain the virus for long periods in the absence of antiretroviral medications *(7)*. Factors that can contribute to a persistently low viral load and a benign disease course include infection with attenuated viruses *(8–10)*, and host genetic factors *(11,12)*. However, these factors are not responsible for all cases of long-term nonprogressive infection, indicating that the host immune response is capable of mediating control of HIV replication.

Both cellular and humoral immune responses have been described in HIV infection; however, the exquisite specificity of neutralizing antibodies for autologous virus has made it difficult to determine the role this arm of the immune system plays in maintenance of the viral setpoint *(13)*. Although HIV-specific antibodies are easily detected after HIV infection, neutralizing antibodies are not commonly generated early after acute infection *(14)*. Neutralizing antibody responses can be detected in some individuals and have been mapped to the V3 loop, which is involved with viral entry, and to the CD4 binding site. One limitation of neutralizing antibodies is that they typically recognize three-dimensional conformations of their epitopes, meaning that they are highly type-specific *(15–17)*. Although a strong neutralizing antibody response might provide the best primary protection against HIV-1 infection, these responses have been extremely difficult to generate with vaccines *(18–22)*. This also has implications for HIV-1 disease progression, in that viruses continue to evolve in the host and escape immune detection.

Elegant studies have demonstrated that the majority of antibodies directed against HIV antigens are directed at nonneutralizing epitopes *(23)*, which have been described as viral debris *(18)*, that are not likely to exert an antiviral effect. This high degree of specificity may also lead to rapid escape from an initially effective neutralizing antibody response. The heavy degree of glycosylation of the viral envelope protein may be another factor that allows the virus to resist antibody-mediated inactivation *(24,25)*. These factors are formidable hurdles to immune-based therapies meant to augment antibody responses.

In a manner similar to other viral infections, CTLs are generated early during the course of acute HIV-1 infection. After infection of CD4+ T-cells, viral proteins that are generated in the cytosol are degraded and presented as epitopic peptides (usually 9–11 amino acids in length) on the cell surface complexed to HLA class I molecules. CTLs recognize infected cells through the interaction of the T-cell receptor (TCR) with the HLA-epitope complex. This occurs prior to the assembly of progeny virions, a process that takes approximately 2.6 days. During this time, an infected cell is vulnerable to attack by CTL; if the cell is eliminated at this time, progeny virus will not be released *(26,27)*.

CTLs are also able to mediate antiviral effects through the elaboration of soluble factors that inhibit viral replication. These include the chemokines RANTES, macrophage inflammatory protein (MIP)-1α and MIP-1β, as well as other factors not yet fully defined. The release of these factors occurs when the TCR recognizes an infected cell. In fact, these factors are released concurrently with the mobilization of the cell's cytolytic machinery when an infected cell is recognized *(28)*, and this probably has an important effect on the microenvironment of the infected cell. RANTES, MIP-1α and MIP-1β have been shown to inhibit HIV infection of cells by competing with the virus for chemokine coreceptors present on the cell surface that are necessary for viral entry. Although the exact contribution of each of these two mechanisms toward suppression of HIV infection in vivo is not clear, it is likely that these mechanisms act synergistically to contain cell-to-cell spread of HIV.

The identification of HIV-1 epitopic peptides recognized by CTLs is an ongoing process and will be important for evaluation of immune responses generated after therapeutic immunization. Over 50 HLA class I alleles have been identified. Each HLA allele contains a binding groove able to present particular peptides that contain the correct binding motif. However, despite the widespread prevalence of some of these alleles in the general population, not all subjects with a particular HLA type will recognize the identical epitope. For example, the HLA-A2 allele has a prevalence of approximately 45% in the North American Causcasoid population. The SLYNTVATL epitope in p17 is recognized by approximately 70% of HLA-A2 subjects and thus far is one of the most immunodominant epitopes recognized. However, a substantial fraction of subjects don't recognize this epitope, and other epitopes are less frequently recognized. For example, an HLA-A2-restricted epitope in RT, ILKEPVHGV, is recognized by approximately 30% of HLA-A2 subjects *(29–32)*. The same holds true for other HLA alleles. Even in subjects matched at three HLA class I alleles, considerable variability in recognition of identified CTL epitopes exists *(33)*. This allows for the prospects of measuring the CTL responses to defined epitopes after therapeutic immunization. The fact that subjects do not target all possible CTL epitopes strengthens the rationale of broadening these responses through therapeutic immunization.

Over the past few years, newer technologies have been developed that allow for easier measurement of immune responses. Elispot assays have allowed direct enumeration of interferon-γ (IFN-γ)-producing T-cells *(3)*, and flow cytometric evaluation of these cells is possible via intracellular cytokine staining *(34)*. HLA class I tetramers allow for the direct visualization of CTLs by flow cytometry. These constructs consist of four HLA class I molecules folded around a peptide in their binding groove and bound to streptavidin. These tetramers are labeled with a fluorescent dye and can directly bind CTLs through the TCR complex *(35)*. In cross-sectional analyses, the viral load setpoint in HLA-A2-positive individuals correlates negatively with HLA-A2-tetramer staining *(36)*.

A more direct example of the antiviral effect of CTLs has been demonstrated in the simian immunodeficiency virus (SIV) macaque model. Acutely infected animals that underwent CD8+ T-cell depletion were unable to control the initial viremia and had higher viral setpoints *(37,38)*. Therefore, the decrease in virus load and establishment of the steady-state viremia appears to be the result of an active CTL-mediated immune response and not antibody responses, or, as others have proposed, exhaustion of susceptible target cells *(39)*.

In a number of viral infections, CD4+ T-helper cells have been shown to be critical for the maintenance of functional CTL (reviewed in ref. *6*). T-helper cells recognize viral proteins processed in the lysosomes of antigen-presenting cells, and that are complexed with HLA class II molecules. T-helper epitopes are typically larger than HLA class 1-restricted epitopes, in the 12–17-amino acid range. They are presented via the exogenous antigen pathway and complexed with HLA class II molecules at the cell surface, where they are recognized by CD4+ T-cells. It is not known exactly what constitutes help, but it is probably composed of released lymphokines and a series of direct cell-cell interactions. The critical role of T-helper cells in response to chronic viral infection has been firmly demonstrated in animal models. For example, after LCMV infection of mice, an LCMV-specific CTL response develops that controls viremia. However, in the absence of CD4+ T-cells, either because of genetic knockout or antibody-mediated depletion, the CTL response cannot be maintained and results in persistent viremia *(40–42)*. In contrast to other infections such as cytomegalovirus (CMV), helper responses in HIV-1 infection are typically low or absent in the presence of persistent viremia.

Cross-sectional studies of subjects with wide ranges of viral loads have demonstrated a negative correlation between HIV-1 Gag-specific helper responses and viral load *(43–46)*. In addition, helper responses are also positively correlated with the magnitude of HIV-1-specific CTL responses *(44)*, further demonstrating that both responses are likely to be important for immune-mediated control of viral replication. The identification and immunologic characterization of subjects with long-term control of HIV replication demonstrates that immune control of HIV is possible, and these subjects typically have robust HIV-specific CTL and helper responses *(47,48)*. These findings suggest that the combination of strong helper and CTL responses is required for control of viremia during HIV infection.

FACTORS LEADING TO LOSS OF CONTROL OF VIREMIA

Immune Exhaustion

A number of longitudinal studies have demonstrated that CTL responses decline with disease progression *(49–52)* and that this decline is probably related to the frequent absence of HIV-1-specific helper responses in infected individuals *(52)*. Immune exhaustion, defined as a disappearance of antigen-specific CTL clones, has been postulated to occur because of sustained high-level viremia. Animal models suggested that CTL could expand maximally and then be deleted in the presence of a high viral load *(53)*. Early studies of Vβ TCR subsets in humans suggested this might also be the case in HIV infection *(54)*. However, more recent studies evaluating antigen-specific CTL clones have demonstrated the persistence of these cells in the face of a high antigen load *(55,56)*. If the defect is not the absence of CTL clones, but rather a lack of function, or a lack of ability to expand in the presence of antigen, these more recent data suggest that efforts to augment these responses could prove beneficial.

This inability to maintain CTL function, despite the physical presence of CTL clones, may be related to inadequate T-helper cell function. More recent studies in LCMV infection show that although deletion of CTLs is possible, the persistence of virus can more often be explained by a silenced phenotype of CTLs that are present (as defined by tetramer staining) but unable to secrete IFN-γ in response to antigenic stimulation *(5,6)*. Although this hypothesis has not yet been confirmed in the setting of HIV-1-infection, it suggests that efforts to restore helper function may increase CTL function.

One hypothesis that would explain the lack of T-helper function after HIV infection would be the deletion of activated CD4+ T-cells during the earliest stages of acute infection. Alternatively, these cells may undergo activation-induced cell death owing to overstimulation at the time of maximum virus load *(57)*. The result would be a lack of CD4 T-cell help, and therefore inadequate help to maintain CTLs with optimal function. In a manner similar to that seen in the LCMV model, CTLs may then be unable to protect against new viral variants that arise, or be unable to expand to sufficient levels to suppress viremia even in the absence of escape mutations *(56,58)*.

Immune Escape

Escape from established immune responses is likely to be a major factor for HIV disease progression, since the infidelity of the viral reverse transcriptase results in rapid generation of viral mutations, and viral diversity may be a substantial hurdle for HIV-specific immunotherapies. Even a single mutation within a defined CTL epitope can be sufficient to abrogate CTL recognition, either by altering residues that are critical for contact with the TCR or that are necessary for peptide binding to the HLA class I molecule. Some longitudinal studies have demonstrated escape from CTL recognition over the course of HIV infection *(59)*, or after adoptive transfer of HIV-specific CTLs *(60)*. Other studies have demonstrated that for some epitopes, lack of HLA binding may be a major reason for the lack of CTL recognition *(61)*. However, this is not a universal finding, and some mutations within CTL epitopes can be cross-recognized by HIV-specific CTLs *(62,63)*. Although mutations within viral regions flanking CTL epitopes may be another potential mechanism for immune escape, this has not been demonstrated in studies thus far *(64)*.

Successful approaches to immune-based therapy may need to target HIV-1 epitopes that are relatively conserved *(65)*; unfortunately, there are few available data describing CTL epitopes that do not tolerate variation. Immune-based therapy may be much more successful in subjects identified shortly after acute infection, when the viral quasispecies diversity is much more limited *(66)*, but this would limit the number of subjects that could be treated. Current approaches will rely on augmenting helper and CTL responses in subjects already suppressed on HAART in the hope that CTL responses able to recognize HIV variants will be able to suppress viral replication in the presence of adequate helper responses, or that in the presence of adequate help new CTL responses able to recognize potential escape variants will be generated.

IMMUNE RECONSTITUTION IN THE ERA OF HAART

Infection with HIV is associated with destruction of the thymic and lymph node architecture *(67)*, and before the advent of HAART there was speculation that irreversible damage might occur early after infection. Since the introduction of HAART, there is now hope that the immune system has the ability to recover after suppression of viral replication, which is reflected in the dramatic decrease in the incidence of opportunistic infections after successful HIV-specific therapy. The immune recovery inflammatory syndromes that have been described reflect the restoration of immunity against opportunistic infections. One report described five subjects with CD4 cell counts below 50 cells/mm^3 who developed fever and severe lymphadenitis 1–3 weeks after beginning indinavir therapy. Lymph node biopsies showed focal lymphadenitis caused by unsuspected *Mycobacterium avium* complex infection, which was probably caused by an increase in memory cells specific for the organism *(68)*. Similar syndromes have been described for CMV-specific immunity (termed immune recovery vitritis) *(69–71)*, and hepatitis C virus infection *(72)*. These clinical responses to the suppression of HIV viremia are consistent with the increases in CD4+ T-cell numbers seen in most subjects.

Dramatic rises in CD4+ T-cell numbers have been documented shortly after the initiation of protease inhibitor-containing regimens *(73–75)*. Although these initial CD4+ T-cell increases were owing to increases in the numbers of circulating memory cells during the first 4 months, there was a subsequent significant increase in the numbers of circulating naive cells. Functional studies revealed increases in proliferative responses to recall antigens and mitogens, but no recovery of HIV-1-specific T-cell responses *(76)*. Other studies have had similar results, with some showing modest recovery of HIV-specific helper responses *(77–79)*. However, other studies have shown declines in preexisting HIV-specific immune responses in the presence of HAART, presumably owing to the lack of ongoing antigenic stimulation needed to maintain these responses over the chronic phase of infection *(80–83)*. Some studies have suggested that there may be restoration of a broader T-cell repertoire with HAART *(84)*, but this has not always been observed *(85)*. The HAART-induced increases in naive cells are an extremely promising result. Naive cell immune reconstitution and the relative lack of recovery of HIV-1-specific immunity strengthen the rationale for pursuing therapeutic vaccination in infected persons.

THYMIC FUNCTION

A widely held view of thymic function was that it decreased with age and that the thymus was either not present or not functional in adults. This was based on observations in humans and animal models showing that the volume of thymic tissue decreased with age and that the production of naive T-cells after myeloablative chemotherapy was delayed in adults versus children *(86,87)*. HIV is thought to cause thymic dysfunction by its ability to infect thymocytes as well as thymic epithelium *(88)*.

A computed tomographic study that evaluated the volume of thymic tissue and its relationship to circulating naive cells in HIV-positive subjects demonstrated abundant thymic tissue in most HIV-1-seropositive adults aged 20–59 years; this was associated with higher CD4 cell counts and numbers of circulating naive T-cells *(89)*. A subsequent study demonstrated an increase in thymic output as measured by TCR excision circles (TRECs) after the initiation of HAART *(90)*, suggesting that the thymus remains active into adult life and that HAART can increase thymic output. Despite the relatively preserved thymic function in adulthood, there are age-related declines in thymic function. A published case of a 55-year-old patient with declining CD4+ T-cell numbers with an undetectable viral load and slow increases in CD4+ T-cell number after the initiation of HAART highlights the fact that there may be limits to thymic function, and therefore to immune reconstitution *(91)*. It remains to be seen how much of a hurdle this will be toward immune reconstitution with HIV-specific immunotherapies.

APPROACHES TO IMMUNE-BASED THERAPY IN HIV INFECTION

Attempts have been made to reconstitute immunity in HIV infection since AIDS was first characterized. These early approaches to immune reconstitution included allogeneic and syngeneic bone marrow transplantation, donor lymphocyte infusions, therapeutic vaccination, cytokine infusions, and various combinations of these. No consistent clinical benefit was found, which was directly related to the inability to control viremia. The prospects for immune reconstitution are more realistic with the advent of HAART, and these approaches can now be viewed from a fresh perspective.

Nonspecific Immunotherapy

Although efforts to augment immune responses are covered elsewhere in other chapters, they may play a role in combination with HIV-specific immunotherapies, so they will be briefly reviewed here. Since one of the major functions of T-lymphocytes is to secrete cytokines, these were natural areas of investigation after the immune deficits associated with AIDS were described. One of the most extensively studied immune-based therapies in HIV-infected persons has been interleukin-2 (IL-2). IL-2 is a cytokine secreted by activated T-lymphocytes that regulates lymphoid proliferation and maturation. An initial pilot study demonstrated increases in viral load caused by immune activation associated with IL-2 infusion *(92)*. However, in the presence of antiretroviral therapy, CD4 cell numbers doubled in subjects with baseline CD4+ T-cell numbers greater than 300 cells/mm^3 without significant increases in viremia *(93)*. Simpler regimens with lower doses have led to similar increases in CD4 cell counts but with less toxicity *(94)*. Trials thus far have been too small to discern a clinical benefit from increased CD4 cell numbers, but two large trials with clinical end points are now enrolling (ESPRIT and SILCAAT) and are designed to detect a decrease in HIV disease progression.

Although these increases in CD4+ cell numbers have not yet translated to clinical efficacy, they may provide a basis for virus-specific immunotherapy. Progressive HIV infection is associated with a greater loss of naive CD4 cells than of memory cells. The immune control of viral infections probably depends on a broad repertoire of virus-specific cells, and it has been shown that HIV leads to deletion of parts of the T-cell repertoire *(54)*. Although IL-2 administration is associated with polyclonal increases in both naive and memory cells in HIV-infected persons, TCR repertoire analysis has shown that defects in the repertoire are not corrected over the short term *(84)*. However, if naive cells are in fact generated by IL-2 administration, HIV-specific immunogens may allow subsets of HIV-specific T-cells to expand and may also permit mediated control of viremia.

IL-12 is another cytokine that is beginning to be tested in clinical trials. IL-12 is predominantly produced by activated antigen-presenting cells and has been shown to augment HIV-specific CTL function in vitro *(95–97)*. In combination with IL-12, HIV-specific immunogens may be much more effective at increasing HIV-specific CTL responses. This has been demonstrated with a DNA vaccine coexpressing IL-12 in a murine model of protective immunity against HSV-2 *(98)*.

Structured Treatment Interruption

One alternative to therapeutic vaccination is the use of the patient's own virus to stimulate virus-specific immune responses. The theory behind this approach relies on the efficacy of current HAART regiments. The ability to achieve substantial inhibition of viral replication allows for a controlled exposure to autologous virus after treatment interruption. An anecdotal case of a patient who was able to control viremia after a series of treatment interruptions sparked interest in this approach as a therapeutic modality. This subject was initially treated with HAART early after acute infection, but an intercurrent illness prompted discontinuation of antiretroviral medications. This was followed by a rise in viremia that was controlled with the reinstitution of HAART. However, subsequent discontinuations of therapy did not result in rebound viremia, and after 24 months off therapy this subject had viral load values persistently below 1000 copies/mL. This control of viremia was associated with persistent and vigorous T-helper cell and CTL responses *(99)*. Another report describing augmented immune responses in subjects with intermittent adherence to HAART also concluded that some subjects were able to control viremia *(100)*.

The philosophy behind this approach in individuals treated early after acute infection is that these subjects tend to have preserved helper T-cell responses *(43)*, a feature typically seen only in chronically infected subjects with control of viremia (sometimes referred to as long-term nonprogressors) *(44)*. The first study of treatment interruptions in this cohort of individuals showed control of viremia (<5000 copies/mL) in 5/9 individuals *(101)*. Evaluation of the immune responses in this cohort of subjects demonstrated augmented helper responses and an increase in the breadth and magnitude of HIV-specific CTL responses over the course of treatment interruptions *(66)*. This study required the reinstitution of antiretroviral therapy at defined times depending on the measured level of viremia. In a subsequent study in SIV-infected macaques, fixed intervals of treatment interruption led to similar control of viremia *(102)*, which would potentially make this approach more feasible in a clinical setting. These data would indicate that all persons with acute or early HIV infection should be considered for treatment with HAART, either for consideration of treatment interruptions, or to increase the likelihood that preserved immune responses would increase the effectiveness of immunotherapy regimens. Although a survival benefit has not yet been shown, the low level of steady-state viremia after successful structured treatment interruptions would predict enhanced survival *(103,104)*.

Despite the success of this approach in acutely infected subjects, efforts to replicate these results in chronically infected subjects have not met with great success *(105,106)*. One major difference in this approach in chronically infected subjects is that helper responses are not usually augmented, and even though naive cells can be generated, the dramatic suppression of HIV in the presence of HAART may not allow these cells to become immunologically active *(76)*. Furthermore, the virus becomes extremely diverse over the course of infection *(66)*, so treatment interruptions could be less effective if a substantial proportion of the quasispecies has escaped immune recognition. Finally, a potential pitfall of this approach is the emergence of drug resistance owing to exposure to suboptimal drug concentrations during the treatment interruptions, which is another reason that such studies should be carried out under carefully controlled conditions.

Therapeutic Vaccination

The prospect of reconstituting specific immune responses with therapeutic vaccines holds a great deal of appeal, but the results of early trials have been disappointing. This is perhaps not surprising since several trials were initiated in the pre-HAART era. HIV infection is associated with immune activation, as is infection with most viral agents. However, HIV is unique in that the very T-cells that are activated to respond to the infecting agent are themselves infected and subsequently either lost, or inactivated. Another possible reason for therapeutic vaccine failures is that cellular activation initiated by these vaccines provides more targets for infection. With the advent of more potent antiretroviral therapy, it is now possible to protect cells from infection after immune activation. The accumulating evidence that a deficiency of HIV-specific immunity exists in subjects unable to control viremia makes this approach to immune reconstitution compelling.

Early trials focused on envelope-based vaccines, with disappointing results. These vaccines have induced HIV-1-specific T-helper cell responses in infected individuals, as well as increased titers of neutralizing antibodies *(107–110)*. However, an analysis of clinical endpoints failed to observe any benefit from vaccination *(111)*. In addition to the difficulty of performing these trials in the absence of HAART, part of the difficulty may also lie in choosing envelope as an immunogen. Envelope-specific proliferative responses have not been shown to correlate with control of viremia in the absence of HAART *(43,44)*. It has also been difficult to demonstrate neutralizing antibody induced by any of the current vaccine candidates, probably because neutralizing antibodies are directed against oligomeric envelopes on cell surfaces, and these cannot be induced with monomeric recombinant envelopes *(15,18,21,112,113)*. Finally, the extreme diversity of envelopes among HIV isolates makes the formulation of an envelope vaccine a challenge.

Remune is one of the most extensively studied therapeutic vaccine candidates. Originally proposed by Jonas Salk, this is an inactivated whole virus vaccine that is inactivated and depleted of the envelope protein during synthesis *(114,115)*. It is derived from a virus originally obtained in Zaire and contains a clade A envelope and clade G gag. Thus far, this vaccine has been administered to over 3000 subjects, with few side effects. Also, in the presence of HAART, Remune has induced significant Gag-specific T-helper cell responses in HIV-infected persons, which were robust in some vaccine recipients *(116)* and have previously only been observed in subjects with long-term nonprogressive HIV infection with control of viremia *(43,44,117)*. A recent trial of over 2500 subjects randomized to receive Remune or placebo failed to detect any evidence of vaccination with Remune on clinical end points. Although there was no benefit to vaccination, this was during the time that PI-containing HAART regimens were becoming the standard of care. In a subgroup analysis of subjects vaccinated in the presence of HAART, subjects that had rebound viremia could not be differentiated from subjects failing because of drug side effects *(118)*. So, although there was no benefit from this intent-to-treat analysis, the possibility remains that a benefit from Remune can be obtained in subjects with relatively intact immune systems in the presence of HAART.

Other approaches are currently being tested or will soon be tested in clinical trials. Canarypox vectors are constructed from an avian virus with limited ability to replicate in mammalian cells. Clinical trials with HIV-negative individuals have shown that vaccines based on these constructs are able to elicit weak HIV-specific CTL responses, T-helper responses, and antibodies *(119–122)*. A small trial has demonstrated the safety of these constructs in HIV-seropositive individuals, but there are no data on the ability of these vaccines to augment HIV-specific immune responses *(123)*. Immunogenicity data from several trials will be available within the next 1–2 years.

Another promising approach toward immune reconstitution will involve the use of mature, monocyte-derived dendritic cells. These are extremely potent antigen-presenting cells that have been shown to generate de novo helper immune responses efficiently, as well as augment memory CTL responses in vivo *(124–126)*. They can be thought of as nature's adjuvant and have already been shown to increase the immunogenicity of Canarypox constructs in HIV-seronegative individuals *(127)*.

Other promising immunogens soon to enter clinical trials include Venezuelan equine encephalitis virus vectors *(128,129)*, DNA vaccines *(130–133)*, and vaccines based on adenovirus vectors *(134)*. It has recently been demonstrated that Tat-specific immune responses are important for the initial containment of SIV replication, so selective augmentation of these responses might also be beneficial *(135)*.

CONCLUSIONS

With the ability to suppress HIV replication with HAART, and with evidence that treatment of infected subjects early after infection allows preservation of immune responses and potential control of HIV replication in the absence of HAART, there is reason to be optimistic that immune control of HIV infection can be achieved. However, there are a number of factors that provide potential hurdles for long-term immune control of HIV, especially in chronically infected persons. With a well-established, diverse quasispecies firmly entrenched, there may be HIV variants present that are not recognized by the host's CTL response, or that contain mutations within CTL epitopes that diminish binding to HLA class I molecules. In either case, augmentation of CTL responses with therapies representing consensus sequences may not be effective. However, it is possible that the ability to stimulate robust helper responses may allow the immune system to evolve continuously, to recognize new virus variants.

These hurdles make the prospect for immune-mediated control of virus replication challenging. However, the recent demonstration that immune-mediated control of HIV is possible, combined with several new constructs now entering clinical trials, provides a strong rationale to pursue HIV-specific immunotherapy for the treatment of HIV infection.

REFERENCES

1. Khanna R, Burrows SR. Role of cytotoxic T lymphocytes in Epstein-Barr virus-associated diseases. Annu Rev Microbiol 2000; 54:19.
2. Rickinson AB, Moss DJ. Human cytotoxic T lymphocyte responses to Epstein-Barr virus infection. Annu Rev Immunol 1997; 15:405.
3. Murali-Krishna K, Altman JD, Suresh M, et al. Counting antigen-specific CD8 T cells: a reevaluation of bystander activation during viral infection. Immunity 1998; 8:177.
4. Butz EA, Bevan MJ. Massive expansion of antigen-specific CD8+ T cells during an acute virus infection. Immunity 1998; 8:167.
5. Zajac AJ, Blattman JN, Murali-Krishna K, et al. Viral immune evasion due to persistence of activated T cells without effector function. J Exp Med 1998; 188:2205.
6. Kalams SA, Walker BD. The critical need for CD4 help in maintaining effective cytotoxic T lymphocyte responses. J Exp Med 1998; 188:2199.
7. Buchbinder SP, Katz MH, Hessol NA, O'Malley PM, Holmberg SD. Long-term HIV-1 infection without immunologic progression. Aids 1994; 8:1123.
8. Alexander L, Weiskopf E, Greenough TC, et al. Unusual polymorphisms in human immunodeficiency virus type 1 associated with nonprogressive infection. J Virol 2000; 74:4361.

9. Daniel MD, Kirchhoff F, Czajak SC, Sehgal PK, Desrosiers RC. Protective effects of a live attenuated SIV vaccine with a deletion in the *nef* gene. Science 1992; 258:1938.

10. Deacon NJ, Tsykin A, Solomon A, et al. Genomic structure of an attenuated quasi species of HIV-1 from a blood transfusion donor and recipients. Science 1995; 270:988.

11. Michael NL, Chang G, Louie LG, et al. The role of viral phenotype and CCR-5 gene defects in HIV-1 transmission and disease progression. Nat Med 1997; 3:338.

12. Smith MW, Dean M, Carrington M, et al. Contrasting genetic influence of CCR2 and CCR5 variants on HIV-1 infection and disease progression. Hemophilia Growth and Development Study (HGDS), Multicenter AIDS Cohort Study (MACS), Multicenter Hemophilia Cohort Study (MHCS), San Francisco City Cohort (SFCC), ALIVE Study. Science 1997; 277:959.

13. Poignard P, Sabbe R, Picchio GR, et al. Neutralizing antibodies have limited effects on the control of established HIV-1 infection in vivo. Immunity 1999; 10:431.

14. Pilgrim AK, Pantaleo G, Cohen OJ, et al. Neutralizing antibody responses to human immunodeficiency virus type 1 in primary infection and long-term-nonprogressive infection. J Infect Dis 1997; 176:924.

15. Fouts TR, Binley JM, Trkola A, Robinson JE, Moore JP. Neutralization of the human immunodeficiency virus type 1 primary isolate JR-FL by human monoclonal antibodies correlates with antibody binding to the oligomeric form of the envelope glycoprotein complex. J Virol 1997; 71:2779.

16. Mo H, Stamatatos L, Ip JE, et al. Human immunodeficiency virus type 1 mutants that escape neutralization by human monoclonal antibody IgG1b12. off. J Virol 1997; 71:6869.

17. Parren PW, Wang M, Trkola A, et al. Antibody neutralization-resistant primary isolates of human immunodeficiency virus type 1. J Virol 1998; 72:10270.

18. Burton DR. A vaccine for HIV type 1: the antibody perspective. [Review] [76 refs]. Proc Natl Acad Sci USA 1997; 94:10018.

19. Belshe RB, Graham BS, Keefer MC, et al. 1994. Neutralizing antibodies to HIV-1 in seronegative volunteers immunized with recombinant gp120 from the MN strain of HIV-1. NIAID AIDS Vaccine Clinical Trials Network. Jama 1994; 272:475.

20. Mascola JR, Snyder SW, Weislow OS, et al. Immunization with envelope subunit vaccine products elicits neutralizing antibodies against laboratory-adapted but not primary isolates of human immunodeficiency virus type 1. The National Institute of Allergy and Infectious Diseases AIDS Vaccine Evaluation Group. J Infect Dis 1996; 173:340.

21. Connor RI, Korber BT, Graham BS, et al. Immunological and virological analyses of persons infected by human immunodeficiency virus type 1 while participating in trials of recombinant gp120 subunit vaccines. J Virol 1998; 72:1552.

22. Letvin NL. Progress in the development of an HIV-1 vaccine. Science 1998; 280:1875.

23. Moore JP, Cao Y, Qing L, et al. Primary isolates of human immunodeficiency virus type 1 are relatively resistant to neutralization by monoclonal antibodies to gp120, and their neutralization is not predicted by studies with monomeric gp120. J Virol 1995; 69:101.

24. Reitter JN, Means RE, Desrosiers RC. A role for carbohydrates in immune evasion in AIDS. Nat Med 1998; 4:679.

25. Wyatt R, Kwong PD, Desjardins E, et al. The antigenic structure of the HIV gp120 envelope glycoprotein. Nature 1998; 393:705.

26. Yang OO, Kalams SA, Rosenzweig M, et al. Efficient lysis of human immunodeficiency virus type 1-infected cells by cytotoxic T lymphocytes. J Virol 1996; 70:5799.

27. Yang OO, Kalams SA, Trocha A, et al. Suppression of human immunodeficiency virus type 1 replication by CD8+ cells: evidence for HLA class I-restricted triggering of cytolytic and noncytolytic mechanisms. J Virol 1997; 71:3120.

28. Wagner L, Yang OO, Garcia-Zepeda EA, et al. Beta-chemokines are released from HIV-1-specific cytolytic T-cell granules complexed to proteoglycans. Nature 1998; 391:908.

29. Brander C, Hartman KE, Trocha AK, et al. Lack of strong immune selection pressure by the immunodominant, HLA-A*0201-restricted cytotoxic T lymphocyte response in chronic human immunodeficiency virus-1 infection. J Clin Invest 1998; 101:2559.
30. Goulder PJ, Sewell AK, Lalloo DG, et al. Patterns of immunodominance in HIV-1-specific cytotoxic T lymphocyte responses in two human histocompatibility leukocyte antigens (HLA)-identical siblings with HLA-A*0201 are influenced by epitope mutation. J Exp Med 1997; 185:1423.
31. Goulder PJR, Altfeld MA, Rosenberg ES, et al. Substantial differences in specificity of HIV-specific cytotoxic T-cells in acute and chronic HIV infection. J Exp Med 2001; 193:181.
32. Betts MR, Casazza JP, Patterson BA, et al. Putative immunodominant human immunodeficiency virus-specific CD8(+) T-cell responses cannot be predicted by major histocompatibility complex class I haplotype. J Virol 2000; 74:9144.
33. Day CL, Shea AK, Altfeld MA, et al. Relative dominance of epitope-specific cytotoxic T-lymphocyte responses in human immunodeficiency virus type 1-infected persons with shared HLA alleles. J Virol 2001; 75:6279.
34. Waldrop SL, Davis KA, Maino VC, Picker LJ. 1998. Normal human CD4+ memory T cells display broad heterogeneity in their activation threshold for cytokine synthesis. J Immunol 1998; 161:5284.
35. Altman JD, Moss PAH, Goulder PJR, et al. Phenotypic analysis of antigen-specific T lymphocytes [published erratum appears in Science 1998;280:1821]. Science 1996; 274:94.
36. Ogg GS, Jin X, Bonhoeffer S, et al. Quantitation of HIV-1-specific cytotoxic T lymphocytes and plasma load of viral RNA. Science 1998; 279:2103.
37. Schmitz JE, Kuroda MJ, Santra S, et al. Control of viremia in simian immunodeficiency virus infection by CD8+ lymphocytes. Science 1999; 283:857.
38. Jin X, Bauer DE, Tuttleton SE, et al. Dramatic rise in plasma viremia after CD8(+) T cell depletion in simian immunodeficiency virus-infected macaques. J Exp Med 1999; 189:991.
39. Phillips AN. Reduction of HIV concentration during acute infection: independence from a specific immune response. Science 1996; 271:497.
40. Matloubian M, Concepcion RJ, Ahmed R. CD4+ T cells are required to sustain CD8+ cytotoxic T-cell responses during chronic viral infection. J Virol 1994; 68:8056.
41. Battegay M, Moskophidis D, Rahemtulla A, Hengartner H, Mak TW, Zinkernagel RM. Enhanced establishment of a virus carrier state in adult CD4+ T-cell-deficient mice. J Virol 1994; 68:4700.
42. von Herrath MG, Yokoyama M, Dockter J, Oldstone MB, Whitton JL. CD4-deficient mice have reduced levels of memory cytotoxic T lymphocytes after immunization and show diminished resistance to subsequent virus challenge. J Virol 1996; 70:1072.
43. Rosenberg ES, Billingsley JM, Caliendo AM, et al. Vigorous HIV-1-specific CD4+ T cell responses associated with control of viremia. Science 1997; 278:1447.
44. Kalams SA, Buchbinder SP, Rosenberg ES, et al. Association between virus-specific cytotoxic T-lymphocyte and helper responses in human immunodeficiency virus type 1 infection. J Virol 1999; 73:6715.
45. Malhotra U, Berrey MM, Huang Y, et al. Effect of combination antiretroviral therapy on T-cell immunity in acute human immunodeficiency virus type 1 infection. J Infect Dis 2000; 181:121.
46. Oxenius A, Price DA, Easterbrook PJ, et al. Early highly active antiretroviral therapy for acute HIV-1 infection preserves immune function of CD8+ and CD4+ T lymphocytes. Proc Natl Acad Sci USA 2000; 97:3382.
47. Harrer T, Harrer E, Kalams SA, et al. Cytotoxic T lymphocytes in asymptomatic long-term nonprogressing HIV-1 infection. Breadth and specificity of the response and relation to in vivo viral quasispecies in a person with prolonged infection and low viral load. J Immunol 1996; 156:2616.

48. Harrer T, Harrer E, Kalams SA, et al. Strong cytotoxic T cell and weak neutralizing antibody responses in a subset of persons with stable nonprogressing HIV type 1 infection. AIDS Res Hum Retroviruses 1996; 12:585.

49. Carmichael A, Jin X, Sissons P, Borysiewicz L. Quantitative analysis of the human immunodeficiency virus type 1 (HIV-1)-specific cytotoxic T lymphocyte (CTL) response at different stages of HIV-1 infection: differential CTL responses to HIV-1 and Epstein-Barr virus in late disease. J Exp Med 1993; 177:249.

50. Klein MR, van Baalen CA, Holwerda AM, et al. Kinetics of Gag-specific cytotoxic T lymphocyte responses during the clinical course of HIV-1 infection: a longitudinal analysis of rapid progressors and long-term asymptomatics. J Exp Med 1995; 181:1365.

51. Rinaldo C, Huang XL, Fan ZF, et al. High levels of anti-human immunodeficiency virus type 1 (HIV-1) memory cytotoxic T-lymphocyte activity and low viral load are associated with lack of disease in HIV-1-infected long-term nonprogressors. J Virol 1995; 69:5838.

52. Miedema F, Meyaard L, Koot M, et al. Changing virus-host interactions in the course of HIV-1 infection [Review] [198 refs]. Immunol Rev 1994; 140:35.

53. Moskophidis D, Lechner F, Pircher H, Zinkernagel RM. Virus persistence in acutely infected immunocompetent mice by exhaustion of antiviral cytotoxic effector T cells [published erratum appears in Nature 1993;364:262]. Nature 1993; 362:758.

54. Pantaleo G, Soudeyns H, Demarest JF, et al. Evidence for rapid disappearance of initially expanded HIV-specific CD8+ T cell clones during primary HIV infection. Proc Natl Acad Sci USA 1997; 94:9848.

55. Brander C, Goulder PJ, Luzuriaga K, et al. Persistent HIV-1-specific CTL clonal expansion despite high viral burden post in utero HIV-1 infection. J Immunol 1999; 162:4796.

56. Islam SA, Hay CM, Hartman KE, et al. Persistence of human immunodeficiency virus type 1-specific cytotoxic T-lymphocyte clones in a subject with rapid disease progression. J Virol 2001; 75:4907.

57. Abbas AK. Die and let live: eliminating dangerous lymphocytes. Cell 1996; 84:655.

58. Hay CM, Ruhl DJ, Basgoz NO, et al. Lack of viral escape and defective in vivo activation of human immunodeficiency virus type 1-specific cytotoxic T lymphocytes in rapidly progressive infection. J Virol 1999; 73:5509.

59. Borrow P, Lewicki H, Wei X, et al. Antiviral pressure exerted by HIV-1-specific cytotoxic T lymphocytes (CTLs) during primary infection demonstrated by rapid selection of CTL escape virus. Nat Med 1997; 3:205.

60. Koenig S, Conley AJ, Brewah YA, et al. Transfer of HIV-1-specific cytotoxic T lymphocytes to an AIDS patient leads to selection for mutant HIV variants and subsequent disease progression. Nat Med 1995; 1:330.

61. Goulder PJ, Phillips RE, Colbert RA, et al. Late escape from an immunodominant cytotoxic T-lymphocyte response associated with progression to AIDS. Nat Med 1997; 3:212.

62. Kalams SA, Johnson RP, Dynan MJ, et al. T cell receptor usage and fine specificity of human immunodeficiency virus 1-specific cytotoxic T lymphocyte clones: analysis of quasispecies recognition reveals a dominant response directed against a minor in vivo variant. J Exp Med 1996; 183:1669.

63. Cao H, Kanki P, Sankale JL, et al. Cytotoxic T-lymphocyte cross-reactivity among different human immunodeficiency virus type 1 clades: implications for vaccine development. J Virol 1997; 71:8615.

64. Brander C, Yang OO, Jones NG, et al. Efficient processing of the immunodominant, HLA-A*0201-restricted human immunodeficiency virus type 1 cytotoxic T-lymphocyte epitope despite multiple variations in the epitope flanking sequences. J Virol 1999; 73:10191.

65. Altfeld MA, Livingston B, Reshamwala N, et al. Identification of novel HLA-A2-restricted human immunodeficiency virus type 1-specific cytotoxic T-lymphocyte epitopes predicted by the HLA-A2 supertype peptide-binding motif. J Virol 2001; 75:1301.

66. Altfeld M, Rosenberg ES, Shankarappa R, et al. Cellular imune responses and viral diversity in individuals treated during acute and early HIV-1 infection. J Exp Med 2001; 193:169.

67. Pantaleo G, Graziosi C, Demarest JF, et al. Role of lymphoid organs in the pathogenesis of human immunodeficiency virus (HIV) infection [Review]. Immunol Rev 1994; 40:105.

68. Race EM, Adelson-Mitty J, Kriegel GR, et al. Focal mycobacterial lymphadenitis following initiation of protease-inhibitor therapy in patients with advanced HIV-1 disease. Lancet 1998; 351:252.

69. Karavellas MP, Lowder CY, Macdonald C, Avila CP, Freeman WR. Immune recovery vitritis associated with inactive cytomegalovirus retinitis: a new syndrome. Arch Ophthalmol 1998; 116:169.

70. Karavellas MP, Plummer DJ, Macdonald JC, et al. Incidence of immune recovery vitritis in cytomegalovirus retinitis patients following institution of successful highly active antiretroviral therapy. J Infect Dis 1999; 179:697.

71. Reed JB, Schwab IR, Gordon J, Morse LS. Regression of cytomegalovirus retinitis associated with protease-inhibitor treatment in patients with AIDS. Am J Ophthalmol 1997; 124:199.

72. John M, Flexman J, French MA. Hepatitis C virus-associated hepatitis following treatment of HIV-infected patients with HIV protease inhibitors: an immune restoration disease? AIDS 1998; 12:2289.

73. Ho DD, Neumann AU, Perelson AS, Chen W, Leonard JM, Markowitz M. Rapid turnover of plasma virions and CD4 lymphocytes in HIV-1 infection. Nature 1995; 373:123.

74. Perelson AS, Neumann AU, Markowitz M, Leonard JM, Ho DD. HIV-1 dynamics in vivo: virion clearance rate, infected cell life-span, and viral generation time. Science 1996; 271:1582.

75. Perelson AS, Essunger P, Cao Y, et al. Decay characteristics of HIV-1-infected compartments during combination therapy. Nature 1997; 387:188.

76. Autran B, Carcelain G, Li TS, et al. Positive effects of combined antiretroviral therapy on CD4+ T cell homeostasis and function in advanced HIV disease. Science 1997; 277:112.

77. Kelleher AD, Carr A, Zaunders J, Cooper DA. Alterations in the immune response of human immunodeficiency virus (HIV)-infected subjects treated with an HIV-specific protease inhibitor, ritonavir. J Infect Dis 1996; 173:321.

78. Angel JB, Kumar A, Parato K, et al. Improvement in cell-mediated immune function during potent anti-human immunodeficiency virus therapy with ritonavir plus saquinavir. J Infect Dis 1998; 177:898.

79. Li TS, Tubiana R, Katlama C, Calvez V, Ait Mohand H, Autran B. Long-lasting recovery in CD4 T-cell function and viral-load reduction after highly active antiretroviral therapy in advanced HIV-1 disease. Lancet 1998; 351:1682.

80. Pitcher CJ, Quittner C, Peterson DM, et al. HIV-1-specific CD4+ T cells are detectable in most individuals with active HIV-1 infection, but decline with prolonged viral suppression. Nat Med 1999; 5:518.

81. Ogg GS, Jin X, Bonhoeffer S, et al. Decay kinetics of human immunodeficiency virus-specific effector cytotoxic T lymphocytes after combination antiretroviral therapy. J Virol 1999; 73:797.

82. Markowitz M, Vesanen M, Tenner-Racz K, et al. The effect of commencing combination antiretroviral therapy soon after human immunodeficiency virus type 1 infection on viral replication and antiviral immune responses. J Infect Dis 1999; 179:527.

83. Kalams SA, Goulder PJ, Shea AK, et al. Levels of human immunodeficiency virus type 1-specific cytotoxic T-lymphocyte effector and memory responses decline after suppression of viremia with highly active antiretroviral therapy. J Virol 1999; 73:6721.

84. Connors M, Kovacs JA, Krevat S, et al. HIV infection induces changes in CD4+ T-cell phenotype and depletions within the CD4+ T-cell repertoire that are not immediately restored by antiviral or immune-based therapies. Nat Med 1997; 3:533.

85. Lederman MM, Connick E, Landay A, et al. Immunologic responses associated with 12 weeks of combination antiretroviral therapy consisting of zidovudine, lamivudine, and ritonavir: results of AIDS Clinical Trials Group Protocol 315. J Infect Dis 1998; 178:70.

86. Mackall CL, Fleisher TA, Brown MR, et al. Lymphocyte depletion during treatment with intensive chemotherapy for cancer. Blood 1994; 84:2221.

87. Mackall CL, Fleisher TA, Brown MR, et al. Age, thymopoiesis, and CD4+ T-lymphocyte regeneration after intensive chemotherapy. N Engl J Med 1995; 332:143.

88. McCune JM. Thymic function in HIV-1 disease. Semin Immunol 1997; 9:397.

89. McCune JM, Loftus R, Schmidt DK, et al. High prevalence of thymic tissue in adults with human immunodeficiency virus-1 infection. J Clin Invest 1998; 101:2301.

90. Douek DC, McFarland RD, Keiser PH, et al. Changes in thymic function with age and during the treatment of HIV infection. Nature 1998; 396:690.

91. Greenough TC, Sullivan JL, Desrosiers RC. 1999. Declining CD4 T-cell counts in a person infected with nef-deleted HIV-1. N Engl J Med 1999; 340:236.

92. Kovacs JA, Vogel S, Albert, JM, et al. Controlled trial of interleukin-2 infusions in patients infected with the human immunodeficiency virus. N Engl J Med 1996; 335:1350.

93. Kovacs JA, Imamichi H, Vogel S, et al. Effects of intermittent interleukin-2 therapy on plasma and tissue human immunodeficiency virus levels and quasi-species expression. J Infect Dis 2000; 182:1063.

94. Davey RT, Jr, Chaitt DG, Albert JM, et al. A randomized trial of high- versus low-dose subcutaneous interleukin-2 outpatient therapy for early human immunodeficiency virus type 1 infection. J Infect Dis 1999; 179:849.

95. McFarland EJ, Harding PA, McWhinney S, Schooley RT, Kuritzkes DR. In vitro effects of IL-12 on HIV-1-specific CTL lines from HIV-1-infected children. J Immunol 1998; 161:513.

96. Landay AL, Clerici M, Hashemi F, Kessler H, Berzofsky JA, Shearer GM. In vitro restoration of T cell immune function in human immunodeficiency virus-positive persons: effects of interleukin (IL)-12 and anti-IL-10. J Infect Dis 1996; 173:1085.

97. Clerici M, Lucey DR, Berzofsky JA, et al. Restoration of HIV-specific cell-mediated immune responses by interleukin-12 in vitro. Science 1993; 262:1721.

98. Kim JJ, Ayyavoo V, Bagarazzi ML, et al. In vivo engineering of a cellular immune response by coadministration of IL-12 expression vector with a DNA immunogen. J Immunol 1997; 158:816.

99. Lisziewicz J, Rosenberg E, Lieberman J, et al. Control of HIV despite the discontinuation of antiretroviral therapy. N Engl J Med 1999; 340:1683.

100. Ortiz GM, Nixon DF, Trkola A, et al. HIV-1-specific immune responses in subjects who temporarily contain virus replication after discontinuation of highly active antiretroviral therapy. J Clini Invest 1999; 104:R13.

101. Rosenberg ES, Altfeld M, Poon SH, et al. Immune control of HIV-1 after early treatment of acute infection. Nature 2000; 407:523.

102. Lori F, Lewis MG, Xu J, et al. Control of SIV rebound through structured treatment interruptions during early infection. Science 2000; 290:1591.

103. Lyles RH, Munoz A, Yamashita TE, et al. Natural history of human immunodeficiency virus type 1 viremia after seroconversion and proximal to AIDS in a large cohort of homosexual men. Multicenter AIDS Cohort Study. J Infect Dis 2000; 181:872.

104. Mellors JW, Rinaldo CR Jr, Gupta P, White RM, Todd JA, Kingsley LA. Prognosis in HIV-1 infection predicted by the quantity of virus in plasma. Science 1996; 272:1167.

105. Ruiz L, Carcelainb G, Martínez-Picadoa J, et al. HIV dynamics and T-cell immunity after three structured treatment interruptions in chronic HIV-1 infection. AIDS 2001; 15:F19.

106. Garcia F, Plana M, Ortiz GM, et al. The virological and immunological consequences of structured treatment interruptions in chronic HIV-1 infection. AIDS 2001; 15:F29.

107. Redfield RR, Birx DL, Ketter N, et al. A phase I evaluation of the safety and immunogenicity of vaccination with recombinant gp160 in patients with early human immunodeficiency

virus infection. Military Medical Consortium for Applied Retroviral Research. N Engl J Med 1991; 324:1677.

108. Sitz KV, Ratto-Kim S, Hodgkins AS, Robb ML, Birx DL. Proliferative responses to human immunodeficiency virus type 1 (HIV-1) gp120 peptides in HIV-1-infected individuals immunized with HIV-1 rgp120 or rgp160 compared with nonimmunized and uninfected controls. J Infect Dis 1999; 179:817.

109. Ratto-Kim S, Sitz KV, Garner RP, et al. Repeated immunization with recombinant gp160 human immunodeficiency virus (HIV) envelope protein in early HIV-1 infection: evaluation of the T cell proliferative response. J Infect Dis 1999; 179:337.

110. Schooley RT, Spino C, Kuritzkes D, et al. Two double-blinded, randomized, comparative trials of 4 human immunodeficiency virus type 1 (HIV-1) envelope vaccines in HIV-1-infected individuals across a spectrum of disease severity: AIDS Clinical Trials Groups 209 and 214. J Infect Dis 2000; 182:1357.

111. Birx DL, Loomis-Price LD, Aronson N, et al. Efficacy testing of recombinant human immunodeficiency virus (HIV) gp160 as a therapeutic vaccine in early-stage HIV-1-infected volunteers. rgp160 Phase II Vaccine Investigators. J Infect Dis 2000; 181:881.

112. Sattentau QJ, Moore JP. Human immunodeficiency virus type 1 neutralization is determined by epitope exposure on the gp120 oligomer. J Exp Med 1995; 182:185.

113. Moore JP, Sodroski J. Antibody cross-competition analysis of the human immunodeficiency virus type 1 gp120 exterior envelope glycoprotein. J Virol 1996; 70:1863.

114. Trauger RJ, Ferre F, Daigle AE, et al. Effect of immunization with inactivated gp120-depleted human immunodeficiency virus type 1 (HIV-1) immunogen on HIV-1 immunity, viral DNA, and percentage of CD4 cells. J Infect Dis 1994; 169:1256.

115. Trauger RJ, Daigle AE, Giermakowska W, Moss RB, Jensen F, Carlo DJ. 1995. Safety and immunogenicity of a gp120-depleted, inactivated HIV-1 immunogen: results of a double-blind, adjuvant controlled trial. J Acquir Immun Defic Syndr 1995; 10 (Suppl 2):S74.

116. Moss RB, Giermakowska W, Wallace MR, Savary J, Jensen F, Carlo DJ. T-helper-cell proliferative responses to whole-killed human immunodeficiency virus type 1 (HIV-1) and p24 antigens of different clades in HIV-1-infected subjects vaccinated with HIV-1 immunogen (Remune). Clin Diagn Lab Immunol 2000; 7:724.

117. Pontesilli O, Carotenuto P, Kerkhof-Garde SR, et al. Lymphoproliferative response to HIV type 1 p24 in long-term survivors of HIV type 1 infection is predictive of persistent AIDS-free infection. AIDS Res Hum Retroviruses 1999; 15:973.

118. Kahn JO, Cherng DW, Mayer K, Murray H, Lagakos S. Evaluation of HIV-1 immunogen, an immunologic modifier, administered to patients infected with HIV having 300 to 549 × 10(6)/L CD4 cell counts: a randomized controlled trial. JAMA 2000; 284:2193.

119. Egan MA, Pavlat WA, Tartaglia J, et al. Induction of human immunodeficiency virus type 1 (HIV-1)-specific cytolytic T lymphocyte responses in seronegative adults by a nonreplicating, host-range-restricted canarypox vector (ALVAC) carrying the HIV-1MN env gene. J Infect Dis 1995; 171:1623.

120. Clements-Mann ML, Weinhold K, Matthews TJ, et al. Immune responses to human immunodeficiency virus (HIV) type 1 induced by canarypox expressing HIV-1MN gp120, HIV-1SF2 recombinant gp120, or both vaccines in seronegative adults. NIAID AIDS Vaccine Evaluation Group. J Infect Dis 1998; 177:1230.

121. Ferrari G, Berend C, Ottinger J, et al. Replication-defective canarypox (ALVAC) vectors effectively activate anti-human immunodeficiency virus-1 cytotoxic T lymphocytes present in infected patients: implications for antigen-specific immunotherapy. Blood 1997; 90:2406.

122. Evans TG, Keefer MC, Weinhold KJ, et al. A canarypox vaccine expressing multiple human immunodeficiency virus type 1 genes given alone or with rgp120 elicits broad and durable CD8+ cytotoxic T lymphocyte responses in seronegative volunteers. J Infect Dis 1999; 180:290.

123. Tubiana R, Gomard E, Fleury H, et al. Vaccine therapy in early HIV-1 infection using a recombinant canarypox virus expressing gp160MN (ALVAC-HIV): a double-blind controlled randomized study of safety and immunogenicity [letter]. AIDS 1997; 11:819.

124. Dhodapkar MV, Krasovsky J, Steinman RM, Bhardwaj N. Mature dendritic cells boost functionally superior CD8(+) T-cell in humans without foreign helper epitopes. J Clin Invest 2000; 105:R9.

125. Dhodapkar MV, Steinman RM, Sapp M, et al. Rapid generation of broad T-cell immunity in humans after a single injection of mature dendritic cells. J Clin Invest 1999; 104:173.

126. Dhodapkar MV, Steinman RM, Krasovsky J, Munz C, Bhardwaj N. Antigen-specific inhibition of effector T cell function in humans after injection of immature dendritic cells. J Exp Med 2001; 193:233.

127. Engelmayer J, Larsson M, Lee A, et al. Mature dendritic cells infected with canarypox virus elicit strong anti-human immunodeficiency virus CD8+ and CD4+ T-cell responses from chronically infected individuals. J Virol 2001; 75:2142.

128. Caley IJ, Betts MR, Irlbeck DM, et al. Humoral, mucosal, and cellular immunity in response to a human immunodeficiency virus type 1 immunogen expressed by a Venezuelan equine encephalitis virus vaccine vector. J Virol 1997; 71:3031.

129. Davis NL, Caley IJ, Brown KW, et al. Vaccination of macaques against pathogenic simian immunodeficiency virus with Venezuelan equine encephalitis virus replicon particles. [erratum appears in J Virol 2000;74:3430]. J Virol 2000; 74:371.

130. Egan MA, Charini WA, Kuroda MJ, et al. Simian immunodeficiency virus (SIV) gag DNA-vaccinated rhesus monkeys develop secondary cytotoxic T-lymphocyte responses and control viral replication after pathogenic SIV infection. J Virol 2000; 74:7485.

131. Lu S, Arthos J, Montefiori DC, et al. Simian immunodeficiency virus DNA vaccine trial in macaques. J Virol 1996; 70:3978.

132. Barouch DH, Santra S, Schmitz JE, et al. Control of viremia and prevention of clinical AIDS in rhesus monkeys by cytokine-augmented DNA vaccination. Science 2000; 290:486.

133. Amara RR, Villinger F, Altman JD, et al. Control of a mucosal challenge and prevention of AIDS by a multiprotein DNA/MVA vaccine. Science 2001; 292:69.

134. Buge SL, Murty L, Arora K, et al. Factors associated with slow disease progression in macaques immunized with an adenovirus-simian immunodeficiency virus (SIV) envelope priming-gp120 boosting regimen and challenged vaginally with SIVmac251. J Virol 1999; 73:7430.

135. Allen TM, O'Connor DH, Jing P, et al. Tat-specific cytotoxic T lymphocytes select for SIV escape variants during resolution of primary viraemia. Nature 2000; 407:386.

11

Passive Immunotherapy for HIV Infection

Jeffrey M. Jacobson

INTRODUCTION

The importance of humoral immunity in the prevention and control of natural HIV infection is unclear. Neutralizing antibody production can be detected soon after acute infection *(1)*. In addition, antibodies capable of neutralization and antibody-dependent cellular cytotoxicity (ADCC) remain present to a greater degree in those patients whose infections remain stable *(2,3)*. Patients with progressing infection tend to lose these antibody activities. Moreover, levels of HIV-directed maternal antibodies are associated with reduced transmission of HIV to the infant *(4–6)*. However, the nature of the relationship between strong humoral responses and control of infection has not been established. Strong HIV-specific cellular immune responses are also seen after acute infection *(7)* and in long-term nonprogressors *(8)*, and there is more compelling evidence of a greater role of these responses in controlling HIV replication *(9)*.

Passive immunization with pathogen-specific antibodies is protective against infection with a number of other organisms. These include rabies virus *(10)*, respiratory syncytial virus *(11)*, cytomegalovirus *(12)*, hepatitis A and B viruses *(13,14)*, varicella-zoster virus *(15)*, poliovirus *(16)*, measles virus *(17)*, rubella virus *(18)*, and mumps virus *(19)*. In addition, this form of treatment has proved effective in the management of established infections with respiratory syncytial virus *(11)*, cytomegalovirus *(20)*, parvovirus B19 *(21)*, hepatitis B virus *(22)*, and Junin arenavirus (Argentine hemorrhagic fever) *(23)*, as well as pneumococcal pneumonia *(24)*, meningococcal meningitis *(23)*, and *Hemophilus influenzae* meningitis *(23)*. The knowledge learned from these interventions contributed to the successful development of effective vaccines against many of these infectious agents *(23)*. Thus, the potential role of passive immunization in preventive and therapeutic strategies against HIV infection deserves further attention.

IN VITRO DATA

HIV Envelope Structure

As a monomer, the gp120 envelope protein of HIV has five variable loops *(V1–V5)* and five constant regions (C1–C5) that are potential targets for antibody binding *(23)*. However, in its natural state on the surface of the virus as a trimer, conformational

From: *Immunotherapy for Infectious Diseases*
Edited by: J. M. Jacobson © Humana Press Inc., Totowa, NJ

changes of gp120 alter the ability of antibodies to bind and neutralize the virus *(23)*. Various envelope sites are also heavily glycosylated, further affecting virus-antibody interactions *(25)*. In general, HIV gp120 is a less effective neutralization target in its natural ("primary viral isolate") state than when laboratory-adapted to grow in immortalized CD4 lymphocyte cell lines. The primary gp120 epitopes sensitive to neutralization are on V2, V3, C4, and the conformationally dependent overlapping regions that make up the CD4 binding site *(26)*. The gp41 glycoprotein, a transmembrane element non-covalently bound to gp120, is involved in virus-cell fusion and also serves as a neutralization target *(27)*.

HIV infection of a cell involves binding to the CD4 receptor, binding to a chemokine coreceptor, fusion with the cell, and then entry into the cell. During each step, the HIV envelope structure undergoes conformational changes. Recent evidence suggests that the transient envelope structures arising during cell binding and fusion may be more susceptible to antibody neutralization and could serve as targets for immunization strategies *(28)*.

Neutralization Epitopes

It has long been known that the V3 loop contains neutralizable epitopes *(29,30)*. Antibodies to this region of the viral envelope are produced early in the course of infection *(31)* and are associated with delayed progression of disease *(32)* and reduced maternal-infant transmission of infection *(33)*. They appear to function by inhibiting coreceptor binding and virus-cell fusion *(34)*. Anti-V3 monoclonal antibodies protect chimpanzees against HIV-1 infection *(35)*, and anti-V3 antibodies elicited by vaccination are associated with protection in animal studies *(36)*. Several anti-V3 monoclonal antibodies have been created (Table 1), but the hypervariability of this region hinders its usefulness as a target for immunologic control by passive or active vaccination strategies *(30,36)*. However, some studies have suggested that some anti-V3 antibodies are more broadly neutralizing *(37,38)*. Nevertheless, clinical HIV isolates appear to be more resistant to the effects of anti-V3 monoclonal antibodies than T-cell laboratory-adapted strains *(36,39)*.

The V2 region and CD4 binding domain on gp120 and the gp41 glycoprotein are better targets for neutralization of clinical viral isolates of HIV *(36)*. Monoclonal antibodies against the CD4 binding domain and V2 region have been created and shown to have neutralizing activity against "primary" viral isolates *(40–43)*. The gp41 molecule is more conserved than gp120 *(44)*. Monoclonal antibody 2F5 binds to the amino acid sequence ELDKWA on the ectodomain of gp41 and is broadly reactive against clinical HIV isolates *(45)*. Seventy-two percent of isolates from different clades contain this amino acid sequence *(45)*. The decapeptide GCSGKLICTT has been identified as another conserved epitope on gp41 that serves as a neutralizing antibody target in laboratory strains of HIV *(44)*. Clinical isolates need to be tested. The monoclonal antibody 2G12 recognizes a discontinuous epitope on gp120 that includes domains in C2, C3, C4, and V4 *(46)*. It also has demonstrated broad neutralizing activity against clinical HIV isolates *(47)*. In a blinded study of a panel of clinical HIV isolates involving several laboratories, the monoclonal antibodies 2F5, 2G12, and b12 showed significant neutralizing activity against almost all isolates tested *(48)*.

Table 1
Targets of Anti-HIV Monoclonal Antibodies

CD4 binding site of gp120
V3 loop of gp120
gp41
Discontinuous gp120 epitopes
CD4
CCR5
CXCR4

Antibody Combinations

Monoclonal antibodies targeting different HIV epitopes can have additive or synergistic neutralizing activity. This was first demonstrated using laboratory-adapted HIV isolates by combining monoclonal antibodies targeting the V3 loop with antibodies against the CD4 binding domain *(49–51)*. Synergy also has been shown using three monoclonal antibody combinations with individual antibody activities against V2, V3, and the CD4 binding domain *(52)*. Li et al. *(53)* studied 14 different anti-HIV monoclonal antibodies and two hyperimmune polyclonal anti-HIV immunoglobulin (HIVIG) preparations individually and in combination for their neutralizing effects on simian/human immunodeficiency virus (SHIV)-vpu$^+$, a chimeric virus that expresses the laboratory-adapted HIV-1$_{IIIB}$ strain envelope glycoproteins on a simian immunodeficiency virus (SIV) backbone *(53)*. Alone, the antibodies 2F5, 2G12, and b12 were the most potent. Synergistic or additive effects were detected when two antibodies targeting different epitopes were combined. Two antibody combinations involving b12, 2F5, 2G12, and 694/98D (anti-V3) were most active. Using the monoclonal antibody F105 as an anti-CD4 binding domain antibody, the monoclonal antibody 694/98D to target V3, the antibody 2F5, and the antibody 2G12, SHIV-vpu$^+$ was found to be synergistically neutralized by three and four antibody combinations *(54)*. The monoclonal antibodies 2F5 and 2G12 combined with a hyperimmune polyclonal anti-HIVIG were demonstrated to be synergistic at neutralizing clinical HIV isolates *(55)*. The hyperimmune anti-HIVIG was created from the plasma of HIV-infected persons with CD4 lymphocyte counts $\geq 400/\mu L$ and high anti-p24 antibody titers *(56)*.

The synergistic effects seen in these studies are probably related to their complementary activities at different epitope targets. In addition, antigen-antibody binding involving one antibody may cause conformational changes in the HIV envelope that makes the second or third epitope target more accessible to neutralization by another antibody *(46,51,57)*. The anti-HIV antibodies are considerably less potent than neutralizing antibodies against other viruses. The anti-CD4 binding domain antibodies are as much as 10^4 less effective than antibodies against poliovirus *(23)*. The b12 antibody is 10-fold less potent than the best antibodies against poliovirus and influenza A *(23)*. Thus, by using combinations of antibodies, neutralization of virus is made more efficient, and the doses of antibodies needed to achieve maximum virus inhibition are reduced. In addition, a broader array of clinical HIV isolates is made susceptible to neutralization, and the likelihood of selecting for antibody-resistant mutants is reduced *(54,55)*. A single amino acid change in an epitope can result in escape from antibody neutralization *(58–60)*. Given the high rate of mutation of HIV, this is a significant risk.

CD4-Immunoglobulin Fusion Compounds

Similar to antibody neutralization, the concentrations of recombinant soluble CD4 (rsCD4) required for in vitro inhibition of clinical HIV-1 isolates are 200–2700 times greater than those required for inhibition of laboratory strains *(61,62)*. Intravenous doses of rsCD4 need to achieve serum concentrations associated with 90–95% in vitro inhibition of the particular clinical isolate to have an in vivo antiviral effect, as measured by quantitative plasma viral cultures *(63)*. One CD4-immunoglobulin product, created by the fusion of rsCD4 with the heavy chain of IgG had no detectable antiviral activity in one clinical study *(64)*, but concentrations able to neutralize most clinical isolates may not have been achieved. A CD4-IgG$_2$ fusion protein, with the Fv portions of both heavy and light chains of the IgG$_2$ molecule replaced by the V1 and V2 domains of CD4, has been found to neutralize most clinical HIV-1 isolates, with inhibitory concentration of 90% (IC$_{90}$) values less than 40 µg/mL for 26 of 28 isolates tested *(47)*. CD4-IgG$_2$ protected 20 of 21 hu-PBL-SCID mice from challenge with the laboratory isolate HIV-1$_{LAI}$ and the clinical isolates HIV-1$_{JR-CSF}$ and HIV-1$_{AD6}$ *(65)*. Phase I clinical studies of this preparation are under way.

Anti-Receptor and Anti-Coreceptor Antibodies

An alternate approach for using antibodies to inhibit HIV replication is to create mono-clonal antibodies targeting the CD4 receptor and the chemokine CCR5 and CXCR4 core-ceptors used by HIV for cell fusion and entry. Anti-CD4 monoclonal antibodies inhibit HIV infection of lymphocytes and macrophages at both CD4-gp120 binding and postbinding steps and block HIV-induced cell-cell fusion and syncytium formation *(66–68)*. A murine monoclonal antibody (mu5A8), subsequently humanized, has been developed against the second domain of CD4 *(69,70)*. Its antiviral activity is synergistic with anti-gp120 anti-bodies *(71)*. The epitope on the second domain of CD4 targeted by this antibody is not involved in MHC class II-mediated immune functions, and the antibody does not promote clearance of CD4 cells in vivo *(69,70)*. Thus, this potential treatment appears safe and is likely to proceed to clinical trials. The monoclonal antibody B4 also targets the CD4 mol-ecule, and its binding to CD4 is enhanced in the presence of chemokine receptor peptides *(72)*. Hence, its binding to the CD4 receptor on the T-cell surface may be affected by core-ceptor interactions *(72)*. It neutralizes against infection with primary HIV-1 isolates *(72)*.

Similarly, it is possible to design anti-CCR5 antibodies that interfere with HIV bind-ing but do not inhibit chemokine binding and intracellular signaling *(73)*. HIV-1 and chemokines bind to different sites on CCR5 *(73)*. Monoclonal antibodies targeting the N-terminus region and the second extracellular loop of CCR5 inhibit HIV infection of cells but not chemokine activity *(73)*. Whether antibodies that target CXCR4 safely can be developed has yet to be shown.

Antibody-Dependent Cellular Cytotoxicity

Another mechanism whereby humoral immunity could affect the course of HIV infection is through ADCC *(74,75)*. This process consists of programming of mononu-clear cells to lyse HIV-infected cells bound to HIV-specific antibody. A different mechanism of ADCC, cell-mediated cytotoxicity (CMC), has been described in which natural killer (NK) cells with anti-HIV antibody bound to their Fc receptors (CD16) target HIV-infected cells coated with HIV envelope antigen (gp120) *(76)*. Lin et al. *(77)* showed that gp120-specific CMC could be augumented by interleukin-2 (IL-2), IL-12, and IL-15 and could be augmented further by combining IL-2 and IL-15. The addition of HIVIG also enhanced CMC *(77)*. The anti-HIV monoclonal antibodies 2G12 and F105 have demonstrated ADCC activity *(46,78)*.

Bispecific Antibodies

Another approach to enhance and broaden the activities of antibodies and effector cells is the creation of bispecific antibodies (BsAbs) *(79)*. One type of BsAb combines two monoclonal antibodies with neutralizing activity against different HIV epitopes. Using the hybridoma cell fusion technique, Gorny et al. *(79)* combined MAbs targeting conserved epitopes of V3 with MAbs against the CD4 binding domain. The BsAbs created had synergistic anti-HIV activity when tested against the HIV-1$_{IIIB}$ laboratory-adapted strain *(79)*. These antibodies presumably would have all the advantages of using combinations of single MAbs.

Another type of BsAb combines anti-HIV and anti-effector cell specificities to mediate ADCC against HIV-infected cells *(79)*. Antibodies against FcγRI, a signaling receptor on monocytes, macrophages, and activated neutrophils, were combined with MAbs against HIV-1 envelope epitopes. The resultant BsAbs were shown to mediate lysis of gp160-transfected CEM cells by FcγRI-expressing U-937 cells, a monocytoid cell line (79). A BsAb containing anti-V3 and anti-FcγRI components had the highest activity. Importantly, these antibodies did not mediate antibody-dependent enhancement of HIV infection.

Other Mechanisms of Anti-HIV Antibody Activity

There are other mechanisms by which antibodies could control HIV infection (Table 2). One is through complement-mediated lysis of free virus or viral-infected cells *(80,81)*. V3 peptides inhibit complement-mediated virolysis by the serum of HIV-infected persons *(82)*, and MAb 694/98D, an anti-V3 antibody has been shown to be complement-activating *(83)*. Antibody binding of gp120 expressed on infected cell surfaces could inhibit fusion of cells, syncytia formation, and cell-to-cell spread to virus *(84)*. In addition, antibodies could serve to clear immunosuppressive HIV proteins, such as gp120. Soluble gp120 is known to impair CD4 lymphocyte function and to promote cell-mediated lysis of uninfected CD4 cells *(85–89)*. Finally, neutralizing antibodies have also been found to inhibit the infection of dendritic cells and the subsequent transmission to T cells, thus potentially interfering with the early events around mucosal HIV transmission *(90)*.

However, some antibodies could have deleterious effects on the course of HIV infection. Anti-gp120 antibodies could mediate lysis of uninfected CD4 cells with free gp120 shed by the virus bound to its surface *(85)*. In addition, some antibodies that bind virus could enhance HIV infection of cells via binding of antibody-HIV complexes to Fc or complement receptors on mononuclear phagocytes or dendritic cells *(91,92)*.

Table 2
Potential Protective Effects of Antibody in HIV Infection

Neutralization
Antibody-dependent cellular cytotoxicity
Complement-mediated lysis of virus and infected cells
Inhibition of cell fusion and cell-to-cell spread of virus through binding of gp120 on infected
   cell surfaces
Clearance of immunosuppressive HIV proteins, such as gp120
Inhibition of HIV infection of dendritic cells

ANIMAL STUDIES

Preexposure Protection Studies
in Monkeys Using Polyclonal Antibody Preparations

Animal models have been used to help define the role of humoral immunity in protection against HIV infection. SIV infection in macaque monkeys mimics HIV infection in humans in that it causes a progressive immunosuppressive illness leading to death. The chimpanzee can be chronically infected with HIV-1, although progressive immunosuppression does not result. The ability of antibodies to protect against infection has been demonstrated in these models, but the results of experiments have not been universally successful. Differences in results may depend on the viral strain tested, the challenge dose, the type of antibody preparation, and the dose of this product.

Putkonen et al. (93) administered 9 mL/kg of anti-SIV$_{sm}$ sera from a clinically healthy SIV-infected cynomolgus macaque to macaques challenged intravenously 6 hours later with 10–100 median mouse infectious doses (MID$_{50s}$) of SIV$_{sm}$. Three of four animals were protected from infection, whereas the two control monkeys who received uninfected monkey serum before challenge became infected. Prechallenge antibody titers in individual animals did not correlate with protection.

An anti-HIV-2 serum was obtained from a macaque that was vaccinated with inactivated whole virus and, as a result, was protected from homologous challenge (93). This product was administered as a low dose (3 mL/kg) to four macaques and as a high dose (9 mL/kg) to three macaques, followed 6 hours later by challenge with 10 MID$_{50}$ of homologous HIV-2. One of four animals receiving the low-dose anti-HIV-2 pool and two of three animals receiving the high-dose pool were protected from infection, whereas all seven animals that received either noninfected serum or no serum became infected when exposed to the same virus dose.

However, when human anti-HIV-2 pools created from five asymptomatic HIV-2-infected individuals were given in the same manner in doses of 12–20 mL/kg before challenge with 10 or 3 MID$_{50}$ of the same HIV-2 strain as the above experiment, all 12 animals became infected (94). This occurred despite neutralizing antibody titers against the challenge viral strain in these animals comparable to those in animals protected by simian-derived anti-HIV-1 serum.

Infection in chimpanzees with the T-cell laboratory-adapted HIV$_{IIIB}$ strain was prevented by the administration 24 hours before virus challenge of a high dose of human HIVIG (95). This HIVIG preparation was pooled from plasma of asymptomatic chronically HIV-infected individuals with neutralizing antibody titers $\geq$ 1:128 (the top 12.5% of virus-neutralizing antibody titers in a cohort of infected persons). A lower dose of the HIVIG preparation failed to provide protection *(96)*.

Lewis et al. *(97)* reported protecting 9 of 11 rhesus macaques from an intravenous challenge with SIV_{mne} (a less pathogenic virus than SIV_{sm}) with plasma from a healthy SIV_{mne}-infected macaque. Plasma from rhesus macaques given an SIV envelope peptide vaccine protected half of the recipient animals from virus challenge *(97)*.

Protection against SIV_{mac} infection with passive immunization has been more difficult to demonstrate. A study by Kent et al. *(98)* showed no protection against challenge with SIV_{mac251} in any of eight cynomolgus macaques receiving pooled plasma (13 or 19 mL/kg) from asymptomatic SIV-infected animals, although high neutralizing antibody activity was detectable at the time of viral challenge.

Gardner et al. *(99)* saw no protection in six macaques given pooled plasma or immunoglobulin containing high titers of SIV neutralizing antibody from asymptomatic, SIV_{mac251}-infected monkeys when they were challenged intravenously with homologous virus 4 or 18 hours later. In fact, five of the six recipient animals had persistent SIV antigenemia, and four died rapidly (<7 months) from AIDS, suggesting that the passive antibody treatment had actually enhanced infection. Elevated antibody titers against a previously described enhancing domain of SIV gp41 were found in these animals *(99)*.

By contrast, a plasma pool from a macaque immunized with human T-cell grown whole SIV_{mac251} vaccine completely protected three of eight macaques from infection and delayed infection in another. This plasma pool had low levels of SIV-neutralizing antibodies but high titers of antibodies against human cell proteins. Thus, the authors concluded that this product was more successful in achieving protection because of the presence of antibodies targeting HLA class I and II antigens *(99)*.

To study passive immunization against maternal-infant transmission, Van Rompay et al. *(100)* prepared an SIV hyperimmune serum by pooling sera from six juvenile and adult rhesus macaques that had been immunized with live attenuated $SIV_{mac1A11}$ and boosted with the same vaccine or whole, inactivated SIV. These animals were then challenged with SIV_{mac251}. They sustained low level viremias for up to 4 years after infection but had no detectable plasma viral load and no clinical illness at the time sera were obtained for the hyperimmune serum pool. This product was given subcutaneously 2 days before an oral SIV_{251} inoculation, and in some animals 1 and 2 weeks later. All six newborn macaques were protected from infection. Untreated neonates all became infected after viral challenge, and most died within 3 months *(100)*.

Siegel et al. *(101)* gave SIV_{agm} immunoglobulin, prepared from a mixture of plasma from African green monkeys either naturally infected or infected with homologous SIV_{agm3}. Although both monkeys became infected, one of them maintained a low virus load, with virus isolation achievable only at one time point 2 weeks after challenge *(101)*.

Monocyte-tropic strains are involved in the transmission of HIV-1. They are more resistant to neutralization by antibodies than T-cell laboratory-adapted strains *(36,39)*. On the other hand, by replicating in antigen-presenting cells, they may induce enhanced immune responses when presented as vaccine. Clements et al. *(102)* immunized rhesus macaques with an attenuated monocyte tropic recombinant of SIV/17E-Cl. These animals developed a low-grade chronic infection with SIV/17E-Cl. Sera taken from the SIV/17E-Cl-infected macaques protected two of four uninfected macaques from challenge with a heterologous monocyte-tropic primary virus isolate, SIV/DeltaB670 *(102)*.

Postexposure Protection Studies
in Monkeys Using Polyclonal Antibody Preparations

Passive immunization has been promoted as a possible strategy for prevention of infection in the immediate postexposure period. Human HIVIG was found to be ineffective at preventing infection with HIV_{IIIB} when given 1 and 4 hours after viral challenge. However, the 1-hour post exposure administration seemed to modify the course of the infection by lowering plasma HIV RNA levels and the frequency of virus isolation (A.M. Prince, personel communication).

Haigwood et al. *(103)* gave immune globulin produced from the plasma of an SIV-infected "long-term nonprogressor" macaque to other macaques 1 and 14 days after acute infection with SIV_{smE660}. Control animals received noninfected immune globulin before challenge with virus. Four of six macaques treated with SIVIG had marked reductions in plasma viral RNA and remained asymptomatic for at least 15 months, whereas 9 of 10 control animals had high and increasing viral loads and progressed to AIDS. The animals with stable disease developed de novo virus-specific antibodies and cytotoxic T-lymphocyte (CTL) activity, responses characteristic of long-term nonprogressors *(103)*.

When the SIV hyperimmune serum prepared by Van Rompay et al. *(100)*, which was effective in the preexposure setting, was administered to three newborn macaques 3 weeks after oral SIV_{mac251} challenge, plasma SIV RNA levels were not affected, and all three animals died within 3 months.

Of course, these studies differ in the nature of the antibody preparation used, the challenge virus, the animal species, and the age of the challenged animals. However, when the studies are taken together, there is clearly a suggestion that the passive administration of antibodies, prepared and dosed properly, could affect the outcome of infection when administered before or immediately after exposure to virus.

Protection Studies in Monkeys Using Monoclonal Antibodies

Monoclonal antibodies have also been evaluated in primate protection models. Emini et al. *(35)* demonstrated protection of chimpanzees against $HIV-1_{IIIB}$ infection with an anti-$HIV-1_{IIIB}$ V3 loop monoclonal antibody administered either before or shortly after (approx. 10 minutes) virus challenge. Kent et al. *(98)* reported the failure of a pool of four neutralizing monoclonal antibodies directed against SIV_{mac} gp120 to protect any of four macaques against challenge with SIV_{mac251}.

Conley et al. *(104)* studied the ability of the anti-HIV gp41 monoclonal antibody 2F5 to protect chimpanzees against an intravenous challenge with a primary monocyte-tropic HIV-1 isolate. This monoclonal antibody has in vitro neutralizing activity against approx. 75% of primary isolates, including the challenge virus, designated 5016. The two control animals became plasma HIV-1 RNA positive within 1 week of virus challenge. The two antibody-treated animals were also infected, but infection was delayed in both animals (first detection of HIV RNA in plasma at weeks 8 and 14), and peak plasma viral RNA was significantly lower in one animal than in the control animals. Thus, although not demonstrating protection, treatment with this monoclonal antibody appeared to alter the course of the HIV infection *(104)*.

The anti-CD4 monoclonal antibody B4 was found to protect all three chimpanzees challenged intravenously with a primary HIV-1 isolate and three of four macaques challenged intravenously with SIV_{mac257} *(72)*.

Mascola et al. *(105)* studied the activity of combinations of antibodies in protecting macaques against intravenous challenge with an SHIV containing the envelope of the primary isolate HIV-89.6. Three of six animals given HIVIG together with the monoclonal antibodies 2F5 and 2G12 were protected from infection; one of three given 2F5 and 2G12 together were protected. The animals that became infected had lower viremias than IVIG-treated controls and maintained near normal CD4 counts. The three monkeys that received 2F5, 2G12, or HIVIG alone, respectively, developed high viremias but had slower falls in their CD4 cell counts and more benign clinical courses than controls *(105)*.

Protection was easier to achieve against vaginal challenge with SHIV89.6 *(106)*. Four of five monkeys receiving HIV IG/2F5/2G12, two of five receiving 2F5/2G12, and two of four receiving 2G12 alone were completely protected from infection. Again, the six animals that became infected had lower plasma viral RNA levels and smaller declines in CD4 lymphocyte counts than control animals. Although the number of animals studied was small, and the progesterone-treated monkey model is not completely comparable to the natural human situation, these experiments suggest that antibody may be more protective against mucosal viral exposure than intravenous challenge *(106)*. This suggestion is supported by the finding that neutralizing antibody inhibits HIV infection of dendritic cells and subsequent spread to T-cells *(90)*. Since dendritic cells in the mucosa are likely to be the initial targets of HIV infection, antibody could play an important role in protecting against the initial establishment of infection *(90)*.

Antibody protection against mucosal infection was also demonstrated in an SHIV-vpu+ study in macaques *(107)*. The triple monoclonal antibody combination of F105, 2F5, and 2G12 given 5 days before cesarean section and immediately after completely protected the infants of four pregnant macaques from an oral SHIV challenge. The four adult macaques were also protected from an intravenous SHIV challenge 3 days post partum. Since the monoclonal antibodies used in this experiment were of the IgG1 type, it appears that antibodies of the secretory IgA type are not necessary for mucosal protection from viral infection *(107)*.

Preexposure Studies in SCID Mice

Severe combined immunodeficient (SCID) mice lack functional T- and B-lymphocytes *(108)*. Human peripheral blood lymphocyte (hu-PBL-SCID) or fetal human thymic or lymph tissue (hu-thy-SCID or SCID-hu) can be engrafted into the peritoneum of these animals *(109,110)*. The intraperitoneal injection of HIV-1 into hu-PBL-SCID mice leads to sustained infection of the human xenograft *(111)*. Antibody given intraperitoneally rapidly distributes into the blood *(112)*. Thus, the hu-PBL-SCID mouse provides a simple, inexpensive animal model to test passive antibody protection strategies. Large numbers of animals can be involved in these studies.

On the other hand, the immunocompromised nature of these animals does not mimic the natural human state when humans are exposed to virus. Furthermore, most human infections occur via the intravenous or mucosal route, not intraperitoneally. Nonetheless, with these limitations in mind, several useful observations have been made.

Several groups have demonstrated the effectiveness of anti-HIV-1 monoclonal antibodies in preventing infection after viral challenges in the hu-PBL-SCD mouse model. A murine monoclonal antibody targeting the principal neutralizing determinant (PND) of the V3 loop of HIV-1$_{IIIB}$ (BAT123) and its mouse-human chimer (CGP 47 439), given in a dose of 40 mg/kg, completely protected six mice each against subsequent challenge with 10 MIDs of HIV-1$_{IIIB}$, a T-cell line (TCLA) strain. Five of the six animals given control murine antibody became infected *(112)*. BAT123 was found to be 100% protective against HIV$_{LAI}$ in doses as low as 1 mg/kg *(113)*.

Another monoclonal antibody with neutralizing activity against the V3 loop of HIV-1, 694/98-D, was found to provide 50% preexposure prophylaxis against HIV$_{LAI}$ (a TCLA strain) when given at a dose of 1.32 mg/kg and 100% protection with a dose of 40 mg/kg *(114)*. The higher concentrations required for complete protection against HIV$_{LAI}$ by MAb694/98-D compared with BAT123 may reflect in vitro neutralization data. Fifty percent in vitro neutralization of HIV$_{LAI}$ against PBL target cells was achieved with 0.6 μg/mL 694/98-D but only 0.09 μg/mL BAT123 *(113,114)*, indicating that BAT123 may be more potent than 694/98D against HIV$_{LAI}$.

Studies of BAT123 were useful in correlating in vitro neutralization data with in vivo anti-HIV protective activity. Complete protection of hu-PBL-SCID mice was achieved with a serum concentration of 16 μg/mL of BAT123, close to the 15 μg/mL concentration needed to achieve >99% in vitro neutralization. Only 43% protection was obtained with a BAT123 concentration of 0.96 μg/mL, three times the 90% in vitro neutralization concentration of 0.32 μg/mL *(113)*. These data suggest that nearly 100% in vitro neutralization concentrations of MAbs may be needed to provide complete protection against HIV-1 infection in vivo *(113)*. However, it should be noted that the dose of HIV-1 that humans are exposed to is usually far less than the 10 MID$_{50}$s usually used to challenge hu-PBL-SCID mice *(115)*. In any event, these concentrations of MAbs are achievable clinically, and certainly the doses employed are more feasible than the 100 to >1000 mg/kg doses of HIVIG required to protect 50% of hu-PBL-SCID mice from HIV-1 infection *(116)*.

It is now known that primary isolates of HIV-1 are not as easily neutralized by antibodies as are TCLA viruses *(36,39)*. For example, BAT123 did not neutralize primary isolates in vitro and failed to protect hu-PBL-SCID mice from infections with primary isolates *(113)*. IgG$_1$b12, a human monoclonal antibody directed against the CD4 binding site (CD4bs) of gp120, has shown neutralizing activity against >75% of primary HIV-1 isolates *(40,48)*. Previously shown to protect hu-PBL-SCID mice against infection with HIV-1$_{LAI}$, this antibody *(117)*, when given in a dose of 50 mg/kg, completely protected hu-PBL-SCID mice from challenge with the primary isolates HIV$_{JR-CSF}$ and HIV$_{AD6}$ *(118)*. Once again, this dose provided serum concentrations corresponding to levels giving 99% in vitro neutralization. Lower doses gave incomplete protection. Similar results were seen for this antibody against the TCLA strain HIV-1$_{LAI}$. Serum concentrations associated with 99% in vitro neutralization, provided by a dose of 10 mg/kg, were required for complete protection of hu-PBL-SCID mice. By contrast, HIVIG showed no effect in protecting hu-PBL-SCID mice in these experiments.

Recently, a monoclonal antibody targeting the V3 loop of gp120 was found to protect hu-PBL-SCID mice and Thy/Liv SCID-hu mice from infection with primary isolates against which the antibody had in vitro neutralizing activity *(119)*. HIV-induced atrophy of the thymic transplants in the SCID-hu mice was prevented by the prior administration of antibody.

It should be noted that in an acute human to mouse xenograft model in which donated human monocytes and lymphocytes are in an activated state, monoclonal antibodies with demonstrated in vitro neutralizing activity against primary isolates failed to provide in vivo protection against infection *(120)*. Since activated cells are more supportive of HIV infection, this animal model is a more difficult one for neutralizing antibodies to demonstrate activity.

Postexposure Studies in SCID Mice

To study the potential role of antibodies in postexposure protection against HIV infection, the antibodies can be administered at several time points after the hu-PBL-SCID mice are challenged with virus. Anti-V3, anti-CD4-BS, anti-gp41, and other antibodies affect the virus-host cell interaction subsequent to gp120-CD4 binding *(121,122)*. Thus, they might be effective at preventing the establishment of infection even after virus challenge. The anti-V3 BAT123 antibody was found to protect hu-PBL-SCID mice from infection when given up to 4 hours after HIV-1$_{LAI}$ challenge *(115)*. It was 62% effective when given 5 hours after challenge and 33% effective when given 6 hours or more after challenge. Anti-CD4-BS IgGb12 provided complete protection against laboratory-adapted (HIV-1$_{LAI}$) and primary (HIV-1$_{JR-CSF}$ and HIV-1$_{AD6}$) isolates when given within 6 hours of HIV-1 challenge and partial protection when given at 8 and 24 hours after challenge *(118)*. When viral breakthrough occurred, both BAT123 and IgGb12 had no effect on subsequent viral burden. By contrast, HIVIG had to be given within 1 hour of viral challenge to be effective *(116)*. The anti-V3 antibody 694/98-D achieved 100% protection when given 15 minutes after HIV$_{LAI}$ challenge and was 50% effective when given 1 hour after challenge *(114)*. The anti-CD4 B4 antibody protected mice for up to 4 hours after challenge with a primary HIV-1 isolate *(72)*.

Role of Antibody-Dependent Cellular Cytotoxicity and Complement

Aside from potency, monoclonal antibodies may differ in their ability to effect ADCC and complement-mediated antiviral effects. BAT123 has been shown to mediate ADCC *(115)*. Replacing the murine Fc domain of BAT123 with a human IgG$_1$ Fc domain eliminated the postexposure prophylactic effectiveness of this antibody in the hu-PBL-SCID mouse model *(123)*. In addition, giving the mice cobra venom factor to inactivate serum complement activity also interfered with the postexposure prophylactic effect of BAT123 (123). Thus, the complement system is important for the anti-HIV activity of BAT123 and probably other antibodies. On the other hand, providing complement did not change 694/98-D's activity in providing postexposure prophylaxis *(114)*.

Escape Mutation

In an important study, HIV-1$_{LAI}$ virus isolated from one hu-PBL-SCID mouse 3 weeks after receiving antibody 694/98-D as preexposure prophylaxis was found to be resistant to neutralization by 694/98-D *(114)*. Sequence analysis of the V3 region of this virus demonstrated amino acid changes in the epitope recognized by 694/98-D and in one amino acid nearby. Thus, mutation leading to escape from neutralization is a risk of therapy with one monoclonal antibody and supports the need for studying combinations of antibodies.

HUMAN STUDIES

Polyclonal Antibody Preparations

A number of preliminary clinical studies have been performed to evaluate HIV-specific passive immunization as treatment for HIV infection. In 1988, Jackson et al. *(124)* reported infusing plasma containing high levels of anti-p24 antibodies into six patients with advanced HIV infection. The infusions resulted in losses of plasma p24 antigen, fewer patients with positive plasma and lymphocyte HIV cultures, a reduction in opportunistic infections, better symptom and Karnofsky performance scores, and gains in weight *(124)*.

Karpas et al. *(125)* gave monthly infusions of anti-HIV hyperimmune plasma to 10 patients with advanced HIV infection. Plasma p24 antigen and HIV DNA were reduced *(125)*. However, the polymerase chain reaction (PCR) assay used to measure plasma HIV DNA was invalidated in a later study *(126)*.

Jacobson et al. *(127)*, in a double-blind, randomized, controlled trial of hyperimmune plasma pools prepared in the same manner as Karpas et al. *(126)*, followed in 63 patients with advanced HIV infection. Plasma donors were asymptomatic HIV-infected individuals who had CD4 cell counts $\geq 400/mm^3$ and were p24 antigen-negative. Plasma recipients received either 250 mL of anti-HIV hyperimmune plasma or control non-HIV-infected plasma every 4 weeks. No effects were seen on CD4 lymphocyte counts or plasma and cell HIV culture titers. However, statistically nonsignificant trends toward delayed time to opportunistic infection and time to death were noted. No effects on weight, Karnofsky performance score, or serum β_2-microglobulin levels were seen *(127)*.

Vittecoq et al. *(128)* infused single-donor plasma containing high titers of p24 antibody at 2-week intervals into nine subjects with advanced HIV infection (CD4 cell counts $<100/mm^3$). This was a nonblinded, randomized controlled study. HIV p24 antigen became nondetectable in all patients receiving hyperimmune plasma. Fewer opportunistic infections were observed in the treated patients. No effects on CD4 lymphocyte count, weight, or Karnofsky performance score were seen *(128)*.

Levy et al. *(129)* performed a double-blind, randomized, controlled study of anti-HIV hyperimmune plasma in 220 patients with advanced HIV disease. These patients received either 250 or 500 mL of the hyperimmune plasma or albumin once a month for 1 year. The hyperimmune plasma was pooled from HIV-infected donors with high titers of anti-p24 antibodies. No benefit of treatment was seen in the study population as a whole. However, subset analysis of patients with CD4 lymphocyte counts between 50 and 200/mm^3 who received the 500-mL/month dose of hyperimmune plasma showed them to have statistically significant improvements in CD4 cell counts and trends toward longer survival and lower serum HIV p24 antigen levels. No effects on the occurrence of opportunistic infections or serum β_2-microglobulin were seen *(129)*.

These studies were performed prior to the availability of the current techniques to measure plasma HIV load by RNA levels. Subsequently, Vittecoq et al. *(130)* performed a double-blind, controlled trial of single-donor hyperimmune plasma versus HIV-negative plasma in 82 patients with CD4 lymphocyte counts <200 cells/mm^3. Plasma was given in doses of 300 mL every 2 weeks for 1 year. Treatment resulted in delayed occurrence of opportunistic infection. A nonsignificant trend toward improved survival was seen. There was no effect of treatment on CD4 lymphocyte counts *(130)*.

No difference between treatment groups in plasma HIV RNA levels was seen, but more patients receiving hyperimmune plasma than those receiving HIV-negative plasma had negative plasma HIV cultures (but not cellular cultures) during the study period *(131)*.

In a different approach, Osther et al. *(132)* infused a porcine hyperimmune globulin, created by immunizing pigs with an HIV lysate, once daily for 5 days into 14 patients with HIV infection. These infusions resulted in loss of p24 antigenemia, enhancement of CD4 cell counts, and improved symptoms *(132)*.

HIVIG was studied in the Pediatric AIDS Clinical Trials Group (PACTG) Protocol 185 for its potential effect on reducing perinatal transmission of HIV. An unexpectedly low overall transmission rate resulting from zidovudine (AZT) treatment caused the trial to be stopped early without determining the effectiveness of HIVIG. However, there were statistically nonsignificant trends toward reduced transmission with HIVIG treatment in women with CD4 lymphocyte counts $<200/mm^3$ and in women who had started receiving zidovudine before they became pregnant. Presumably, these were women with more advanced disease and greater risks of transmitting infection to their newborns. In addition, none of the 9 infected neonates in the HIVIG arm of the study had positive HIV cultures at birth compared with 5 (38%) of 13 infected neonates in the IVIG arm, a statistically significant difference *(133)*. Thus, passive immunization with HIVIG may have been effective in reducing transmission in the subset of patients at greatest risk to do so, and this may have affected the degree of viral replication in those infants who did become infected. However, an effect on plasma HIV RNA levels was not seen in PACTG Protocol 273 when 30 HIV-infected children aged 2–11 years on stable anti-retroviral therapy were given 6 monthly infusions of 200, 400, or 800 mg/kg of the same HIVIG preparation *(134)*.

Monoclonal Antibodies

Hinkula et al. *(135)* studied two different murine monoclonal antibodies, F58 and P4/D10, targeting the V3 loop of HIV-1$_{IIIB}$, a TCLA strain. One of the antibodies was given twice a month for 3 months to 11 patients with AIDS. The antibody administered neutralized the primary virus isolate of 9 of the 11 recipient patients. Plasma HIV RNA decreased in four patients, remained stable in another four, and increased in three patients. There were no changes in CD4 cell counts, but mitogen- and non-HIV antigen-induced lymphoproliferative responses improved in 9 of 11 patients *(135)*.

Gunthard et al. *(136)* studied a chimeric mouse-human monoclonal antibody (CGP-47-439) against the V3 loop of HIV-1$_{IIIB, MN}$ laboratory-adapted strains. This chimeric antibody was derived from the murine BAT123 monoclonal antibody. Various doses were given to 12 patients at 3-week intervals for 24 weeks. Plasma HIV RNA levels decreased in two patients and increased in one *(136)*.

In sum, although a number of these human studies suggested a clinical benefit from the administration of various passive immunization products, no clear antiviral effect has been demonstrated to date.

CONCLUSIONS

There is now a body of evidence showing that antibodies have the ability to prevent and control HIV infection. Antibodies with neutralizing activity against strains of HIV in vitro are able to protect animals against infection with those strains. These include clinical isolates, which are more resistant than laboratory-adapted strains to neutralization by antibodies.

Successful animal protection studies usually have utilized 10 MID_{50}s of virus as the challenge inoculum to be neutralized. It is likely that natural human exposures consist of inocula far smaller, probably on the order of ≤ 1 MID_{50} *(115)*. On the other hand, natural host antibody responses are usually inadequate to protect and control HIV infection durably. Exogenous administration of protective quantities of more potent targeted antibodies seems to be technically feasible and practical in the clinical setting.

Undoubtedly, the doses of anti-HIV antibodies required for treatment must be greater than those required for prevention, perhaps 2–3 logs greater *(23)*. A Pediatrics AIDS Foundation-sponsored workshop on HIV passive immunization recommended that the criteria for advancing candidate anti-HIV monoclonal antibodies to human trials include a requirement for 90% in vitro neutralization of most clinical isolates at concentrations of 5–10 µg/mL. It was felt that these concentrations could be safely reached in the sera of patients after administration of monoclonal antibody preparations *(137)*. Comparable levels have been associated with protection in animal studies. However, several hu-PBL-SCID mouse experiments have demonstrated that doses associated with >99% in vitro neutralization activity are required for successful protection *(115)*. Treatment of infection, as opposed to prevention of infection, is likely to require even higher doses and/or potency. No clear therapeutic antiviral benefit has been seen with the antibody preparations studied to date, but monoclonal antibodies with potent neutralizing activity against clinical isolates have not yet gone into clinical trials.

In addition to neutralizing activity, the ability of antibodies to activate complement-mediated lysis of free virus and infected cells, as well as ADCC against infected cells, would be attractive features. These activities were found to be important in hu-PBL-SCID mouse protection studies *(114, 123)*.

Monoclonal antibodies will need to be administered in combination to obtain synergistic potency, reduce dosage requirements, counteract any infection enhancement activity of any antibodies in the combination, and prevent the emergence of mutant viral strains resistant to neutralization.

The host immune response to natural infection with HIV involves both humoral and cellular components. The response is partially effective in controlling viral replication but not in eradicating infection in most circumstances. Enhancing either arm of the immune response should prove beneficial. Passively administered antibodies might prove to be particularly useful in protection against the initial infection of dendritic cells, as well as monocytes and lymphocytes and might thus protect against the establishment of the infection. In addition, research in this area should identify HIV epitopes targeted by antibodies and cytotoxic T lymphocytes that will aid in the design of effective vaccines.

REFERENCES

1. Albert J, Abrahamsson B, Nagy K, et al. Rapid development of isolate-specific neutralizing antibodies after primary HIV-1 infection and consequent emergence of virus variants which resist neutralization by autologous sera. AIDS 1990; 4:107–112.
2. Robert-Guroff M, Goedert JJ, Naugle CL, Jennings AM, Blattner WA, Gallo RC. Spectrum of HIV-1 neutralizing antibodies in a cohort of homosexual men: results of a 6 year prospective study. AIDS Res Hum Retroviruses 1989; 5:343–350.

3. Tyler DS, Lyerly HK, Weinhold KJ. Anti-HIV-1 ADCC. AIDS Res Hum Retroviruses 1989; 5:557–563.
4. Ugen KE, Goedert JJ, Boyer J, et al. Vertical transmission of human immunodeficiency virus (HIV) infection. Reactivity of maternal sera with glycoprotein 120 and 41 peptides from HIV type 1. J Clin Invest 1992; 89:1923–1930.
5. Goedert JJ, Mendez H, Drummond JE, et al. Mother-to-infant transmission of human immunodeficiency virus type 1: association with prematurity or low anti-gp120. Lancet 1989; 2:1351–1354.
6. Devash Y, Calvelli TA, Wood DG, Reagan KJ, Rubinstein A. Vertical transmission of human immunodeficiency virus is correlated with the absence of high-affinity/avidity maternal antibodies to the gp120 principal neutralizing domain. Proc Natl Acad Sci USA 1990; 87:3445–3449.
7. Safrit JT, Andrew CA, Zhu T, Ho DD, Koup RA. Characterization of human immunodeficiency virus type 1-specific cytotoxic T lymphocyte clones isolated during acute seroconversion: recognition of autologous virus sequences within a conserved immunodominant epitope. J Exp Med 1994; 179:463–472.
8. Harrer T, Harrer E, Kalams SA, et al. Strong cytotoxic T cell and weak neutralizing responses in a subset of persons with stable nonprogressing HIV type 1 infection. AIDS Res Hum Retroviruses 1996; 12:585–592.
9. Schmitz JE, Kuroda MJ, Santra S, et al. Control of viremia in simian immunodeficiency virus infection by CD8+ lymphocytes. Science 1999; 283:857–860.
10. Bahmanyar M, Fayaz A, Nour-Salehi S, Mohammadi M, Koprowski H. Successful protection of humans exposed to rabies infection: postexposure treatment with the new human diploid cell rabies vaccine and antirabies serum. JAMA 1976; 236: 2751–2754.
11. Groothius JR, Stimoes EAF, Levin MJ, et al. Prophylactic administration of respiratory syncytial virus immune globulin to high-risk infants and young children. N Engl J Med 1993; 329:1524–1530.
12. Snydman DR, Werner BG, Heinze-Lacey B, et al. Use of cytomegalovirus immune globulin to prevent cytomegalovirus disease in renal transplant recipients. N Engl J Med 1987; 317:1049–1054.
13. Stokes J, Jr, Neefe JR. The prevention and attenuation of infectious hepatitis by gamma globulin. JAMA 1945; 127:144–145.
14. Beasley RP, Hwang LY, Steven CE. Efficacy of hepatitis B immune globulin for prevention of perinatal transmission of the hepatitis B virus carrier state: final report of a randomized double-blind, placebo-controlled trial. Hepatology 1983; 3:135–141.
15. Ross AH. Modification of chicken pox in family contacts by administration of gamma globulin. N Engl J Med 1962; 267:369–376.
16. Hammon WM, Coriel LL, Wehrie PF. Evaluation of Red Cross gamma globulin as a prophylactic agent for poliomyelitis. JAMA 1953; 151:1272–1285.
17. Janeway CA. Use of concentrated human serum gamma globulin in the prevention and treatment of measles. Bull NY Acad Med 1945; 21:202–220.
18. Korns RF. Prevention of German measles with immune serum globulin. J Infect Dis 1952; 90:183–189.
19. Gellis SS, McGuinnes AC, Peters M. Study of prevention of mumps orchitis by gamma globulin. Am J Med Sci 1945; 210:661–664.
20. Emanuel D, Cunningham I, Jules-Elysee K, et al. Cytomegalovirus pneumonia after bone marrow transplantation successfully treated with the combination of ganciclovir and high-dose intravenous immune globulin. Ann Intern Med 1988; 109:777–782.
21. Frickhofen N, Abkowitz JL, Safford M, et al. Persistent B19 parvovirus infection in patients infected with human immunodeficiency virus type 1 (HIV-1): a treatable cause of anemia in AIDS. Ann Intern Med 1990; 113:926–933.

22. Beasley RP, Hwang LY, Stevens CE, et al. Efficacy of hepatitis B immune globulin for prevention of perinatal transmission of hepatitis B virus carrier state: final report of randomized double-blind, placebo-controlled trial. Hepatology 1983; 3:135–141.

23. Krause RM, Dimmock NJ, Morens DM. Summary of antibody workshop: The Role of Humoral Immunity in the Treatment and Prevention of Emerging and Extant Infectious Diseases. J Infect Dis 1997; 176:549–559.

24. Casedevall A. Crisis in infectious disease: time for a new paradigm? Clin Infect Dis 1996; 23:790–794.

25. Reitter JN, Means RE, Desrosiers RC. A role for carbohydrates in immune evasion in AIDS. Nat Med. 1998; 4:679–684.

26. Hairharan K, Nara PL, Caralli VM, Norton FL, Haigwood N, Kang CY. Analysis of the cross-reactive anti-gp120 antibody population in human immunodeficiency virus-infected asymptomatic individuals. J Virol 1993; 67:953–960.

27. Muster T, Steindl F, Purtscher M, et al. A conserved neutralizing epitope on gp41 of human immunodeficiency virus type 1. J Virol 1993; 67:6642–6647.

28. LaCasse RA, Follis KE, Trahey M, Scarborough JD, Littman DR, Nunberg JH. Fusion-competent vaccines: broad neutralization of primary isolates of HIV. Science 1999; 283:357–362.

29. Matsushita S, Robert-Guroff M, Rusche J, et al. Characterization of a human immunodefiency virus neutralizing monoclonal antibody and mapping of the neutralizing epitope. J Virol 1998; 62:2107.

30. Moore JP, Nara PL. The role of the V3 loop in HIV infection. AIDS 1991; 5(Suppl 2):S21.

31. Rusche JR, Javaherian K, McDanal C, et al. Antibodies that inhibit fusion of human immunodeficiency virus-infected cells bind a 24-amino-acid sequence of the viral envelope gp120. Proc Natl Acad Sci USA 1988; 85:3198–3202.

32. Yamanaka T, Fujimura Y, Ishimoto S, et al. Correlation of titer of antibody to principal neutralizing domain of HIV_{MN} strain with disease progression in Japanese hemophiliacs seropositive for HIV type 1. AIDS Res Hum Retroviruses 1997; 13:317.

33. Devash Y, Calvelli TA, Wood DG, Reagan KJ, and Rubinstein A.Vertical transmission of HIV is correlated with the absence of high affinity/avidity maternal antibodies to the gp120 principal neutralizing domain. Proc Natl Acad Sci USA 1990; 87:3445–3449.

34. Cocchi F, DeVico AL, Demo AG, Cara A, Gallo RC, Lusso P. V3 domain of HIV-1 envelope glycoprotein gp120 is critical for chemokine-mediated blockade of infection. Nat Med 1996; 2:1244.

35. Emini EA, Schleif WA, Nunberg JH, et al. Prevention of HIV-1 infection in chimpanzees by gp120 V3 domain-specific monoclonal antibody. Nature 1992; 355:728–730.

36. Girard M, Barre-Sinoussi F, van der Ryst E. Vaccination of chimpanzees against HIV-1. Antibiot Chemother 1996; 48:121–124.

37. Gorny MK, Conley AJ, Karwowska S, et al. Neutralization of diverse HIV-1 variants by an anti-V3 human monoclonial antibody. J Virol 1992; 66:7538–7542.

38. Jahaverian K, Langlois AJ, LaRosa FJ, et al. Broadly neutralizing antibodies elicited by the hypervariable neutralizing determinant of HIV-1. Science 1990; 250:1590–1593.

39. Moore JP, Cao Y, Quing L, et al. Primary isolates of human immunodeficiency virus type 1 are relatively resistant to neutralization by monoclonal antibodies to gp120 and their neutralization is not predicted by studies with monomeric gp120. J Virol 1995; 69:101.

40. Burton DR, Pyati J, Koduri R, et al. Efficient neutralization of primary isolates of HIV-1 by a recombinant human monoclonal antibody. Science 1994; 266:1024–1027.

41. Posner MR, Cavacini LA, Emes CL, Power J, Byrn RA. Neutralization of HIV-1 by F105, a human monoclonal antibody to the CD4 binding site of gp120. J Acquir Immune Defic Syndr 1993; 6:7–14.

42. Fevrier M, Boudet F, Deslandres A, Theze J. Two new monoclonal antibodies against HIV type 1 glycoprotein gp120: characterization and neutralizing activities against HIV type 1 strains. AIDS Res Hum Retroviruses 1995; 11:491–500.

43. Gorny MK, Moore JP, Conley AJ, et al. Human anti-V2 monoclonal antibody that neutralizes primary but not laboratory isolates of human immunodeficiency virus type 1. J Virol 1994; 68:8312–8320.

44. Cotropia J, Ugen KE, Kliks S, et al. A human monoclonal antibody to HIV-1 gp41 with neutralizing activity against diverse laboratory isolates. J Acquir Immune Defic Syndr 1996; 12:221–232.

45. Muster T, Guinea R, Trkola A, et al. Cross-neutralizing activity against divergent human immunodeficiency virus type 1 isolates induced by the gp41 sequence ELDKEAS. J Virol 1994; 68:4031–4034.

46. Trkola A, Purtscher M, Muster T, et al. Human monoclonal antibody 2G12 defines a disinctive neutalization epitope on the gp120 glycoprotein of human immunodeficiency virus type 1. J Virol 1996; 70:1100–1108.

47. Trkola A, Pomales AB, Yuan H, et al. Cross-clade neutralization of primary isolates of human immunodeficiency virus type 1 by human monoclonal antibodies and tetrameric CD4-IgG. J Virol 1995; 69:6609–6617.

48. D'Souza MP, Milman G, Bradac JA, McPhee D, Hanson CV, Hendry RM. Neutralization of primary HIV-1 isolates by anti-envelope monoclonal antibodies. AIDS 1995; 9:867–874.

49. Laal S, Burda S, Gorny MK, Karwowska S, Buchbinder A, Zolla-Pazner S. Synergistic neutralization of human immunodeficiency type 1 by combinations of human monoclonal antibodies. J Virol 1994; 68:4001–4008.

50. Thali M, Furman C, Wahren B, et al. Cooperativity of neutralizing antibodies directed against the V3 and CD4 binding regions of the human immunodeficiency virus gp120 envelope glycoprotein. J Acquir Immune Defic Syndr 1992; 5:591–599.

51. Tilley SA, Honnen WJ, Racho ME, Chou T-C, Pinter A. Synergistic neutralization of HIV-1 by human monoclonal antibodies against the V3 loop and the CD4-binding site of gp120. AIDS Res Hum Retroviruses 1992; 8:461–467.

52. Vijh-Warrier S, Pinter A, Honnen WJ, Tilley S. Synergistic neutralization of human immunodeficiency virus type 1 by a chimpanzee monoclonal antibody against the V2 domain of gp120 in combination with monoclonal antibodies against the V3 loop and the CD4-binding site. J Virol 1996; 70:4466–4473.

53. Li A, Baba TW, Sodroski J, et al. Synergistic neutralization of a chimeric SIV/HIV type 1 virus with combinations of human anti-HIV type 1 envelope monoclonal antibodies or hyperimmune globulins. AIDS Res Hum Retroviruses 1997; 13:647–656.

54. Li A, Katinger H, Posner MR, et al. Synergistic neutralization of simian-human immunodeficiency virus SHIV-vpu+ by triple and quadruple combinations of human monoclonal antibodies and high-titer anti-human immunodeficiency virus type 1 immunoglobulins. J Virol 1998; 72:3235–3240.

55. Mascola JR, Louder MK, Van Cott TC, et al. Potent and synergistic neutralization of human immunodeficiency (HIV) type 1 primary isolates by hyperimmune anti-HIV immunoglobulin combined with monoclonal antibodies 2F5 and 2G12. J Vir 1997; 71: 7198–7206.

56. Cummins LM, Weinhold KJ, Matthews TJ, et al. Preparation and characterization of an intravenous solution of IgG from human immunodeficiency virus-seropositive donors. Blood 1991; 77:1111–1117.

57. Cavacini LA, Emes CI, Power J, et al. Human monoclonal antibodies to the V3 loop of HIV-1 gp120 mediate variable and distinct effects on binding and viral neutralization by a human monoclonal antibody to the CD4 binding site. J Acquir Immune Defic Syndr 1993; 6:6353–6358.

58. McKeating JA, Bennett J, Zolla-Pazner S, et al. Resistance of a human serum-selected human immunodeficiency virus type 1 escape mutant to neutralization by CD4 binding site monoclonal antibodies is conferred by a single amino acid change in gp120. J Virol 1993; 67:5216–5225.

59. Yoshiyama H, Mo H, Moore JP, Ho DD. Characterization of mutants of human immun-odeficiency virus type 1 that have escaped neutralization by a monoclonal antibody to the gp120 V2 loop. J Virol 1994; 68:974–978.

60. Shotton C, Arnold C, Sattentau Q, Sodroski J, McKeating JA. Identification and charac-terization of monoclonal antibodies specific for polymorphic antigenic determinants within the V2 region of the human immunodeficiency virus type I. J Virol 1995; 69:222–230.

61. Daar ES, Li XL, Mougdil T, Ho DD. High concentrations of recombinant soluble CD4 are required to neutralize primary human immunodeficiency virus type 1 isolates. Proc Natl Acad Sci USA 1990; 87:6574–6578.

62. Daar ES, Ho DD. Relative resistance of primary HIV-1 isolates to neutralization by solu-ble CD4. Am J Med 1991; 90(Suppl 4A):22S–26S.

63. Schacker T, Coombs RW, Collier AC, et al. The effects of high-dose recombinant soluble CD4 on human immunodeficiency virus type 1 viremia. J Infect Dis 1994; 169:37–40.

64. Hodges TL, Kahn JO, Kaplan LD, et al. Phase I study of recombinant human CD4-immunoglobulin G therapy of patients with AIDS and AIDS-related complex. Antimicrob Agents Chemother 1991; 35:2580–2586.

65. Gauduin MC, Allaway GP, Maddon PJ, Barbas CF, Burton DR, Koup RA. Evaluation of the protective role of two recombinant immunoglobulin molecules in passive protection against primary isolates of HIV-1. Keystone Symposium: Immunopathogenesis of HIV Infection 1996; Hilton Head Island, South Carolina.

66. Dalgleish AG, Beverley PCL, Clapham PR, Crawford DH, Greaves MF, Weiss RA. The CD4 (T4) antigen is an essential component of the receptor for the AIDS retrovirus. Nature 1984; 312:763–767.

67. Klatzman D, Champagne E, Chamaret S, et al. T-lymphocytes T4 molecule behaves as the receptor for human retrovirus LAV. Nature 1984; 312:767–768.

68. McDougal JS, Kennedy MS, Sligh JM, Cort SP, Mawle A, Nicholson JKA. (1986) Bind-ing of HTL-III/LAV to T4+ T cells by complex of the 110K viral protein and the T4 mol-ecule. Science 1986; 231:382–385.

69. Reimann KA, Burkly LC, Burrus B, Waite BCD, Lord CI, Letvin NL. (1993) *In vivo* administration to rhesus monkeys of a CD-4 specific monoclonal antibody capable of blocking AIDS virus replication. AIDS Res Hum Retroviruses 1993; 9:199–207.

70. Reimann KA, Lin WU, Bixler S, et al. A humanized form of a CD4-specific monoclonal antibody exhibits decreased antigenicity and prolonged plasma half-life in rhesus mon-keys while retaining its unique biological and antiviral properties. AIDS Res Hum Retro-viruses 1997; 13:933–943.

71. Burkly L, Mulrey L, Blumenthal R, Dimitrov DS. Synergistic inhibition of human immun-odeficiency virus type 1 envelope glycoprotein-mediated cell fusion and infection by an antibody to CD4 domain 2 in combination with anti-gp120 antibodies. J Virol 1995; 69: 4267–4273.

72. Chang YW, Sawyer LSW, Murthy KK, et al. Postexposure immunoprophylaxis of primary isolates by an antibody to HIV receptor complex. Proc Natl Acad Sci USA 1999; 96:10367–10372.

73. Olson W, Nagashima K, Tran D, et al. HIV-1 and chemokine-inhibitory activities of anti-CCR5 antibodies map to distinct CCR5 epitopes [Abstract]. In: Programs and Abstracts, 6th Conference on Retroviruses and Opportunistic Infections 1999; Chicago.

74. Murayama T, Cai Q, Rinaldo CR. Antibody-dependent cellular cytotoxicity mediated by CD16+ lymphocytes from HIV-seropositive homosexual men. Clin Immunol Immunopathol 1990; 55:297–304.

75. Ahmad A, Morriset R, Thomas R, Menezes J. Evidence for a defect of antibody-dependent cellular cytotoxicity (ADCC) effector function and anti-HIV gp120/gp41-specific ADCC mediating antibody titers in HIV-infected individuals. J Acquir Immune Defic Syndr 1994; 7:428–437.

76. Tyler DS, Nastala CL, Stanley SD, et al. Gp120 specific cellular cytotoxicity in HIV-1 seropositive individual: evidence of circulating CD16$^+$ effector cells armed in vivo with cytophilic antibody. J Immunol 1990; 142:1177–1182.

77. Lin S-J, Roberts RL, Ank BJ, Nguyen QH, Thomas EK, Stiehm ER. Human immunodeficiency virus (HIV) type-1 gp120-specific cell-mediated cytotoxicity (CMC) and natural killer (NK) activity in HIV-infected (HIV+) subjects: enhancement with interleukin-2 (IL-2), IL-12, and IL-15. Clin Immunol Immunopathol 1997; 82:163–173.

78. Posner MR, Elboim HS, Cannon T, Cavacini L, Hideshima T. Functional activity of an HIV-1 neutralizing IgG monoclonal antibody: ADCC and complement mediated lysis. AIDS Res Hum Retroviruses 1992; 5:553–558.

79. Gorny MK, Keler T, Burda S, et al. Functional studies of bispecific antibodies directed against HIV-1 and the Fcγ 1 receptor type 1. Antibiot Chemother 1996; 48:173–183.

80. Gregersen JP, Mehdi S, Baur A, Hilfenhaus J. Antibody- and complement-mediated lysis of HIV-infected cells and inhibition of viral replication. J Med Virol 1990; 30:287–293.

81. Spear GT, Sullivan BL, Landay AL, Lint TF. Neutralization of human immunodeficiency virus type 1 by complement occurs by viral lysis. J Virol 1990; 64:5869–5873.

82. Spear GT, Takefman DM, Sharpe S, Ghassemi M, Zolla-Pazner S. Antibodies to the HIV-1 V3 loop in serum from infected persons contribute a major proportion of immune effector functions including complement activation, antibody binding, and neutralization. Virology 1994; 204:609–615.

83. Spear GT, Takefman DM, Sullivan BL, Landay AL, Zolla-Pazner S. Complement activation by human monoclonal antibodies to human immunodeficiency virus. J Virol 1993; 67:53–59.

84. Fung MSC, Sun C, Sun NC, et al. Monoclonal antibodies that neutralize HIV-1 virions and inhibit syncytium formation by infected cells. Biotechnology 1987; 5:940–946.

85. Lyerly HK, Matthews TJ, Langlois AJ, Bolognesi DP, Weinhold KJ. Human T-cell lymphotropic virus IIIB glycoprotein (gp120) bound to CD4 on normal lymphocytes and expressed by infected cells serves as target for immune attack. Proc Natl Acad Sci USA 1987; 84:4601–4605.

86. Siliciano RF, Lawton T, Knall C, et al. Analysis of host-virus interactions in AIDS with anti-gp120 T cell clones: effects of HIV sequence variation and a mechanism for CD4+ cell depletion. Cell 1988; 54:561–575.

87. Orentas RJ, Hildreth JE, Obah E, et al. Induction of CD4+ human cytolytic T cells specific for HIV-infected cells by a gp160 subunit vaccine. Science 1990; 248:1234–1237.

88. Liegler TJ, Stites DP. HIV-1gp120 and anti-gp120 induce reversible unresponsiveness in peripheral CD4 T lymphocytes. J Acquir Immune Defic Syndr 1994; 7:340–348.

89. Theodore AC, Kornfield H, Wallace RP, Criukshank WW. CD4 modulation of noninfected human T lymphocytes by HIV-1 envelope glycoprotein gp120 contributions to the immunosuppression seen in HIV-1 infection by induction of CD4 and CD4 unresponsiveness. J Acquir Immune Defic Syndr 1994; 7:899–907.

90. Frankel SS, Steinman RM, Michael NL, et al. Neutralizing monoclonal antibodies block human immunodeficiency virus type 1 infection of dendritic cells and transmission to T cells. J Virol 1998; 72(12):9788–9794.

91. Takeda A, Tuazon CV, Ennis FA. Antibody-enhanced infection by HIV-1 via Fc receptor-mediated entry. Science 1988; 86:8055–8058.

92. Robinson WE, Montefiore DC, Gillespie DH, Mitchell WM. Complement mediated, antibody dependent enhancement of HIV-1 infection in vitro is characterized by increased protein and RNA synthesis and infectious virus release. J Acquir Immune Defic Syndr 1989; 2:33–42.

93. Putkonen P, Thorstensson R, Ghavamzadeh L, et al. Prevention of HIV-2 and SIVsm infection by passive immunization in cynomolgus monkeys. Nature 1991; 352:436–438.

94. Biberfeld G, Thorstensson R, Putkonen P. HIV-2 vaccine trials in cynomolgus monkeys. Antibiot Chemother 1996; 48:113–120.

95. Prince AM, Reesink H, Pascual D, et al. Prevention of HIV infection by passive immunization with HIV immunoglobulin. AIDS Res Hum Retroviruses 1991; 7:971–973.

96. Prince AM, Horowitz B, Baker L, et al. Failure of a human immunodeficiency virus (HIV) immune globulin to protect chimpanzees against experimental challenge with HIV. Proc Natl Acad Sci USA 1988; 85:6944–6948.

97. Lewis MG, Elkins WR, McCutchan FE, et al. Passively transferred antibodies directed against conserved regions of SIV envelope protect macaques from SIV infection. Vaccine 1993; 11:1347–1355.

98. Kent KA, Kitchin P, Mills KH, et al. Passine immunization of cynomolgus macaques with immune sera or a pool of neutralizing monoclonal antibodies failed to protect against challenge with SIV_{mac251}. AIDS Res Hum Retroviruses 1994; 10:189–194.

99. Gardner M, Rosenthal A, Jennings M, Yee J, Antipa L, Robinson E Jr. Passive immunization of rhesus macaques against SIV infection and disease. AIDS Res Hum Retroviruses 1995; 111:843–854.

100. Van Rompay KKA, Berardi CJ, Dillard-Telm S, et al. Passive immunization of newborn rhesus macaques prevents oral simian immunodeficiency virus infection. J Infect Dis 1998; 177:1247–1259.

101. Siegel F, Kurth R, Norley S. Neither whole inactivated virus immunogen nor passive immunoglobulin transfer protects against SIV_{agm} infection in the African green monkey natural host. J Acquir Immune Defic Syndr 1995; 8:217–226.

102. Clements JE, Montelaro RC, Zink MC, et al. Cross-protective immune responses induced in rhesus macaques by immunization with attenuated macrophage-tropic simian immunodeficiency virus. J Virol 1995; 69:2737–2744.

103. Haigwood NL, Watson A, Sutton WF, et al. Passive immune globulin therapy in the SIV/macaque model: early intervention can alter disease profile. Immunol Lett 1996; 51:107–114.

104. Conley AJ, Kessler JA II, Boots LJ, et al. The consequence of passive administration of an anti-human immunodeficiency virus type 1 neutralizing monoclonal antibody before challenge of chimpanzees with a primary virus isolate. J Virol 1996; 70:6751–6758.

105. Mascola JR, Lewis MG, Stiegler G, et al. Protection of macaques against pathogenic simian/human immunodeficiency virus 89.6PD by passive transfer of neutralizing antibodies. J Virol 1999; 73:4009–4018.

106. Mascola JR, Gabriela S, VanCott TC, et al. Protection of macaques against vaginal transmission of a pathogenic HIV-1/SIV chimeric virus by passive infusion of neutralizing antibodies. Nat Med 2000; 6:207–210.

107. Baba TW, Liska V, Hofmann-Lehmann R, et al. Human neutralizing monoclonal antibodies of the IgG1 subtype protect against mucosal simian-human immunodeficiency virus infection. Nat Med 2000; 6:200–206.

108. Custer RP, Bosma GC, Bosma MJ. Severe combined immunodeficiency (SCID) in the mouse. Pathology, reconstitution, neoplasms. Am J Pathol 1985; 120:464–477.

109. McCune JM, Namikawa R, Kaneshima H, Schultz LD, Lieberman M, Weissman IL. The SCID-hu mouse: murine model for the analysis of human hematolymphoid differentiation and function. Science 1988; 241:1632–1639.

110. Mosier DE, Gulizia RJ, Baird SM, Wilson DB. Transfer of a functional human immune system to mice with severe combined immunodeficiency. Nature 1988; 335:256–259.

111. Mosier DE, Gulizia RJ, Baird SM, Wilson DB, Spector DH, Spector SA. Human immunodeficiency virus infection of human-PBL-SCID mice. Science 1991; 251:791–794.

112. Safrit JT, Fung MSC, Andrews CA, et al. Hu-PBL-SCID mice can be protected from HIV-1 infection by passive transfer of monoclonal antibody to the principal neutralizing determinant of the envelope gp120. AIDS 1993; 7:15–21.

113. Gauduin MC, Safrit JT, Weir R, Fung MS, Koup RA. Pre- and post-exposure protection against human immunodeficiency virus type 1 infection mediated by a monoclonal antibody. J Infect Dis 1995; 171:1203–1209.

114. Andrus L, Prince AM, Bernal I, et al. Passive immunization with a human immunodeficiency virus type 1-neutralizing monoclonal antibody in Hu-PBL-SCID mice; isolation of a neutralization escape variant. J Infect Dis 1998; 177:889–897.

115. Koup RA, Safrit JT, Weir R, Gauduin M-C. Defining antibody protection against HIV-1 transmission in Hu-PBL-SCID mice. Semin Immunol 1996; 8:263–268.

116. Andrus L, McCarthy M, Cobb KE, et al. Passive immunization against HIV-1 infection. In: Girard M, Valette L (eds). Retroviruses of Human AIDS and Related Animal Diseases. Paris: Foundation Merieux, 1993, pp. 251–257.

117. Parren PW, Ditzel HJ, Gulizia RJ, et al. Protection against HIV-1 infection in hu-PBL-SCID mice by passive administration with a neutralizing monoclonal antibody against the gp120-binding site. AIDS 1995; 9:F1–F6.

118. Gauduin M-C, Parren PWHI, Weir R, Barbas CF, Burton DR, Koup RA. Passive immunization with a human monoclonal antibody protects hu-PBL-SCID mice against challenge by primary isolates of HIV-1. Nat Med 1997; 3:1389–1393.

119. Okamoto Y, Eda Y, Ogura A, et al. In SCID-hu mice, passive transfer of a humanized antibody prevents infection and atrophic change of medulla in human thymic implant due to intravenous inoculation of primary HIV-1 isolate. J Immunol 1998; 160:69–76.

120. Schutten M, Tenner-Racz K, Racz P, van Bekkum DW, Osterhaus AD. Human antibodies that neutralize primary human immunodeficiency virus type 1 in vitro do not provide protection in an in vivo model. J Gen Virol 1996; 77:1667–1675.

121. Moore JP, Nara PL. The role of the V3 loop of gp120 in HIV infection. AIDS 1994; 5:S21–S33.

122. Trkola A, Dragic T, Arthos J, et al. CD4-dependent, antibody-sensitive interactions between HIV-1 and its co-receptor CCR-5. Nature 1996; 384:184–187.

123. Gauduin M-C, Weir R, Fung MSC, Koup RA. Involvement of the complement system in antibody-mediated post-exposure protection against human immunodeficiency virus type 1. AIDS Res Hum Retroviruses 1998; 14:205–211.

124. Jackson GG, Perkins JT, Rubenis M, et al. Passive immunoneutralization of human immunodeficiency virus in patients with advanced AIDS. Lancet 1988; 2:647–654.

125. Karpas A, Hill F, Youle M, et al. Effects of passive immunization in patients with the acquired immunodeficiency syndrome-related complex and acquired immunodeficiency syndrome. Proc Natl Acad Sci USA 1988; 85:9234–9237.

126. Busch MP, Henrard DR, Hewlett IK, et al. Poor sensitivity, specificity, and reproducibility of detection of HIV-1 DNA in serum by polymerase chain reaction. The Transfusion Safety Study Group. J Acquir Immune Defic Syndr 1992; 5:872–877.

127. Jacobson JM, Colman N, Ostrow NA, et al. Passive immunotherapy in the treatment of advanced human immunodeficiency virus infection. J Infect Dis 1993; 168:298–305.

128. Vittecoq D, Mattlinger B, Barre-Sinoussi F, et al. Passive immunotherapy in AIDS: a randomized trial of serial human immunodeficiency virus-positive transfusions of plasma rich in p24 antibodies versus transfusions of seronegative plasma. J Infect Dis 1992; 165:364–368.

129. Levy J, Youvan T, Lee ML. Passive hyperimmune plasma therapy in the treatment of acquired immunodeficiency syndrome: results of a 12 month multicenter double-blind controlled trial. Blood 1994; 84:2130–2135.

130. Vittecoq D, Chevret S, Morand-Joubert L, et al. Passive immunotherapy in AIDS: a double-blind randomized study based on transfusions rich in anti-human immundeficiency virus 1 antibodies vs transfusions of seronegative plasma. Proc Natl Acad Sci USA 1995; 92:1195–1199.

131. Morand-Joubert L, Vittecoq D, Roudot-Thoraval F, et al. Virological and immunological data of AIDS patients treated by passive immunotherapy (transfusions of plasma rich in HIV-1 antibodies). Vox Sang 1997; 73:149–154.

132. Osther K, Wiik A, Black F, et al. PASSHIV-1 treatment of patients with HIV-1 infection. A preliminary report of a phase 1 trial of hyperimmune porcine immunoglobulin to HIV-1. AIDS 1992; 6:1457–1464.

133. Stiehm ER, Lambert JS, Mofenson LM, et al. Efficacy of zidovudine and human immunodeficiency virus (HIV) hyperimmune immunoglobin for reducing perinatal HIV transmission from HIV-infected women with advanced disease: results of Pediatric AIDS Clinical Trials Group Protocol 185. J Infect Dis 1999;179:567–575.

134. Stiehm ER, Lambert JS, Mofenson LM, et al. Use of human immunodeficiency virus (HIV) human hyperimmune immunoglobulin in HIV type 1-infected children (Pediatric AIDS Clinical Trials Group Protocol 273). J Infect Dis 2000; 181:548–554.

135. Hinkula J, Bratt G, Gilljam G, et al. Immunological and virological interactions in patients receiving passive immunotherapy with HIV-1 neutralizing monoclonal antibodies. J Acquir Immune Defic Syndr 1994; 7:940–951.

136. Gunthard HF, Gowland PL, Schupback J. A phase I/IIA clinical study with a chimeric mouse-human monoclonal antibody to the V3 loop of human immunodeficiency virus type 1 gp120. J Infect Dis 1994; 170: 1384–1393.

137. Stiehm ER, Mofenson L, Zolla-Pazner S, Jackson B, Martin NL, Ammann AJ. Summary of the workshop on passive immunotherapy in the prevention and treatment of HIV infection. The Passive Antibody Workshop Participants. Clin Immunol Immunopathol 1995; 75:84–93.

12

Host Cell-Directed Approaches for Treating HIV and Restoring Immune Function

J. Michael Kilby and R. Pat Bucy

INTRODUCTION

Despite a number of recent therapeutic advances, there remains an urgent need for new approaches to treat HIV infection, the causative agent of AIDS. In this chapter, treatment strategies are reviewed that target host cell interactions or immune responses, rather than acting as direct antiviral agents. Certain treatments that target host factors—such as cytokines, chemokines, immunomodulators, or therapeutic vaccination—will probably prove to be effective adjuvants to conventional antiviral therapy in the future and may even hold the potential to alter the natural history of HIV infection in some individuals.

The demonstration of persistent high levels of HIV replication within the untreated host, even during the often prolonged asymptomatic course of early HIV infection (1), has led to a logical therapeutic emphasis on the development of more potent antiviral drugs. Ground-breaking studies evaluating the responses to antiretroviral regimens revealed the dynamic nature of viral replication along with the potential to suppress the amount of viral genetic material (HIV RNA or viral load) in the plasma by 1000-fold or more (2,3). The critical role of the plasma viral load was further emphasized by the observation that this measurement is also tightly linked to the rate of disease progression in untreated patients (4). Larger randomized clinical trials later demonstrated that individuals treated with highly active antiretroviral therapy (HAART) regimens had decreases in opportunistic infections and death compared with those treated with less potent therapies (5,6). Improved clinical outcomes have been well documented outside of the clinical trial setting as well (7), and for the first time in the history of the epidemic, a decline in AIDS-related mortality has been noted in the United States. The dramatic reduction in plasma viral load after HAART treatment is associated with an apparent halt in disease progression and substantial functional improvement in the immune system, but such treatment does not bring about complete eradication of the pathogen. Understanding the host factors that keep viral replication in check during the prolonged steady-state phase will provide key mechanistic insights, which may be critical for devising novel therapeutic interventions that will potentially synergize with antiretroviral regimens to eliminate chronic active infection.

From: *Immunotherapy for Infectious Diseases*
Edited by: J. M. Jacobson © Humana Press Inc., Totowa, NJ

Although clinical outcomes have improved considerably in the HAART era, many individuals cannot tolerate long-term therapy with the complex drug regimens involved. The selection for drug-resistant viruses continues to be a major problem in clinical practice. Although there is clearly a significant improvement in the absolute number of circulating CD4 T-cells for most HAART-treated patients, CD4 counts rarely approach normal levels even when dramatic and sustained declines in viral replication rates are seen. Finally, when individuals who have achieved prolonged plasma viral load suppression discontinue HAART, there is typically a rapid rebound in viral replication, resulting in a return to high plasma viral load levels *(8)*. Residual HIV infection persists following prolonged effective HAART and has been detected in both blood and tissue biopsies *(9–13)*. Thus, although HAART has provided unprecedented benefits for many HIV-infected patients, many barriers remain if we are to rely on this approach alone in the struggle against AIDS.

Previous investigations revealed several host factors that influence the risk of HIV acquisition or disease progression, often in the context of evaluating atypical clinical cases. The same viral strain may lead to extremely different rates of disease progression in different hosts *(14)*. Conversely, the clinical courses of genetically identical triplets infected perinatally were strikingly uniform *(15)*. These observations suggest that the viral load set point (and the corresponding rate of disease progression) for an individual may be determined primarily by host factors that control viral replication, rather than the virologic characteristics of the original inoculum. Although viral variants exist that play a role in some cases, understanding which host effects account for the substantial differences in progression rate between individuals should provide critical insights into the development of new therapeutic targets. Many investigations have focused on unique hosts who have been repeatedly exposed to HIV and yet have not shown evidence of productive viral infection. Subjects with defective expression of CCR5, a receptor utilized by most sexually transmitted HIV strains, appear to be overrepresented among this group of exposed, noninfected individuals *(16,17)*.

However, these rare host phenotypes do not account for the majority of differences in disease progression between individuals. Additional investigations of subjects with repeated exposure to HIV who have remained seronegative reveal that such individuals frequently have detectable HIV-specific immune responses *(18–20)*. These data suggest that some individuals may become infected (perhaps with a very low viral dose) and mount an immune response sufficient to control the infection prior to the development of an antibody response and established chronic infection. Another approach has been to concentrate on long-term nonprogressors, subjects who are infected with HIV yet do not develop immunodeficiency over many years in the absence of antiretroviral treatment. Generally, these investigations demonstrate a combination of virologic (attenuated or defective viral strains) and host (strong HIV-specific immune responses) factors that contribute to slowed disease progression *(21,22)*.

Another line of evidence strongly implicating the magnitude of antiviral immune responses in controlling infection is the association between alleles related to immune responsiveness, such as HLA classes I and II, and the clinical course of HIV infection *(23–25)*. Recent studies have focused more specifically on the impact of HIV-specific CTL responses, which are determined by HLA class I antigen presentation, on the rate of clinical progression across the spectrum of HIV disease *(26,27)*. The critical role of

CD8 T-cells in the control of viral load is also supported by a recent investigation involving SIV-infected rhesus macaques. Deletion of CD8+ cells via the administration of monoclonal antibodies prompted a rapid increase in viremia *(28,29)*, strongly implying that an active immune response is maintaining the viral load set point.

All currently approved therapies for HIV infection target a viral enzyme (either reverse transcriptase or protease). If viral replication could be safely inhibited by targeting a host element, this would provide several theoretical advantages. In many instances, host factors in general may be more conserved throughout the population compared with the highly variable and changeable nature of viral proteins. Unlike the rapidly growing and genetically unstable virus quasispecies, host factors would not be predicted to respond quickly to drug pressure in the selection process for drug-resistant variants. Treatment strategies directed at host cells have the potential to be synergistic with antiviral regimens, while minimizing risks of cross-resistance or shared toxicities with drugs from the currently available therapeutic classes. A key unanswered question is which host factors, if any, can be successfully targeted by therapeutic interventions. We describe several potential approaches to host cell-based therapies: blocking host cell entry, modulating the immune activation state, increasing absolute lymphocyte cell counts, increasing the clearance of the latently infected cell pool, and enhancing immune control over viral replication. Based on the diverse lines of evidence outlined above and the suggestion that viral suppression alone is insufficient in the quest for a cure, researchers have recently focused particular attention on the latter strategy: stimulation of HIV-specific cellular immune responses in addition to striving for complete viral suppression with HAART *(30–32)*.

TARGETING CELL ENTRY

A logical therapeutic strategy is to intervene at the level of the initial interactions between HIV and target cells. Theoretically, successfully targeting the process of viral entry into host cells would provide certain advantages over drugs that inhibit viral enzymes brought into play in the later steps of the viral life cycle. For more than a decade, it has been known that a critical initial step in the viral entry process is the binding of portions of the HIV surface glycoprotein (gp120) to the CD4 receptor, expressed primarily on T-helper lymphocytes. In 1988, in vitro data suggested that recombinant, soluble CD4 could competitively inhibit HIV infection and syncytium formation, presumably by acting as a decoy and binding to gp120 in place of susceptible CD4-expressing T-cells *(33–36)*. However, clinical trials did not demonstrate any antiviral effects in vivo *(37)*. Another series of in vitro studies in 1988 suggested the potential for sulfated polyanionic substances to interfere nonspecifically with the binding of HIV to T-cells, resulting in potent inhibition of viral replication *(38–40)*. Unfortunately, clinical trials were unsuccessful owing to poor absorption of oral dextran *(41,42)* and severe adverse events related to intravenous dextran *(43)*.

Between 1995 and 1997, a number of investigative groups reported that β-chemokines and their derivatives had a significant inhibitory effect on viral replication in vitro *(44–47)*. The initial observations occurred at a time when the CD4 receptor was the only well-characterized cell entry mechanism for HIV. More than a decade after the identification of the key interactions between HIV and the CD4 receptor, it is now clear that HIV must bind to two distinct molecules on the cell surface before it can infect human cells. HIV isolates categorized as non-syncytium-inducing (NSI) are most often implicated in the sexual transmission of infection. NSI viruses typically require the presence of the β-chemokine receptor CCR5 in addition to CD4 *(48,49)*. CCR5 is the natural receptor for RANTES, macrophage inflammatory protein (MIP)-1α, and MIP-β, mediators of inflammatory reactions and chemotaxis. Syncytium-inducing (SI) or T-tropic viral strains, often associated with more rapid disease progression in the setting of advanced HIV infection and AIDS, tend to utilize the α-chemokine receptor CXCR4 (also called fusin) *(50)*. The natural ligand for CXCR4 is stromal-derived factor (SDF-1), a protein constituitively expressed in many tissues that may mediate cellular trafficking such as the homing of lymphocytes into inflamed tissues or the repopulation of transplanted stem cells into bone marrow *(51,52)*.

It may be possible to alter host expression of the chemokine receptors. For example, a gene therapy strategy involving expression of a modified CXCR4 molecule (an intrakine) demonstrated antiviral effects against T-tropic HIV in vitro, possibly because the altered CXCR4 was effectively trapped in the endoplasmic reticulum and not appropriately expressed on the cell surface for HIV binding *(53)*. At the present time, there is insufficient information about the normal role chemokines play in inflammatory responses and other physiologic processes. The discovery of the role of CCR5 receptors in HIV was owing in part to the recognition of a relatively common mutation in the CCR5 gene, a 32-bp deletion (Δ32) that results in lack of cell surface expression of the chemokine receptor among individuals who have been multiply exposed to HIV yet not infected with the virus *(17,49,54)*. Thus there is evidence that individuals homozygous for the Δ32CCR5 mutation are substantially protected from becoming infected, although these individuals do not have an obvious deleterious phenotype associated with the defective expression of CCR5.

However, evidence related to the effects of alterations in the CXCR4 pathway raises theoretical concerns. Knockout mice that cannot express SDF-1, the ligand for CXCR4, undergo abnormal fetal development (cardiac and B-cell lymphopoesis defects) and die perinatally *(55)*. Another theoretical concern is that effectively blocking one of the chemokine receptors may provide selection pressure for the outgrowth of viruses utilizing alternative receptors. One undesirable scenario is that selectively inhibiting NSI viruses, by administering one of the β-chemokines, for example, may ultimately drive the evolution of viral strains within an individual to SI CXCR4-utilizing viruses, which are associated with more rapid clinical progression and CD4 depletion.

However, the most straightforward approach to blocking chemokine receptors would be to administer the natural ligands or other small molecules that may serve as competitive inhibitors. A recent in vitro study demonstrates that a specific isoform of MIP-1α may be the most potent CCR5 agonist and may be a candidate for clinical studies *(56)*. Recent in vitro investigations involving the bicyclam AMD3100 provide further data to support the feasibility of blocking HIV-1 entry via the the CCR5 receptor *(57)*. An example of a synthetic compound that appears to block HIV-1 entry via CXCR4 receptor inhibition is T22, an 18-amino acid peptide *(58)*. A smaller derivative, termed T134 (14 amino acids), exhibits greater potency and less cytotoxicity in vitro *(59)*.

The subsequent step in the viral entry process, gp41-mediated membrane fusion, has potential as a more universal therapeutic target because it may be utilized by all HIV isolates regardless of cellular tropism or antigenic variations. Synthetic peptides corresponding to segments of gp41 have been shown to disrupt the folding and unfolding of the gp41 tertiary structure necessary for membrane fusion to occur. A 36-amino acid peptide, T-20, was found to be a particularly potent inhibitor of HIV-1 in vitro. This agent demonstrated a 50% inhibitory concentration (IC_{50}) of 1.7 ng/mL in T-cell lines *(60)*. In the first clinical trial of a peptide fusion inhibitor, intravenous T-20 resulted in significant, dose-related declines in plasma HIV RNA levels *(25)*. There was an approx. 99% reduction in viral load during short-term T-20 administration in the four subjects in the highest dose group tested (100 mg twice daily). An analysis of viral dynamics showed that the initial slope of virus decline, a measure of antiretroviral potency, was comparable to that achieved with other approved HIV therapies including three- and four-drug combinations of reverse transcriptase and protease inhibitors. The second clinical trial of T-20, recently completed, involved 78 subjects enrolled at multiple sites around the United States *(61)*. This trial allowed heavily pretreated patients to add T-20 therapy to their preexisting oral antiretroviral regimens. Over a 28-day administration period, dose-related reductions in plasma HIV RNA levels were demonstrated that confirmed the findings in the phase I trial. Thus, these findings provide proof of concept that therapeutics targeting a viral entry event can result in safe and clinically meaningful inhibition of viral replication. However, this approach to blocking viral entry is not directly aimed at a conserved host target, as exemplified by the suggestion that selection for resistant viral variants is possible *(62,63)*.

TARGETING CELL ACTIVATION STATE

Closely related to direct inhibition of HIV cell entry is the concept of modulating host cell activation status, to influence the progression of disease favorably. It has been recognized for many years that activated lymphocytes are more susceptible to HIV infection than resting or quiescent cells *(64)*. Nonspecific T-cell stimulation factors, such as phytohemagglutinin and interleukin-2 (IL-2), are routinely utilized in the laboratory to increase HIV infectivity in cell culture experiments. Clinical trials evaluating IL-2 infusions as a strategy to increase absolute CD4 numbers (see below) demonstrated that some patients receiving inadequate antiretroviral therapy had bursts of viremia corresponding to the immunoactivation state induced by potent T-cell stimulation *(65)*. Possible clinical correlates include observations that nonspecific antigenic stimulation, such as routine influenza *(66)*, pneumococcal *(67)*, or tetanus toxoid *(68)* vaccinations, may transiently stimulate HIV replication in the absence of adequate antiretroviral suppression. Such effects have not been demonstrated among patients effectively suppressed on HAART. Similarly, there appear to be temporary increases in plasma viral load when patients develop opportunistic infections, despite adherence to antiretroviral medications *(69,70)*. These bursts of viral activity subside as concomitant infections are treated.

Although immunosuppressive therapy is obviously not an attractive option for widespread use among patients with acquired T-cell deficiency, preliminary studies have been carried out to explore the potential for limiting T-cell activation as a therapeutic strategy. Particularly in the pre-HAART era, such approaches were frequently a last resort for palliative reasons when conventional therapeutic options had been exhausted. Pilot studies explored the safety and feasibility of using agents such as pentoxyfylline *(71,72)* and thalidomide *(56,73)* as inhibitors of tumor necrosis factor (TNF) to limit the proinflammatory cytokine cascade that stimulates cycles of HIV replication. When we administered tapering doses of prednisone to advanced AIDS patients with wasting syndrome, a decline in markers of immunoactivation (neopterin and TNF receptor II levels) was followed by a dose-related decline in plasma viral load *(74)*. In a large clinical study involving less advanced HIV infection, patients receiving corticosteroids had prolonged moderate elevations in their absolute circulating CD4 counts while on therapy compared with individuals receiving reverse transcriptase inhibitor therapy alone *(75)*. A multicenter trial in the United States is now being planned to evaluate the effects of low-dose prednisone when administered to patients with partial but not complete viral load suppression on HAART. A pilot study evaluating the effects of low-dose cytotoxic chemotherapy to limit the availability of susceptible target cells is also currently nearing completion.

The evidence that inflammatory events adversely affect blood CD4 counts and the apparent paradox of prednisone increasing circulating lymphocyte numbers in less advanced HIV-infected patients are quite compatible with evidence regarding the T-cell redistribution phenomenon between tissues and peripheral blood. Based on blood analysis alone, Pakker et al. *(76)* surmised that the initial rise in circulating CD4 cells following initiation of HAART was due to a redistribution of memory cells from tissues to the periphery. To explore these issues further, we analyzed blood and lymph node tissues obtained concurrently from patients before and after the initiation of HAART *(77)*. Ten weeks after HAART, the number of lymphocytes per excised cervical lymph node had decreased, whereas the number of blood lymphocytes tended to increase. The expression levels of several proinflammatory cytokines (interferon-γ [IFN-γ], IL-1β, IL-6, and MIP-1α) declined following HAART. After therapy, the expression of adhesion molecules known to mediate lymphocyte sequestration into inflamed tissues (vascular cell adhesion molecule [VCAM]-1 and intracellular cell adhesion molecule [ICAM]-1) was also significantly reduced. These data support the hypothesis that the abrupt rise in blood CD4 cells immediately after therapy is related to redistribution and that this redistribution is mediated by a resolution of immunoactivation that had sequestered T-cells within inflamed tissues. This inverse relationship between blood and inflamed tissues has also been described for other infectious diseases. For example, a recent report suggests that the reversal of anergy in patients receiving therapy for tuberculosis corresponds to the release into the bloodstream of tuberculosis-specific T-cells previously sequestered in infected tissues *(78)*.

TARGETING T-CELL NUMBERS

Another logical approach to ameliorate the consequences of HIV infection would be to stimulate increases in absolute CD4 cell counts. The aim of this strategy is to reverse the best characterized immunodeficiency of AIDS without necessarily getting at the underlying cause of lymphocyte depletion. Controversy remains about the exact pathogenesis of CD4 cell depletion in AIDS; it has never been conclusively demonstrated that CD4 cells are killed by a direct HIV cytopathic effect. The frequency of infected CD4 T-cells is generally very low, so that even though infected cells are quickly cleared in active infection (via either a cytopathic effect or direct lysis by immune viral-specific CTL), this mechanism alone may not account for depletion of the entire population of CD4 T-cells. CD4 cell decline over the natural history of HIV infection may also be caused by cell death of uninfected cells induced by toxic viral products or a failure of lymphocyte regenerative capacity. The mechanism of CD4 depletion over the long natural history of the infection may not be the same process that accounts for the partial rebound in CD4 T-cells (and other lymphocyte subsets) that occurs within weeks of HAART induction.

As described above, evidence suggests that at least part of the improvement in CD4 cell counts on therapy is a trafficking phenomenon rather than a reflection of new T-cell production. This model is consistent with the general understanding that T-cells are long lived and not rapidly replaced by the body when depleted in other clinical situations *(79,80)*. On the other hand, recent studies suggest that there may be a very gradual return of naive T-cells from unknown regenerative sites after several months of therapy *(81)*. Despite impressive T-cell gains in some treated patients, the absolute CD4 cell numbers rarely approach normal levels following HAART alone.

Recently, investigators from a large clinical trial made up of a mixture of zidovudine-experienced and treatment-naive subjects concluded that patients with the largest increases in absolute CD4 counts on HAART were at higher risk for virologic breakthrough on therapy *(82)*. The authors proposed the hypothesis that the higher number of target cells detected following combination therapy in some cases helped to fuel the fire of viral replication. Other clinical trials, which enrolled fewer previously treated subjects, did not suggest that the rise in CD4 cells is predictive of virologic breakthrough *(83,84)*. It is conceivable that patients with more advanced disease tend to have more dramatic rises in CD4 counts when HAART is initiated and that these more advanced patients may be less able to control viral replication via an immune mechanism.

Investigators at the National Institutes of Health (NIH) have conducted a series of trials to evaluate the use of recombinant human IL-2 as a T-cell growth factor in HIV-infected patients *(65,85)*. Although occasional transient increases in viral load were seen during IL-2 infusions, many subjects with baseline CD4 cell counts >200 cells/mm^3 had significant boosts in CD4 cell counts without apparent long-term changes in the viral load set point. Some patients experienced rises to normal ranges (approx. 800–2000), which is virtually unprecedented in the setting of antiretroviral therapy alone. Patients with lower CD4 cell counts at baseline generally had less impressive responses, and the risk/benefit ratio appeared to be less favorable in this setting. The IL-2 infusions are associated with frequent adverse symptoms including flu-like aches and pains, fevers, headaches, and occasionally more severe sequelae. Other ongoing investigations are exploring the possibility of low-dose (and therefore more tolerable) daily IL-2 therapy rather than high-dose intermittent therapy, and preliminary responses in CD4 counts have been less dramatic but generally encouraging *(86,87)*. Larger randomized clinical trials are in progress to evaluate responses in combination with HAART and to determine whether increased CD4 cell numbers correlate with improved clinical outcomes.

Other experimental approaches have been evaluated in small clinical trials to increase T-cell numbers. Recent debate has focused on the importance of residual thymus activity in some adults with HIV infection *(88)*, and pilot studies exploring the possibilities of thymic implants as therapy for HIV-infected adults are under way. Carroll et al. *(89)* have performed a series of clinical studies in which plasmapheresis is performed on HIV-infected individuals, isolated CD4 T-cells are costimulated ex vivo with

CD3/CD28, and then the amplified CD4 cell population is reinfused into the host. In addition to the potential benefits of increased absolute CD4 cell counts, these reinfused CD4 cells may result in less susceptibility to M-tropic virus disease progression because the costimulation process downregulates cellular CCR5 expression *(89)*. Through this intensive technique, these patients have achieved infusion-related rises in absolute CD4 cell numbers.

TARGETING ENHANCED CLEARANCE OF THE LATENT POOL

The demonstration that cells containing potentially infectious, integrated provirus persist following prolonged undetectable plasma viral loads on HAART has prompted discussions about strategies that might complement HAART by stimulating the clearance of the latently infected cell pool. The population of latently infected cells appears to be established quite early in the process of HIV infection and then persists for many years regardless of therapy *(11,12,90,91)*. In support of this general concept, in our own unpublished observations the total complement of viral DNA in a cohort of HIV-infected patients remains relatively stable for periods of follow-up of up to a decade.

Because the immune system probably does not target resting T-cells with integrated provirus, the best strategy to induce clearance of the latently infected pool may be to activate viral replication in the presence of HAART. This approach would have been difficult to comprehend several years ago, when any attempt to activate viral replication, even transiently, was considered counterproductive. However, after improvements in therapy resulted in dramatic and sustained declines in plasma viral load, more radical approaches seemed justifiable in the quest for viral eradication. Investigational agents that could serve as potent T-cell stimuli have been proposed, but there are uncertainties about the relative safety and tolerability of administration. For example, infusion of OKT3 generates a transient potent stimulus for T-cell activation, although administration over several days results in immunosuppressive effects. Although this drug has been utilized with relative safety in the transplantation setting, there are anecdotal reports of severe systemic reactions to OKT3 in HIV-infected subjects. Less toxic possibilities might include growth factors that are capable of stimulating multiple leukocyte cell lines. Granulocyte/macrophage colony-stimulating factor (GM-CSF), for example, has been shown in some but not all in vitro studies to upregulate HIV expression in the absence of potent antiretroviral therapy *(9)*. HIV-infected cells appear to have a reduced capacity to produce GM-CSF and IL-2, and GM-CSF administration may partially restore cellular IL-2 production *(92)*. Retrospective studies suggest the possibility that GM-CSF has a beneficial effect on survival not entirely explained by the avoidance of neutropenia *(93,94)*. Further studies are in planning stage or under way to explore the prognostic implications of the relative responses to these agents as well as the overall therapeutic role of granulocyte growth factors in AIDS.

As described above, several trials have been conducted to evaluate the effects of intermittent recombinant human IL-2 infusions. A preliminary report relating to this experience suggested that some patients who had undergone several cycles of IL-2 in addition to HAART had extremely low levels of proviral DNA or latently infected cells despite analysis of large amounts of blood obtained through plasmapheresis *(95)*. In a few patients, analysis of lymph node tissue also did not show cells with integrated viral DNA. Although these findings remain to be confirmed and corroborated, the suggestion is that T-cell stimulation has the potential to trigger clearance of the latently infected cell pool. This could occur because cells reactivating viral replication are eliminated either by virus-mediated destruction or targeted immune surveillance. Both retrospective analyses and prospective clinical trials are under way to clarify our understanding of the role of IL-2 in the clearance of latent infection.

TARGETING ENHANCED
IMMUNE CONTROL OF VIRAL REPLICATION

As described above, there is accumulating circumstantial evidence that host factors, specifically the cytotoxic T-lymphocyte (CTL) response to HIV, play a significant role in determining the extent of viral replication. The initial decline in plasma HIV RNA following acute infection coincides with the appearance of HIV-specific CTLs (and not neutralizing antibody) *(96)*. There is evidence that a highly specific CTL response may induce selective pressure on the viral quasispecies early on in the course of infection but that virologic escape can occur later if viral variants evolve that no longer correspond with the predominant HIV-specific CTL population *(97)*. The relative frequency of HIV-specific CTLs appears to be inversely proportional to the plasma viral load, in both recently infected individuals *(27)* and those with more established disease *(26)*. In a simian model of AIDS, eliminating CD8+ lymphocytes from monkeys with chronic SIV infection resulted in marked increases in plasma viral load *(29)*. When SIV-specific CD8+ cells reappeared, viral replication was again suppressed. These observations led to a hypothesis that the viral load set point, the plasma HIV RNA steady state achieved when the rate of viral replication is held at a relatively constant level by host factors controlling replication, is determined primarily by the degree of antigen-driven CTL activity *(31)*.

If the viral load set point is primarily determined by the extent of antigen-driven host immune responses, this phenomenon may help to explain the complex nature of latent HIV infection. Latently infected cells are established very early in the process of HIV infection, at a time when the HIV-specific cellular immune response has not fully matured. High levels of viral antigen ultimately stimulate a viral-specific CTL response, which coincides with the substantial decrease in plasma viral load that accompanies the resolution of the acute infection syndrome *(96)*. Most patients who never receive potent antiretroviral therapy eventually succumb to progressive disease and are not able to control viral replication in the long term. However, exceptional individuals who have long-term nonprogression of HIV disease, as already described, appear to maintain some degree of HIV-specific CD4+ *(98)* and CD8+ T-cell responses *(21)* over extended periods. Because T-helper (CD4+) function is necessary for a fully effective CTL (CD8+) response, these two cellular responses are interdependent. Once patients are treated with potent antiretroviral therapy, however, viral antigen may eventually fall below the threshold necessary to maintain adequate CTL responses. A patient with acute symptomatic HIV infection prior to seroconversion, for example, developed HIV-specific CTLs that were attenuated as HAART was administered. When the patient abruptly discontinued therapy, a high plasma viral load and severe symptoms returned, followed by the reappearance of HIV-specific CTLs *(99)*. If indeed the limited duration of HIV-specific CTL activity in most treated patients is caused by the lack of sustained, antigen-driven CTL responses, then a reappraisal of the therapeutic vaccination strategy is indicated. Once an individual has successfully achieved potent suppression of viral replication and an increase in general immune responsiveness (owing in part to a change in the cytokine milieu and lymphocyte redistribution) on HAART, restimulating HIV-specific CD4 and CD8 T cell immunity may be critical for achieving prolonged immunologic containment of viral replication.

The most promising strategy being explored for preventive HIV vaccines is to combine a prime immunogen (often incorporating HIV antigens within an attenuated viral vector) with boost peptide immunogens (gp120, gp160, or portions thereof) to induce CTL and neutralizing antibody, respectively *(100,101)*. The ideal immunogen for therapeutic vaccination strategies, once chronic viral infection has already been established, may be an agent from the former category (designed to present antigens via a class I- or CTL-mediated mechanism rather than the more conventional aim of stimulating neutralizing antibody). Multicenter randomized clinical trials have been designed to evaluate the effects of combining HAART with HIV therapeutic vaccinations. One trial in development will compare the effects of different immune-based strategies (cycles of IL-2, a canarypox HIV immunogen, or both) in addition to HAART on the extent of virologic rebound when therapy is temporarily interrupted after 1 year.

Another intriguing line of evidence regarding the influence of host immune responses on the viral load set point derives from observations of intermittent therapy. Generally, adherence to combination drug regimens has been one of the tenets of HIV therapy, and there is evidence that incomplete suppression (such as with inappropriately low drug doses or frequently skipped doses) leads to a higher incidence of drug resistance over time. However, individual patients who intermittently received moderately potent but not complete suppression on the combination of didanosine and hydroxyurea, for example, appear to maintain HIV-specific CTL responses that correlate with strikingly delayed and attenuated viral rebound when treatment is held *(102,103)*. Similarly, in studies of acutely infected patients who received antiretroviral therapy very early in the disease course, those patients who had abrupt, self-limited interruptions in HAART tended to develop strong HIV-specific CTL responses corresponding to very limited viral rebound on discontinuation of therapy *(104)*. These anecdotal observations suggest the possibility that, under the right circumstances, strategic interruptions in therapy may result in restimulation of waning host immune responses that can mediate control of viral replication rates after therapy becomes intolerable or is no longer effective. Pilot studies are under way to determine the effects of different therapeutic strategies involving experimental vaccines and planned HAART interruptions as synergistic exogenous and endogenous immunizations, respectively.

Although complete viral eradication remains a worthy goal of HIV treatment, these preliminary observations and studies suggest that long-term immunologic control over HIV replication may be more eminently achievable and just as beneficial in the long run. Analogous to other common human viral pathogens (cytomegalovirus, Epstein-Barr virus, varicella-zoster virus, and so on) that maintain some form of clinical latency following a temporary or subclinical illness, it is conceivable that immune-based therapies can induce a life-long truce with HIV that falls short of a complete cure. Avoidance of damaging high levels of viral replication without the need for costly and complex ongoing therapies would result in a dramatic change in the natural history of HIV infection for each infected individual and could potentially alter our perspective on the overall AIDS epidemic.

REFERENCES

1. Piatak M, Saag MS, Yang LC, et al. High levels of HIV-1 in plasma during all stages of infection determined by competitive PCR. Science 1993; 259:1749–1754.
2. Wei X, Ghosh SK, Taylor ME, et al. Viral dynamics in human immunodeficiency virus type 1 infection. Nature 1995; 373:117–122.
3. Ho DD, Neumann AU, Perelson AS, Chen W, Leonard JM, Markowitz M. Rapid turnover of plasma virions and CD4 lymphocytes in HIV-1 infection. Nature 1995; 373:123–126.
4. Mellors JW, Rinaldo CR, Gupta P, White RM, Todd JA, Kingsley LA. Prognosis in HIV-1 infection predicted by the quantity of virus in plasma. Science 1996; 272:1167–1170.
5. Hammer SM, Squires KE, Hughes MD, et al. A controlled trial of two nucleoside analogues plus indinavir in persons with human immunodeficiency virus infection and CD4 cell counts of 200 per cubic millimeter or less. AIDS Clinical Trials Group 320 Study Team. N Engl J Med 1997; 337:725–733.
6. Gulick RM, Mellors J, Havlir D, et al. Treatment with indinavir, zidovudine, and lamivudine in adults with human immunodeficiency virus infection and prior antiretroviral therapy. N Engl J Med 1997; 337:734–739.
7. Palella FJ Jr, Delaney KM, Moorman AC, et al. Declining morbidity and mortality among patients with advanced human immunodeficiency virus infection. HIV Outpatient Study Investigators. N Engl J Med 1998; 338:853–860.
8. Wong JK, Gunthard HF, Havlir DV, et al. Reduction of HIV-1 in blood and lymph nodes following potent antiretroviral therapy and the virologic correlates of treatment failure. Proc Natl Acad Sci USA 1997; 94:12574–12579.
9. Hockett RD, Kilby JM, Derdeyn CA, et al. Constant mean viral copy number per infected cell in tissues regardless of high, low, or undetectable plasma HIV RNA. J Exp Med 1999; 189:1545–1554.
10. Zhang L, Ramratnam B, Tenner-Racz K, et al. Quantifying residual HIV-1 replication in patients receiving combination antiretroviral therapy. N Engl J Med 1999; 340:1605–1613.
11. Wong JK, Hezareh M, Gunthard HF, et al. Recovery of replication-competent HIV despite prolonged suppression of plasma viremia. Science 1997; 278:1291–1295.
12. Finzi D, Hermankova M, Pierson T, et al. Identification of a reservoir for HIV-1 in patients on highly active antiretroviral therapy. Science 1997; 278:1295–1300.
13. Derdeyn CA, Kilby JM, Miralles GD, et al. Detection of HIV-1 latent and persistent active infection in blood lymphocytes in HIV-1 infection. J Infect Dis 1999; 180:1851–1862.
14. Michael NL, Brown AE, Volgt RF, et al. Rapid disease progression without seroconversion following primary HIV-1 infection—evidence for highly susceptible human hosts. J Infect Dis 1997; 24:175.
15. Saulsbury FT. The clinical course of HIV infection in genetically identical children. J Infect Dis 1997; 24:971–974.
16. Liu R, Paxton WA, Choe S, et al. Homozygous defect in HIV-1 coreceptor accounts for resistance of some multiply-exposed individuals to HIV-1 infection. Cell 1996; 86:367–377.
17. Paxton WA, Martin SR, Tse D, et al. Relative resistance to HIV-1 infection of CD4 lymphocytes from persons who remain uninfected despite multiple high-risk sexual exposure. Nat Med 1996; 2:412–417.
18. Bernard NF, Yannakis CM, Lee JS, Tsoukas CM. Human immunodeficiency virus (HIV)-specific cytotoxic T lymphocyte activity in HIV-exposed seronegative persons. J Infect Dis 1999; 179:538–547.
19. Goh WC, Markee J, Akridge RE, et al. Protection against human immunodeficiency virus type 1 infection in persons with repeated exposure: evidence for T cell immunity in the absence of inherited CCR5 coreceptor defects. J Infect Dis 1999; 179:548–557.
20. Rowland-Jones SL, Dong T, Fowke KR, et al. Cytotoxic T cell responses to multiple conserved HIV epitopes in HIV-resistant prostitutes in Nairobi. J Clin Invest 1998; 102:1758–1765.

21. Cao Y, Qin L, Zhang L, Safrit J, Ho DD. Virologic and immunologic characterization of long-term survivors of human immunodeficiency virus type 1 infection. N Engl J Med 1995; 332:201–208.

22. Pantaleo G, Menzo S, Vaccarezza M, et al. Studies in subjects with long-term nonprogressive human immunodeficiency virus infection. N Engl J Med 1995; 332:209–216.

23. Kaslow RA, Carrington M, Apple R, et al. Influence of combinations of human major histocompatibility complex genes on the course of HIV-1 infection. Nat Med 1996; 2:405–411.

24. Keet IP, Tang J, Klein MR, et al. Consistent associations of HLA class I and II and transporter gene products with progression of HIV type 1 infection in homosexual men. J Infect Dis 1999; 180:299–309.

25. Kilby JM, Hopkins S, Venetta TM, et al. Potent suppression of HIV-1 replication in humans by T-20, a peptide inhibitor of gp41-mediated virus entry. Nat Med 1998; 4:1302–1307.

26. Ogg GS, Jin X, Bonhoeffer S, et al. Quantitation of HIV-1-specific cytotoxic T lymphocytes and plasma load of viral RNA. Science 1998; 279:2103–2106.

27. Musey L, Hughes J, Schacker T, Shea T, Corey L, McElrath MJ. Cytotoxic-T-cell responses, viral load, and disease progression in early human immundeficiency virus 1 infection. N Engl J Med 1997; 337:1267–1274.

28. Jin X, Bauer DE, Tuttleton SE, et al. Dramatic rise in plasma viremia after CD8(+) T cell depletion in simian immunodeficiency virus-infected macaques. J Exp Med 1999; 189:991–998.

29. Schmitz JE, Kuroda MJ, Santra S, et al. Control of viremia in simian immunodeficiency virus infection by CD8(+) lymphocytes. Science 1999; 283:857–860.

30. Ho DD. Toward HIV eradication or remission: the tasks ahead. Science 1998; 280:1866–1867.

31. Bucy RP. Immune clearance of HIV-1 replication active cells: a model of two patterns of steady state HIV infection. AIDS Res Hum Retroviruses 1999; 15:223–227.

32. Richman D. The challenge of immune control of immunodeficiency virus. J Clin Invest 1999; 104:677–678.

33. Fisher RA, Bertonis JM, Meier W. HIV infection is blocked in vitro by recombinant soluble CD4. Nature 1988; 331:76–78.

34. Hussey RE, Richardson NE, Kowalski M. A soluble CD4 protein selectively inhibits HIV replication and syncytium formation. Nature 1988; 331:78–81.

35. Deen KC, McDougal JS, Inacker R. A soluble form of CD4 (T4) protein inhibits AIDS virus infection. Nature 1988; 331:82–84.

36. Traunecker A, Luke W, Karajalainen K. Soluble CD4 molecules neutralize HIV-1. Nature 1988; 331:84–86.

37. Kahn JO, Allan JD, Hodges TL. The safety and pharmacokinetics of recombinant soluble CD4 (rCD4) in subjects with AIDS and AIDS-related complex. Ann Intern Med 1990; 112:254–261.

38. Baba M, Pauwels R, Balzarini J. Mechanisms of inhibitory effect of dextran sulfate and heparin on replication of HIV in vitro. Proc Natl Acad Sci USA 1988; 85:6132–6136.

39. Baba M, Snoeck R, Pauwels R. Sulfated polysaccharides are potent and selective inhibitors of various enveloped viruses, including HSV, CMV, VSV, and HIV. Antimicrob Agents Chemother 1988; 32:1742–1745.

40. Mitsuya H, Looney DJ, Kuno S. Dextran sulfate suppression of viruses in the HIV family: inhibition of virion binding to CD4+ cells. Science 1988; 240:646–649.

41. Abrams DI, Kuno S, Wong R. Oral dextran sulfate (UA001) in the treatment of the acquired immunodeficiency syndrome (AIDS) and AIDS-related complex. Ann Intern Med 1989; 110:183–188.

42. Lorentsen KJ, Hendrix CW, Collins JM. Dextran sulfate is poorly absorbed after oral administration. Ann Intern Med 1989; 111:561–566.

43. Flexnor C, Barditch-Crovo PA, Kornhauser DM. Pharmacokinetics, toxicity, and activity of intravenous dextran sulfate in human immunodeficiency infection. Antimicrob Agents Chemother 1991; 35:2544–2550.
44. Cocchi F, Devico AL, Garzino-Demo A, Arya SK, Gallo RC, Lusso P. Identification of RANTES, MIP-1 alpha, and MIP-1 beta as the major HIV-suppressive factors produced by CD8+ T cells. Science 1995; 270:1811–1815.
45. Pal R, Garzino-Demo A, Markham PD, et al. Inhibition of HIV-1 infection by the beta chemokine MDC. Science 1997; 278:695–698.
46. Arenzana-Seisedos F, Virelizier JL, Rousset D. HIV blocked by chemokine antagonist. Nature 1996; 383:400.
47. Simmons G, Clapham PR, Picard L. Potent inhibition of HIV-1 infectivity in macrophages and lymphocytes by a novel CCR5 antagonist. Science 1997; 276:276–279.
48. Dragic T, Litwin V, Allaway GP, et al. HIV-1 entry into CD4+ cells is mediated by the chemokine receptor CC-CKR-5. Nature 1996; 381:667–673.
49. Deng H, Liu R, Ellmeier W, et al. Identification of a major co-receptor for primary isolates of HIV-1. Nature 1996; 381:661–666.
50. Oberlin E, Amara A, Bachelerie, F, et al. The CXC chemokine SDF-1 is the ligand for LESTR/fusin and prevents infection by T-cell-line-adapted HIV-1. Nature 1996; 382:833–835.
51. Bleul CC, Farzan M, Choe H, et al. The lymphocyte chemoattractant SDF-1 is a ligand for LESTR/fusin and blocks HIV-1 entry. Nature 1996; 382:829–833.
52. Derdeyn CA, Costello C, Kilby JM, et al. Correlation between circulating SDF-1 levels and CD4 cell count in human immunodeficiency virus type-1 infected individuals. AIDS Res Hum Retroviruses 1999; 15:1063–1071.
53. Chen JD, Bai X, Yang AG. Inactivation of HIV-1 chemokine co-receptor CXCR-4 by a novel intrakine strategy. Nat Med 1997; 3:1110–1116.
54. Dean M, Carrington M, Winkler C, et al. Genetic restriction of HIV-1 infection and progression to AIDS by a deletion allele of the CKR5 structural gene. Science 1996; 273:1856–1862.
55. Nagasawa T, Hirota S, Tachibana K, et al. Defects of B-cell lymphopoiesis and bone-marrow myelopoiesis in mice lacking the CXC chemokine PBSF/SDF-1. Nature 1996; 382:635–638.
56. Klausner JD, Makonkawkeyoon L, Akarasewi P, et al. The effect of thalidomide on the pathogenesis of HIV-1 and M. tuberculosis infection. J Acquir Immun Defic Syndr Hum Retrovirol 1996; 11:247–257.
57. Donzella G, Schols D, Lin S. AMD3100, a small molecule inhibitor of HIV-1 entry via the CXCR4 co-receptor. Nat Med 1998; 4:72–77.
58. Murakami T, Nakajima T, Koyanagi Y. A small molecule CXCR4 inhibitor that blocks T cell line-tropic HIV-1 infection. J Exp Med 1997; 186:1389–1393.
59. Arakaki R, Tamamaura H, Premanathan M. T134, a small-molecule CXCR4 inhibitor, has no cross-drug resistance with AMD3100, a CXCR4 antagonist with a different structure. J Virol 1999; 73:1719–1723.
60. Wild C, Greenwell T, Matthews T. A synthetic peptide from HIV-1 gp41 is a potent inhibitor of virus-mediated cell-cell fusion. Aids Res Hum Retroviruses 1993; 9:1051–1053.
61. Lalezari J, Eron J, Carlson M. Safety, pharmacokinetics, and antiviral activity of T-20 as a single agent in heavily pre-treated patients. In: 6th Conference on Retroviruses and Opportunistic Infections, 1999 (Abstract LB13).
62. Rimsky LT, Shugar DC, Matthews T. Determinants of HIV-1 resistance to gp41-derived inhibitory peptides. J Virol 1998; 72:986–992.
63. Wei X, Kilby JM, Hopkins S, Saag MS, Shaw G. HIV-1 selection in response to inhibition of virus fusion and entry. In: 6th Conference on Retroviruses and Opportunistic Infections, 1999 (Abstract 611).

64. Pantaleo G, Graziosi C, Fauci AS. The immunopathogenesis of human immunodeficiency virus infection. N Engl J Med 1993; 328:327–335.
65. Kovacs JA, Baseler M, Dewar RJ, et al. Increases in CD4 T lymphocytes with intermittent courses of interleukin-2 in patients with human immunodeficiency virus infection. A preliminary study. N Engl J Med 1995; 332:567–575.
66. O'Brien WA, Grovit-Ferbas K, Namazi A, et al. Human immunodeficiency virus-type 1 replication can be increased in peripheral blood of seropositive patients after influenza vaccination. Blood 1995; 86:1082–1089.
67. Brichacek B, Swindells S, Janoff EN, Pirruccello S, Stevenson M. Increased plasma human immunodeficiency virus type 1 burden following antigenic challenge with pneumococcal vaccine. J Infect Dis 1996; 174:1191–1199.
68. Stanley SK, Ostrowski MA, Justement JS, et al. Effect of immunization with a common recall antigen on viral expression in patients infected with human immunodeficiency virus type 1. N Engl J Med 1996; 334:1222–1230.
69. Donovan RM, Bush CE, Markowitz NP, Baxa DM, Saravolatz LD. Changes in virus load markers during AIDS-associated opportunistic diseases in HIV-infected persons. J Infect Dis 1996; 174:401–403.
70. Sulkowski MS, Chaisson RE, Karp CL, Moore RD, Margolick JB, Quinn TC. The effect of acute infectious diseases on plasma HIV-1 viral load and the expression of serologic markers of immune activation among HIV-infected adults. J Infect Dis 1998; 178:1642–1648.
71. Dezube BJ, Lederman MM, Spritzler JG, et al. High-dose pentoxifylline in patients with AIDS: inhibition of tumor necrosis factor production. J Infect Dis 1995; 171:1628–1632.
72. Landman D, Sarai A, Sathe SS. Use of pentoxifylline therapy for patients with AIDS-related wasting: pilot study. Clin Infect Dis 1994; 18:97–99.
73. Reyes-Teran G, Sierra-Madero JG, Martinez del Cerro V, et al. Effects of thalidomide on HIV-associated wasting syndrome: a randomized, double-blind, placebo-controlled clinical trial. AIDS 1996; 10:1501–1507.
74. Kilby JM, Tabereaux PB, Mulanovich V, Shaw GM, Bucy RP, Saag MS. Effects of tapering doses of oral prednisone on viral load among HIV-infected patients with unexplained weight loss. AIDS Res Hum Retroviruses 1997; 13:1533–1537.
75. Andrieu JM, Lu W, Levy R. Sustained increases in CD4 cell counts in asymptomatic human immunodeficiency virus type 1-seropositive patients treated with prednisolone for 1 year. J Infect Dis 1995; 171:523–530.
76. Pakker NG, Notermans DW, deBoer RJ, et al. Biphasic kinetics of peripheral blood T cells after triple combination therapy in HIV-1 infection: a composite of redistribution and proliferation. Nat Med 1998; 2:208–214.
77. Bucy RP, Hockett RD, Derdeyn CA, et al. Initial increase in blood CD4(+) lymphocytes after HIV antiretroviral therapy reflects redistribution from lymphoid tissues. J Clin Invest 1999; 103:1391–1398.
78. Dieli F, Friscia G, Di Sano C, et al. Sequestration of T lymphocytes to body fluids in tuberculosis: reversal of anergy following chemotherapy. J Infect Dis 1999; 180:225–228.
79. Mackall CL, Fleisher TA, Brown MR, et al. Age, thymopoiesis, and CD4+ T-lymphocyte regeneration after intensive chemotherapy. N Engl J Med 1995; 332:143–149.
80. Moreland LW, Bucy RP, Koopman WJ. Regeneration of T cells after chemotherapy. N Engl J Med 1995; 332:1651–1652.
81. Autran B, Carcelain G, Li TS, et al. Positive effects of combined antiretroviral therapy on CD4+ T cell homeostasis and function in advanced HIV disease. Science 1997; 277:112–116.

82. Lewin SR, Vesanen M, Kostrikis L, et al. Use of real-time PCR and molecular beacons to detect virus replication in human immunodeficiency virus type 1-infected individuals on prolonged effective antiretroviral therapy. J Virol 1999; 73:6099–6103.

83. Pialoux G, Raffi F, Brun-Vezinet F, et al. A randomized trial of three maintenance regimens given after three months of induction therapy with zidovudine, lamivudine, and indinavir in previously untreated HIV-1-infected patients. N Engl J Med 1998; 339:1269–1276.

84. Reijers MH, Weverling GJ, Jurriaans S, et al. Maintenance therapy after quadruple induction therapy in HIV-1 infected individuals. Lancet 1998; 352:185–190.

85. Kovacs JA, Vogel S, Albert JM, et al. Controlled trial of interleukin-2 infusions in patients infected with the human immunodeficiency virus. N Engl J Med 1996; 335:1350–1356.

86. Jacobson EL, Pilaro F, Smith KA. Rational interleukin-2 therapy for HIV positive individuals: daily low doses enhance immune function without toxicity. Proc Natl Acad Sci USA 1996; 93:10405–10410.

87. Arno A, Ruiz L, Juan M, et al. Efficacy of low-dose subcutaneous interleukin-2 to treat advanced HIV-1 in persons with <250 CD4 T cells and undetectable viral load. J Infect Dis 1999; 180:56–60.

88. McCune JM, Loftus R, Schmidt DK, et al. High prevalence of thymic tissue in adults with HIV-1 infection. J Clin Invest 1998; 101:2301–2308.

89. Carroll RG, Riley JL, Levine BL, et al. Differential regulation of HIV-1 fusion cofactor expression by CD28 costimulation of CD4+T cells. Science 1997; 276:273–276.

90. Chun TW, Stuyver L, Mizell SB, et al. Presence of an inducible HIV-1 latent reservoir during highly active antiretroviral therapy. Proc Natl Acad Sci USA 1997; 94: 13193–13197.

91. Chun TW, Engel D, Berrey MM, Shea T, Corey L, Fauci AS. Early establishment of a pool of latently infected, resting CD4(+) T cells during primary HIV-1 infection. Proc Natl Acad Sci USA 1998; 95:8869–8873.

92. Hartung T, Pitrak DL, Foote MA, Shatzen EM, Verral SC, Wendel A. Filgrastim restores interleukin-2 production in blood from patients with advanced HIV infection. J Infect Dis 1998; 178:686–692.

93. Miles SA. Hematopoietic growth factors as adjuvants to antiretroviral therapy. AIDS Res Hum Retroviruses 1992; 8:1073–1080.

94. Szelc CM, Mitcheltree C, Roberts RL Stiehm ER. Deficient polymorphonuclear cells and mononuclear cell antibody-dependent cellular cytotoxicity in pediatric and adult HIV infection. J Infect Dis 1992; 166:486–493.

95. Chun TW, Engel D, Mizell SB, et al. Effect of interleukin-2 on the pool of latently infected, resting CD4+ T cells in HIV-1-infected patients receiving highly active antiretroviral therapy. Nat Med 1999; 5:651–655.

96. Koup RA, Safrit JT, Cao Y, et al. Temporal association of cellular immune responses with the initial control of viremia in primary human immunodeficiency virus type 1 syndrome. J Virol 1994; 68:4650–4655.

97. Borrow P, Lewicki H, Wei X, et al. Antiviral pressure exerted by HIV-1-specific cytotoxic T lymphocytes (CTLs) during primary infection demonstrated by rapid selection of CTL escape virus. Nat Med 1997; 3:205–211.

98. Rosenberg ES, Billingsley JM, Caliendo AM, et al. Vigorous HIV-1-specific CD4+ T cell responses associated with control of viremia. Science 1997; 278:1447–1450.

99. Daar ES, Bai J, Hausner MA, Majchrowicz M, Tamaddon M, Giorgi JV. Acute HIV syndrome after discontinuation of antiretroviral therapy in a patient treated before seroconversion. Ann Intern Med 1998; 128:827–829.

100. Corey L, McElrath MJ, Weinhold K, et al. Cytotoxic T cell and neutralizing antibody responses to HIV-1 envelope with a combination vaccine regimen. J Infect Dis 1998; 177:301–309.

101. Clements-Mann ML, Weinhold K, Matthews TJ, et al. Immune responses to HIV-1 induced by canarypox expressing HIV-1MN gp120, HIV-1SF2 recombinant gp120, or both vaccines in seronegative adults. J Infect Dis 1998; 177:1230–1246.

102. Vila J, Nugier F, Bargues G, et al. Absence of viral rebound after treatment of HIV-infected patients with didanosine and hydroxycarbamide. Lancet 1997; 352:635–636.

103. Lisziewicz J, Jessen H, Finzi D, Siliciano RF, Lori F. HIV-1 suppression by early treatment with hydroxyurea, didanosine, and a protease inhibitor. Lancet 1998; 352:199–200.

104. Ortiz GM, Nixon DF, Trkola A, et al. HIV-1-specific immune responses in subjects who temporarily contain virus replication after discontinuation of highly active antiretroviral therapy. J Clin Invest 1999; 104:R13–R18.

13

Gene Therapy for HIV-1 Infection

Ralph Dornburg and Roger J. Pomerantz

INTRODUCTION

Since the discovery that AIDS is caused by a retrovirus, HIV-1, enormous efforts have been made to develop new drugs that will combat this infectious disease. Although new conventional drugs have been found to block the replication of this virus efficiently, new mutant strains continuously arise, which escape the inhibitory effect of such drugs. Furthermore, since HIV-1 integrates its genome into that of the host cell, dormant viruses persist in infected individuals over long periods. Thus, great efforts are currently being made in many laboratories to develop alternative genetic approaches to inhibit the replication of this virus. With growing insight into the mechanism and regulation of HIV-1 replication, in the past decade, many strategies have been developed and proposed for clinical application to block HIV-1 replication inside the cell. Such strategies use either antiviral RNAs or proteins (for some recent reviews, see refs. *1–4*). Antiviral strategies that employ RNAs have the advantage that they are less likely to be immunogenic than protein-based antiviral agents. However, protein-based systems have been engineered using inducible promoters that only become active upon HIV-1 infection. Although such antivirals have been proved to be very effective in vitro, their beneficial effect in vivo is very difficult to evaluate and still remains to be shown. In particular, the long latent period from infection to the onset of AIDS (up to 10 years or longer) makes it very difficult to evaluate the efficacy of a new drug.

Another obstacle is the transduction of therapeutic genes into the patient's immune cells. Although a large variety of gene transfer tools exist, which allow efficient transduction of genes in tissue culture, it becomes more and more evident that ex vivo transduced cells do not survive long in vivo. No efficient gene delivery tools are available at this point that would allow robust delivery to the actual target cell in vivo. This chapter summarizes experimental genetic approaches toward blocking HIV-1 replication and current gene delivery techniques for transducing therapeutic genes into the precise target cells.

HIV-1 LIFE-CYCLE AND POTENTIAL TARGETS FOR GENETIC ANTIVIRALS

HIV-1 primarily infects and destroys cells of the human immune system, in particular CD4+ T-lymphocytes and macrophages. The destruction of such cells leads to a severe immunodeficiency, e.g., the inability to fight other infectious agents or tumor

From: *Immunotherapy for Infectious Diseases*
Edited by: J. M. Jacobson © Humana Press Inc., Totowa, NJ

cells *(5)*. Thus, AIDS patients usually die from secondary infections (e.g., tuberculosis, pneumonia) or cancer (e.g., Kaposi's sarcoma). To prevent the destruction of the cells of the immune system, a diverse array of efforts is now under way to make such cells resistant to HIV-1 infection. This approach has been termed *intracellular immunization (6)*.

HIV-1 replicates via a classic retroviral life cycle (Fig. 1). Virus entry is mediated by the binding of the viral envelope protein to a specific receptor, termed CD4, which is expressed on the cell surface of T-lymphocytes and certain monocyte/macrophage populations. However, in contrast to other retroviruses, other receptors are also required for cell entry. Such coreceptors (e.g., CXCR-4 and CCR5) have been found to be chemokine receptors. Efforts are being made to develop genetic antivirals, which interfere with the first step of viral infection (Fig. 2).

After entry into the cell, the viral RNA is reverse-transcribed into viral DNA by the viral reverse transcriptase (RT). The resulting preintegration complex is then actively transported across the nuclear membrane. Thus, in contrast to C-type retroviruses, HIV-1 is capable of infecting quiescent cells. Many attempts are now also under way to endow immune cells with genes that would prevent reverse transcription and/or integration (Fig. 2).

Lentiviruses also express a number of critical regulatory genes from multiply-spliced mRNAs. Thus, a series of studies are currently under way to test the potential of genetic antivirals directed not only against the structural core and envelope proteins (e.g., matrix proteins, RT, integrase, protease) but also against some regulatory proteins, which are specific and essential for the life cycle of lentiviruses. HIV-1 contains six regulatory genes, which are involved in the complex pathogenesis. For example, the *Tat* gene is the major transcriptional transactivator of HIV-1 and is essential for activity of the long terminal repeat (LTR) promoter. The Tat protein stimulates HIV-1 transcription via an RNA intermediate called the transactivation response (TAR) region, which is found just downstream of the 5' LTR. The product of the *Rev* gene ensures the transport of unspliced viral RNA from the nucleus to the cytoplasm. *Tat* and *Rev* are absolutely essential for HIV-1 replication, and therefore became major targets for the development of genetic antivirals. Such antivirals attack the virus after integration into the chromosomes of the host and are aimed at preventing or reducing particle formation and/or release from infected cells (Fig. 2).

Other critical accessory proteins include Vpr (which leads to G2 arrest in the cell cycle of infected cells), Nef (which stimulates viral production and activation of infected cells), Vpu (which stimulates viral release), and Vif (which seems to augment viral production in either early or late steps in the viral life cycle). These regulatory proteins may be somewhat less crucial to viral load and replication in comparison with Tat and Rev. Consequently, antiviral agents, which attack these proteins, are less likely to significantly prevent infection and/or the spread of the virus.

Potential genetic inhibitors of virus replication should have four features, which overcome the shortcomings of conventional treatments: First, they should be directed against a highly conserved moiety in HIV-1, which is absolutely essential for virus replication, eliminating the chance that new mutant variants may arise that can escape this attack. Second, they must be highly effective and must greatly reduce or, ideally, completely block the production of progeny virus. Third, they must be nontoxic. A

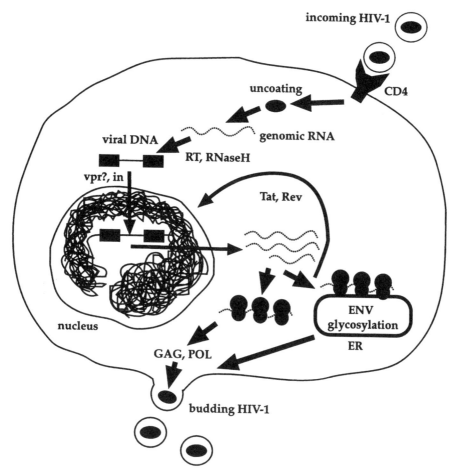

Fig. 1. Life cycle of HIV-1, which is similar to that of all retroviruses studied. HIV-1 attaches to the target cell mainly by binding to the CD4 molecule. After fusion of the viral and cellular membranes, retroviral core particles are released into the cytoplasm. The RNA genome is converted into a double-stranded DNA by the viral reverse transcriptase (RT) and ribonuclease H (RNaseH) and actively transported into the nucleus, probably aided by the viral protein Vpr. The viral DNA is integrated into the genome of the host cell by the viral integrase (in). The integrated DNA form of the virus is called the provirus. In contrast to other retroviruses, transcription and RNA splicing of the provirus is regulated by viral accessory proteins. For example, the viral protein Tat must bind to a specific sequence in the HIV genome (termed TAR) to enable highly efficient transcription of the provirus. Rev is required to control RNA splicing and the transport of RNAs into the cytoplasm. Finally, in the cytoplasm, virus core particles are assembled by encapsidating full-length genomic viral RNAs (recognized by specific encapsidation sequences). At the cell membrane, virus particle assembly is completed by the interaction of the core with the viral membrane proteins, and new particles "bud" (are released) from the infected cell. For more details regarding regulatory proteins, see also Figure 5. Env, envelope; ER, endoplasmatic reticulum.

fourth criteria, is that the antiviral agent has to be tolerated by the immune system. It would not make much sense to endow immune cells with an antiviral agent that elicits an immune response against itself, leading to the destruction of the HIV-1-resistant cell after a short period.

VIRUS LIFE-CYCLE   MOLECULAR INTERCEPTION

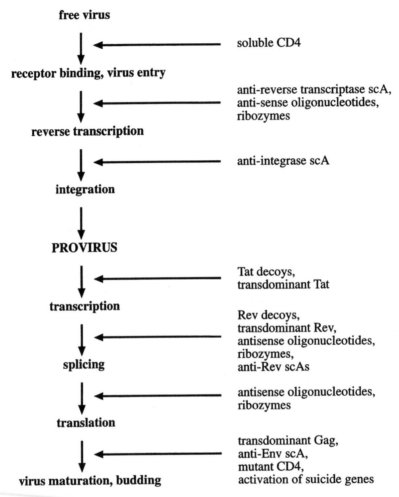

Fig. 2. Overview of possible genetic targets to block HIV-1 replication. The different approaches are described in detail in the text.

GENETIC ANTIVIRALS TO BLOCK HIV-1 REPLICATION

Protein-Based Inhibitors

Transdominant Negative Mutant Proteins

Replication of the HIV-1 virus depends on several regulatory proteins. Replication, however, is greatly impaired when certain mutant forms of such proteins are present. Thus, mutant viral proteins have been used to block HIV-1 replication. Transdominant (TD) negative mutants still bind to their targets but are unable to perform their actual function. They compete with the corresponding native, wild-type protein inside the cell and greatly reduce virus replication, especially when they are expressed from strong promoters (e.g., the cytomegalovirus immediate early promoter [CMV-IE]) *(1)*.

Transcription from the HIV-1 LTR promoter is dependent on the Tat protein. Mutant Tat proteins, which still bind to the nascent viral RNA but are unable to further trigger RNA elongation of transcription, greatly reduce the production of HIV-1 RNAs and consequently the production of progeny virus *(7)*. In addition, mutant Gag proteins lead to abnormal virus core assembly and have also been shown to inhibit HIV-1 replication *(8)*.

In a similar way, mutant Rev proteins interfere with regulated posttranscriptional events and also greatly reduce the efficiency of virus replication in an infected cell. In particular, one Rev mutant, termed RevM10, has been shown to efficiently block HIV-1 replication and has become a standard to measure the inhibitory effect of other anti-HIV-1 genetic antivirals. Clinical trials are now under way to test long-term expression and therapeutic effects of RevM10 in AIDS patients (see also Clinical Trials below).

Toxic Genes

The production of progeny virus can also be reduced by endowing HIV-1 target cells with toxic genes. Such genes were inserted downstream of the HIV-1 LTR promoter and only become activated immediately upon HIV-1 infection, when the viral Tat protein is expressed. The activation of the toxic gene leads to immediate cell death, and therefore no new progeny virus particles can be produced. In vitro experiments have shown that the production of HIV-1 virus particles was indeed reduced, if target cells were endowed with genes coding for the herpes simplex virus (HSV) thymidine kinase or a mutant form of the bacterial diphtheria toxin protein *(9)*.

CD4 and HIV-1 Coreceptors as Decoys

Efforts have been made to block HIV-1 replication by modifying the main envelope docking molecules CD4, CXCR-4, or CCR-5. For example, a chimeric CD4 coding gene has been constructed, which contained an endoplasmatic reticulum (ER) retention sequence, derived from the T-cell receptor (TCR) CD3-ε chain. Thus, this mutant CD4 molecule remained inside the endoplasmatic reticulum (ER) and was able to prevent HIV-1 envelope maturation by binding to the HIV-1 envelope in the ER and blocking its transport to the cell surface. Consequently, formation of infectious particles could not take place. In other experiments, soluble CD4 has been used to block the envelope of free extracellular virus particles and to prevent binding to fresh target cells *(5)*.

It has been reported that individuals who have a mutant form of CCR-5, a coreceptor used by macrophage-tropic strains of HIV-1, are naturally protected against HIV-1 infection. Such mutant CCR-5 appears to be retained in the ER and therefore is not available at the cell surface for HIV-1 entry. Thus, efforts are being made to phenotypically knock out wild-type CCR-5 in HIV-1-infected individuals to make their macrophages resistant to CCR-5-tropic HIV-1 infection. Macrophages have been transduced with a genetically modified chemokine gene, which expresses a modified protein targeted to the ER. In the ER, the modified chemokine binds to CCR-5, preventing its transport to the cell surface.

Single-Chain Antibodies

Single-chain antibodies (scA, also termed single-chain variable fragments [scFv]) were originally developed for *E. coli* expression to bypass the costly production of monoclonal antibodies in tissue culture or mice. They comprise only the variable domains of both the heavy and light chain of an antibody and are expressed from a single gene. The resulting single-chain antibody can bind to its antigen with similar affinity as an Fab fragment of the authentic antibody molecule.

sFvs against viral proteins (e.g., the envelope, integrase, RT, matrix, Rev, and Tat proteins) that lack a hydrophobic signal peptide are expressed intracellularly and are retained in the cytoplasm. They are capable of binding to specific domains of HIV-1 proteins and have been shown to prevent integration of the HIV-1 into the host chromosome or to block virus maturation. Some intracellular sFvs have been found to greatly reduce the ability of HIV-1 to replicate; other sFvs have had moderate success *(4,10,11)*.

RNA-Based Inhibitors

Antisense RNAs and Ribozymes

Artificial antisense oligonucleotides (RNAs or single-stranded DNAs) have been successfully used to selectively suppress the expression of various genes. Furthermore, the presence of double-stranded RNA inside the cell can induce the production of interferon and/or other cytokines, stimulating an immune response. Indeed, it has also been reported that the expression of RNAs capable of forming a double-stranded RNA molecule with the HIV-1 RNA (antisense RNAs) can significantly reduce the expression of HIV-1 proteins and consequently the efficiency of progeny virus production *(12–18)*.

Ribozymes are very similar to antisense RNAs. They bind to specific RNA sequences, but they are also capable of cleaving their target at the binding site catalytically (Fig. 3). Thus, they may not need to be overexpressed to fulfill their biologic function. Many sites in the HIV-1 genome have been successfully targeted. However, several questions are being asked, e.g., can an efficient subcellular colocalization be obtained, in particular in vivo? Will the target RNA be efficiently recognized owing to secondary and tertiary folding of the target RNA? Will RNA binding proteins prevent efficient binding? Experimentation in several laboratories has addressed these problems, and clinical trials have been initiated to test the therapeutic effect of ribozymes in AIDS patients.

RNA Decoys

RNA decoys are mutant RNAs that resemble authentic viral RNAs that have crucial functions in the viral life cycle. They mimic such RNA structures and decoy viral and/or cellular factors required for the propagation of the virus *(8)*. For example, HIV-1 replication largely depends on the two regulatory proteins Tat and Rev. These proteins bind to specific regions in the viral RNA, the TAR loop and the Rev response element (RRE), respectively. Tat binding to TAR is crucial in the initiation of RNA transcription, and Rev binding to RRE is essential in controlling splicing, RNA stability, and the transport of the viral RNA from the nucleus to the cytoplasm. These two complex secondary RNA structures within the HIV-1 genome appear to be unique for the HIV-1 virus, and no cellular homologous structures have been identified. Thus, such structures appear to be valuable targets for the attack with genetic antivirals.

HIV-1 target cells have been endowed with genes that overexpress short RNAs containing TAR or RRE sequences. These RNA molecules capture Tat or Rev proteins, preventing the binding of such proteins to their actual targets. Consequently, HIV-1 replication is markedly impaired. This strategy has the advantage over antisense RNAs

HAMMERHEAD RIBOZYME

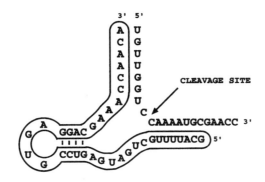

HAIRPIN RIBOZYME

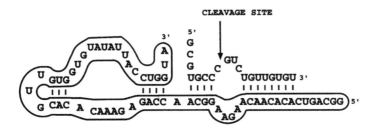

Fig. 3. Schematic representation of two ribozymes to block HIV-1 replication. The structures shown are paired with actual HIV-I target sequences. (Top) A hammerhead ribozyme pairs specifically with a sequence in the gag region of the HIV-1 genome. (Bottom) A hairpin ribozyme designed to bind to and cleave the 5′ end of the viral genome, abolishing the reverse transcription and integration of progeny virus.

and ribozymes in that mutant Tat or Rev, which will not bind to the RNA decoys, will also not bind to their actual targets. Thus, the likelihood that mutant strains would arise that would bypass the RNA decoy trap is low.

Combination Therapies

The question still needs to be addressed of whether mutant forms of the HIV-1 virus could arise that would eventually escape the blocking genetic antiviral. In addition, increased multiplicities of infection seem to overwhelm most gene therapeutic approaches toward inhibiting HIV-1 replication. Thus new approaches toward augmenting the anti-HIV-1 activities of single genetic antivirals are being developed, and experiments are under way in many laboratories to test the therapeutic effect of a combination of two or more anti-HIV-1 antivirals. For example, combinations of different ribozymes (i.e., an RRE decoy with RevM10 and a ribozyme) were more efficient blockers of HIV-1 replication than either genetic antiviral alone. Furthermore, it has been reported that a combination of conventional anti-HIV-1 drugs with genetic antivirals inhibits HIV-1.

GENETIC "GUNS" TO DELIVER GENETIC ANTIVIRALS

In all the therapeutic approaches described above, the corresponding genes have to be transduced into the appropriate target cell to express the therapeutic agent of interest. Since HIV-1 remains and replicates in the body of an infected person for many years, it will be essential to stably introduce therapeutic genes into the genome of target cells for either continuous expression or for availability on demand. Thus, gene delivery tools such as naked DNA, liposomes, or adenoviruses, which are highly effective for transient expression of therapeutic genes, may not be useful for gene therapy of HIV-1 infection.

The most efficient tools for stable gene delivery are retroviral vectors, which stably integrate into the genome of the host cell, as this is a part of the retroviral life cycle (Fig. 1). This is why virus-based gene delivery systems have been derived from this class of viruses. This is also why they are being used in almost all current human gene therapy trials, including on-going clinical AIDS trials *(19–24)*.

Retroviral vectors are basically retroviral particles that contain a genome in which all viral protein coding sequences have been replaced with the gene(s) of interest. As a result, such viruses cannot further replicate after one round of infection. Furthermore, infected cells do not express any retroviral proteins, which makes cells that carry a vector provirus (the integrated DNA form of a retrovirus) invisible to the immune system.

Retroviral Vectors Derived from C-Type Retroviruses

All current retroviral vectors used in clinical trials have been derived from murine leukemia virus (MLV), a C-type retrovirus with a rather simple genomic organization (Fig. 4). The MLV-derived gene delivery system consists of two components: the retroviral vector, which is a genetically modified viral genome containing the gene of interest and replacing retroviral protein coding sequences, and a helper cell that supplies the retroviral proteins for the encapsidation of the vector genome into retroviral particles (Fig. 4). Retrovirus helper cells can produce gene transfer particles for very long periods (e.g., several years).

Retroviral Vectors Derived from HIV-1

Retroviral vectors derived from MLV have been shown to be very useful in transferring genes into a large variety of human cells. However, they infect human hematopoietic cells poorly, because such cells lack the receptor, which is recognized by the MLV envelope protein. Furthermore, retroviral vectors derived from C-type retroviruses are unable to infect quiescent cells: such viruses (and their vectors) can only establish a provirus after one cell division, during which the nuclear membrane is temporarily dissolved. Thus, efforts are under way in many laboratories to develop retroviral vectors from lentiviruses, e.g., HIV-1 or the simian immunodeficiency virus (SIV), which are able to establish a provirus in nondividing cells *(25–31)*.

Figure 5 shows plasmid constructs used to create HIV-1-derived packaging cells. Vector virus can be harvested from the transfected cells for a limited period and can be used to infect fresh target cells. Although this gene transfer system was shown to be functional initially, it was not highly efficient, and efforts are under way to develop better packaging to make it suitable for broad clinical applications. However, many questions regarding the safety of such vectors still need to be addressed.

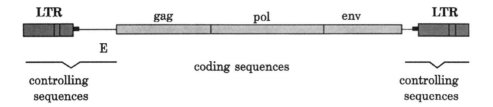

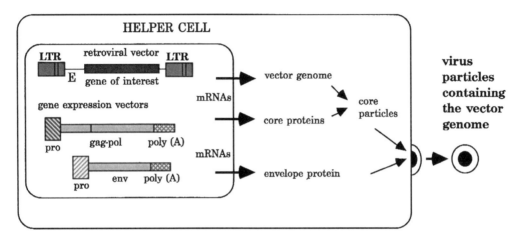

Fig. 4. Retroviral helper cells derived from C-type retroviruses. A C-type retroviral provirus. (Top) The DNA intermediate of a retrovirus. The protein-coding genes (*gag-pol* and *env*) are flanked by *cis*-acting or controlling sequences, which play essential roles during replication. (Bottom) In a retroviral helper cell, the retroviral protein coding genes, which code for all virion proteins, are expressed (ideally) from heterologous promoters (pro) and polyadenylated via a heterologous polyadenylation signal sequence (poly A). To minimize reconstitution of a full-length provirus by recombination, the *gag-pol* and *env* genes are split to different gene expression vectors. In the retroviral vector, the viral protein coding sequences are completely replaced by the gene(s) of interest. Since the vector contains specific encapsidation sequences (E), the vector genome is encapsidated into retroviral vector particles, which bud from the helper cell. The virion contains all proteins necessary to reverse transcribe and integrate the vector genome into that of a newly infected target cell. However, since there are no retroviral protein coding sequences in the target cell, vector replication is limited to one round of infection. LTR, long terminal repeat.

Unanswered Questions

Even if we can transduce enough cells in vivo with anti-HIV-1 genes to inhibit virus replication significantly, many other questions remain to be answered. For example, it is not clear whether a cell that has been endowed with a certain HIV-1 resistance gene will be able to fulfill its normal biologic function in vivo. Will the body be able to eliminate all HIV-1-infected cells or will the infected person become a life-long carrier of the virus, which is still replicating in the body although at levels that cause no clinical symptoms owing to the presence of HIV-1 resistance genes? Will the patient be capable of infecting new individuals? Finally, because genetic therapies can all be overcome with in vitro challenges using very high amounts of HIV-1, will there be a difference in antiviral effects in peripheral blood versus lymphoid tissues?

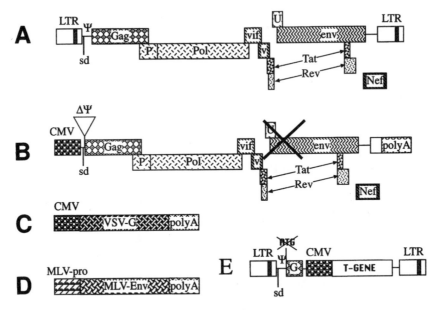

Fig. 5. Retroviral packaging system derived from HIV-1. **(A)** A provirus of HIV-1. **(B–D)** Plasmid constructs to express pseudotyped HIV-1 retroviral particles. **(E)** A plasmid construct to encapsidate and transduce genes with a HIV-1 vector (the plasmid sequences to propagate such constructs in bacteria are not shown). Besides the genes encoding for HIV-1 proteins, which form the core of the virus (e.g., Gag: structural core proteins; P, protease; Pol, reverse transcriptase and integrase) and the envelope (e.g., env [envelope protein]), the HIV-1 genome also codes for several regulatory proteins (termed Vif, U [= Vpu], V [= Vpr], Tat, Rev, and Nef), which are expressed from spliced mRNAs and which have important functions in the viral life cycle. **(B)** Plasmid construct to express the core and regulatory proteins. To avoid encapsidation and transduction of genes coding for such proteins, the following modifications have been made: the 5′ long terminal repeat (LTR) promoter of the HIV-1 provirus has been replaced with the promoter of cytomegalovirus (CMV) to enable constitutive gene expression; the 3′ LTR has been partially replaced with the polyadenylation signal sequence of simian virus 40 (polyA); the encapsidation signal has been deleted (ΔΨ); the reading frames for the envelope and vpu genes have been blocked. **(C), (D)** Plasmid constructs used to express the envelope proteins of the vesicular stomatitis virus (VSV-G) or the envelope protein of murine leukemia virus (MLV), respectively. In the absence of HIV-1 envelope proteins, which are rather toxic to the cell, HIV-1 efficiently incorporates the envelope proteins of VSV or MLV into virions. The use of such envelopes also further reduces the risk of the reconstitution of a replication-competent HIV-1 by homologous recombination between the plasmid constructs. **(E)** A retroviral vector used to package and transduce a gene of interest (T-gene) with HIV-1-derived vectors. Since the encapsidation sequence extends into the Gag region, part of the gag gene (G) has been conserved in the vector. However, the ATG start codon has been mutated. The gene of interest is expressed from an internal promoter, since the HIV-1 LTR promoter is silent without Tat. sd, splice donor site.

ANIMAL MODEL SYSTEMS

One of the major problems with any therapeutic agent against HIV-1 infection is the lack of an appropriate and inexpensive animal model system to test the efficiency of an antiviral agent. Since HIV-1 only causes AIDS in humans, it is very difficult to test and evaluate the therapeutic effect of novel antiviral agents in vivo. In addition, the evaluation of the efficacy of a new drug is further complicated by the very long clinical latency period of the virus until the onset of AIDS (which can be 10 years or more). Although a virus similar to HIV-1 has been found in monkeys SIV, results obtained with this virus do not necessarily reflect the onset of AIDS in humans caused by HIV-1. Furthermore, many antivirals that block HIV-1 are ineffective in blocking SIV. Thus, other animal model systems need to be developed to study the effect of anti-HIV-1 therapies *(32,33)*.

In the past decade, many strains of laboratory mice have been bred, which lack components of the immune system. Severe combined immunodeficient (SCID) mice are deficient in functional B- and T-lymphocytes. Thus, they are unable to reject allogeneic organ grafts. SCID mice have been used extensively to study human leukemia and other malignancies and for modeling human retroviral pathogenesis including antiviral gene therapy. Furthermore, in the past few years, much progress has been made in transplanting hematopoietic stem cells into SCID mice to mimic and study human hematopoiesis. It has been shown that transplantation of human hematopoietic cells into such mice can lead to the repopulation of the mouse's blood with human CD4- and CD8-positive T-lymphocytes. Thus, SCID mice also appear to be good candidates for developing mouse model systems for HIV-1 infection *(33)*.

CLINICAL TRIALS

G. Nabel's group has recently conducted initial in vivo studies on intracellular immunization against primate lentiviruses: a trans-dominant negative Rev protein (RevM10) was studied in humans infected with HIV-1. It was demonstrated that T-cells transduced with RevM10 had a significant longer half-life, compared with control T-cells, when reinfused into patients in different stages of disease. These early initial phase I trials were performed using MLVs, as well as microparticulate bombardment with a gene gun. In another approach, clinical trials have just begun to test the therapeutic effect of anti-HIV-1 ribozymes in AIDS patients.

An exciting study has recently been reported by R. Morgan's group in which an antisense construct to Tat and Rev genes in SIV was used to transduce T-lymphocytes from rhesus macaques. The monkeys were then challenged with SIV intravenously. The animals with the transduced cells had significantly lower viral loads and higher CD4 counts, compared with control monkeys, suggesting for the first time that gene therapy against lentiviruses may have significant efficacy in vivo. Clearly, these are both very preliminary studies in humans and in primates, which require more detailed evaluation. Other trials using a variety of different complementary approaches are ongoing in initial phase I studies *(32)*.

REFERENCES

1. Bitton N, Gorochov G, Debre P, Eshhar Z. Gene therapy approaches to HIV-infection: immunological strategies: use of T bodies and universal receptors to redirect cytolytic T-cells. Front Biosci 1999; 4:D386–D393.
2. Kohn DB, Sarver N. Gene therapy for HIV-1 infection. Adv Exp Med Biol 1996; 394:421–428.
3. Palu G, Bonaguro R, Marcello A. In pursuit of new developments for gene therapy of human diseases. J Biotechnol 1999; 68:1–13.
4. Pomerantz RJ, Trono D. Genetic therapies for HIV infections: promise for the future. AIDS 1995; 9:985–993.
5. Smith C, Sullenger BA. AIDS and HIV infection. Mol Cell Biol Hum Dis Ser 1995; 5:195–236.

6. Baltimore D. Intracellular immunization. Nature 1988; 235:395–396.
7. Caputo A, Grossi MP, Rossi C, et al. The tat gene and protein of the human immunodeficiency virus type 1. N Microbiol 1995; 18:87–110.
8. Lisziewicz J. Tar decoys and trans-dominant gag mutant for HIV-1 gene therapy. Antibiot Chemother 1996; 48:192–197.
9. Tiberghien P. Use of suicide genes in gene therapy. J Leukoc Biol 1994; 56:203–209.
10. Marasco WA. Intrabodies: turning the humoral immune system outside in for intracellular immunization. Gene Ther 1997; 4:11–15.
11. Rondon IJ, Marasco WA. Intracellular antibodies (intrabodies) for gene therapy of infectious diseases. Annu Rev Microbiol 1997; 51:257–283.
12. Earnshaw DJ, Gait MJ. Progress toward the structure and therapeutic use of the hairpin ribozyme. Antisense Nucleic Acid Drug Dev 1997; 7:403–411.
13. Hampel A. The hairpin ribozyme: discovery, two-dimensional model, and development for gene therapy. Prog Nucleic Acid Res Mol Biol 1998; 58:1–39.
14. James W. The use of ribozymes in gene therapy approaches to AIDS. Recent Results Cancer Res 1998; 144:139–146.
15. Kijima H, Ishida H, Ohkawa T, Kashani-Sabet M, Scanlon KJ. Therapeutic applications of ribozymes. Pharmacol Ther 1995; 68:247–267.
16. Macpherson JL, Ely JA, Sun LQ, Symonds GP. Ribozymes in gene therapy of HIV-1. Front Biosci 1999; 4:D497–D505.
17. Rossi JJ. Therapeutic applications of catalytic antisense rnas (ribozymes). Ciba Found Symp 1997; 209:195–204.
18. Sun LQ, Ely JA, Gerlach W, Symonds G. Anti-HIV ribozymes. Mol Biotechnol 1997; 7:241–251.
19. Dornburg R. Reticuloendotheliosis viruses and derived vectors. Gene Ther 1995; 2:301–310.
20. Gunzburg WH, Salmons B. Development of retroviral vectors as safe, targeted gene delivery systems [review]. J Mol Med 1996; 74:171–182.
21. Miller AD. Retrovirus packaging cells. Hum Gene Ther 1990; 1:5–14.
22. Mitani K, Caskey CT. Delivering therapeutic genes—matching approach and application. Trends Biotechnol 1993; 11:162–166.
23. Turchetto L, Benati C, Mattei S, et al. An approach to HIV gene therapy by transduction of multifunctional retroviral vectors in primary human t lymphocytes. J Biol Regul Homeost Agents 1997; 11:79–81.
24. Warner JF, Jolly D, Mento S, Galpin J, Haubrich R, Merritt J. Retroviral vectors for HIV immunotherapy. Ann NY Acad Sci 1995; 772:105–116.
25. Dull T, Zufferey R, Kelly M, et al. A third-generation lentivirus vector with a conditional packaging system. J Virol 1998; 72:8463–8471.
26. Klimatcheva E, Rosenblatt JD, Planelles V. Lentiviral vectors and gene therapy. Front Biosci 1999; 4:D481–D496.
27. Naldini L, Blomer U, Gallay P, et al. In vivo gene delivery and stable transduction of nondividing cells by a lentiviral vector. Science 1996; 272:263–267.
28. Parolin C, Sodroski J. A defective HIV-1 vector for gene transfer to human lymphocytes. J Mol Med 1995; 73:279–288.
29. Poeschla E, Corbeau P, Wong-Staal F. Development of HIV vectors for anti-HIV gene therapy. Proc Natl Acad Sci USA 1996; 93:11395–11399.
30. Zufferey R, Dull T, Mandel RJ, et al. Self-inactivating lentivirus vector for safe and efficient in vivo gene delivery. J Virol 1998; 72:9873–9880.
31. Zufferey R, Nagy D, Mandel RJ, Naldini L, Trono D. Multiply attenuated lentiviral vector achieves efficient gene delivery in vivo. Nat Biotechnol 1997; 15:871–875.
32. Amado RG, Mitsuyasu RT, Zack JA. Gene therapy for the treatment of AIDS: animal models and human clinical experience. Front Biosci 1999; 4:D468–D475.
33. Jamieson BD, Aldrovandi GM, Zack JA. The SCID-hu mouse: an in-vivo model for HIV-1 pathogenesis and stem cell gene therapy for AIDS. Semin Immunol 1996; 8:215–221.

IV
Immunotherapy for Infectious Diseases Other than HIV

14

Immunotherapy of Viral Infections Other than HIV

Michelle Onorato and Richard B. Pollard

INTRODUCTION

Our understanding of the immune system's role in eliminating acute viral infections, in suppressing latent viral pathogens, and in the pathogenesis of chronic viral infection has grown in the past decade, leading to strategies for modulating the immune response as a potential adjunct to existing antiviral therapy when it exists or as stand-alone therapy in infections for which effective antiviral agents do not yet exist. Administration of antibody, both to prevent acute infection (as in the case of respiratory syncytial virus [RSV]) and to ameliorate chronic infection (as in the case of hepatitis B) is but one example of specifically targeted immunobased therapy. Administration of cytokines, such as interleukin-12 (IL-12), is a more innovative approach to modulating immune responses in general and suppressing chronic infection. The adoptive transfer of pathogen-specific cytotoxic T-cells has been effective in prevention of Epstein-Barr virus (EBV)-related disease post transplant.

RESPIRATORY SYNCYTIAL VIRUS

RSV is a common pathogen, infecting nearly all children by 6 years of age (1). Although most infections are mild, the ubiquitous nature of the virus means that the total number of serious cases is still large. In the United States, RSV is thought to be responsible for up to 50% of admissions for bronchiolitis and 25% of admissions for pneumonia among pediatric patients (2). Serious RSV infections tend to occur in infants younger than 6 months; children with underlying pulmonary or cardiac disease; and children with chronic or transient immunodeficiency (3–5). However, the most serious illness and the highest mortality rates are found in posttransplant patients (both adult and pediatric) and in those undergoing chemotherapy for leukemia; mortality rates in this population exceed 50% even in those treated with ribavirin (6). Thus, the morbidity and mortality from RSV infections, together with the lack of an effective vaccine, have led to the use of respiratory syncytial virus immunoglobulin (RSVIG) for immunoprophylaxis in high-risk populations. Randomized trials in various pediatric populations at risk have shown reductions in hospitalizations, hospital days, and intensive care unit days among the groups receiving the highest dose of RSVIG (7).

From: *Immunotherapy for Infectious Diseases*
Edited by: J. M. Jacobson © Humana Press Inc., Totowa, NJ

However, the strategy of immunoprophylaxis with RSVIG-enhanced immune glob-ulin has flaws. The high volume of immunoglobulin that must be administered carries risks, as well as the need for prolonged infusion in a monitored setting. The high cost of the infusions is also prohibitive. For these reasons, a variety of monoclonal anti-bodies to RSV have been developed that can be administered in small volumes by intra-muscular injection. Of these, palivizumab (MedImmune, Gaithersburg, MD) has been shown to have efficacy in the prevention of RSV-associated disease in at-risk children. Palivizumab is a humanized immunoglobulin G-1 with affinity for the F protein of RSV and has good activity against clinical isolates of both type A and type B RSV. In in vitro neutralization assays, palivizumab is 20 times more potent than RSVIG *(8)*.

A clinical trial conducted over the 1996–1997 RSV season showed efficacy of this antibody in RSV disease in high-risk pediatric populations. At 139 centers in the United States, United Kingdom, and Canada, 1502 children with either prematurity or bronchopulmonary dysplasia were enrolled and randomized to receive five injections of either palivizumab at 15 mg/kg or placebo. Palivizumab prophylaxis resulted in a 55% reduction in hospitalization attributable to RSV infection. The benefit was great-est in children with prematurity alone as a risk factor, compared with children who had bronchopulmonary dysplasia. The incidence of adverse events was similar in the treat-ment and placebo groups *(9)*. Not surprisingly, the monoclonal antibody to RSV did not seem to have the same protective effect with regard to otitis media and respiratory infections other than RSV that the pooled RSVIG provides, since the latter probably contains antibodies to multiple pathogens. Current guidelines for pediatric prophylaxis with palivizumab or RSVIG are in Table 1 *(10)*. Prophylaxis should be administered from the beginning to the end of RSV season.

EBV-ASSOCIATED LYMPHOPROLIFERATIVE DISORDERS

EBV-associated lymphoproliferations arise as complications of organ and marrow allografts. Rates of EBV lymphoproliferative disorders approaching 10% are seen in cardiac and cardiopulmonary transplants, probably owing to the intensity of immuno-suppression *(11)*. EBV-associated lymphomas seen after marrow allograft are usually diffuse large cell lymphomas of B-cell origin, involving both nodal and extranodal sites, and are oligoclonal or monoclonal. In further contrast, they are of donor rather than host origin and develop within the window between initial engraftment (3–60 days post transplant) and return of T-cell function (6–8 months post transplant). These char-acteristics suggest absence of host EBV-specific T-cell response as the factor responsi-ble for the proliferation of donor EBV-transformed B cells *(12)*. Other evidence for the importance of intact T-cell response comes from in vitro analyses of immune responses in patients recovering from infectious mononucleosis, which suggest that HLA-restricted, virus-specific T-cells are capable of killing EBV-transformed B-cells and that HLA-restricted virus-specific CD8+ T-cells are likely to be the dominant contrib-utors to sustained resistance *(13–15)*.

In light of this, transfer of peripheral blood mononuclear cells (PBMCs) from the respective EBV-seropostive marrow donors to treat EBV-associated lymphoma in mar-row allograft recipients has been attempted. Small numbers are infused (on the order of 10^5–10^6 T-cells/kg) PBMCs or HLA partially matched T cells from in vitro expanded T-cell lines derived from an EBV-seropositive marrow donor. In the largest series of

Table 1
Recommendations for Prophylaxis of Respiratory Syncytial Virus (RSV) Infections in Children

Population	Method of prophylaxis
<2 years old with chronic lung disease requiring therapy in last 6 months	Palivizumab preferred
Born at ≤32 weeks gestational age	Palivizumab preferred
Born at 32–35 weeks gestational age	Palivizumab only if other underlying condition present
<2 years old with chronic lung disease requiring therapy in last 6 months *or* born at ≤32 weeks gestational age with congenital heart defect	RSVIG contraindicated in presence of cyanotic congenital heart defects; consider Palivizumab
Severely immunocompromised children (severe combined immunodeficiency or AIDS)	Consider RSVIG in RSV season in place of IVIG

patients treated with this adoptive cell therapy, clinical and pathologic resolution of the EBV-associated lymphoma was observed in 20 of the 22 patients; reduction or eradication of lymphoma cells with replacement by a T-cell infiltrate was noted as early as 8 days following infusion. Thirteen of the 22 patients treated have survived in sustained remission for 3–42 months following lymphocyte infusion; no patient has experienced relapse of lymphoma. Of the 22 patients from Memorial Sloan-Kettering, 3 patients developed acute graft-versus-host disease, and 9 patients developed chronic graft-versus-host disease, which was a cause of death in 1 patient. However, the results with regard to eradication of EBV-associated lymphoma by donor cell transfer are less consistent at centers where T-cell-specific monoclonal antibody and pharmacologic interventions are routine for the prevention of graft-versus-host disease (16). Such interventions may prevent or delay an effective response by the donor-derived EBV-specific cells.

The infusion of donor-derived EBV-specific T-cells has also been used prophylactically to prevent immunoblastic lymphoma in children undergoing allogenic bone marrow tranplant who were felt to be at high risk for the development of lymphoma post transplant. No EBV-related lymphomas were diagnosed in the 39 children so treated; additionally, in those children who had high levels of EBV-DNA detected before entry, 2–4 log decreases in EBV DNA levels were seen (17).

Alterations in the lymphoid populations of the recipients have been observed after infusion of donor-derived PMBCs. Expansion of CD4+ and CD8+ populations of T-cells are common. Lymphocyte responses to mitogens and antigens to which the donor has been exposed also increase in the recipients (18).

A similar strategy has been applied to therapy of EBV-related lymphoma complicating organ allograft. Emanuel and colleagues (19) have reported complete pathologic remission of a multifocal monoclonal EBV+ B-cell lymphoma of the central nervous system complicating lung allograft. The patient received a total of three infusions of PMBCs from his HLA-matched sibling over 8 months; biopsies done 6 weeks after the third infusion did not demonstrate residual lymphoma (19). A variation on this approach involves the activation of autologous PBMC with IL-2 prior to reinfusion in four patients with EBV-related lymphoproliferative disease. Functional assays of these activated cells demonstrated preferential cytotoxicity against autologous EBV-transformed cells and some activity against allogenic EBV+ targets. All four patients treated with these activated PMBCs had durable regressions of the lymphoma *(20)*.

Another approach to the treatment of EBV-related lymphoproliferative disorders, as well as other types of lymphoma and leukemias, has been the administration of monoclonal antibody to CD20 antigen (rituximab) found on normal and malignant B-lymphocytes, producing antibody-dependent and complement-mediated cytotoxicity in these cells. Although the utility of this approach extends beyond EBV-associated lymphoma, it has been used along with infusions of irradiated donor-derived lymphocytes with some success in treatment of EBV-related lymphoproliferative disorders following allogenic stem cell transplantation. The two patients treated experienced disappearance of the monoclonal B-cell populations and normalization of elevated EBV DNA titers *(21)*. A report of three patients treated with rituximab for lymphoproliferative disease following lung transplant suggests some efficacy in this population as well, with two complete remissions in the three patients treated *(22)*.

IMMUNE-BASED APPROACHES TO HEPATITIS B

Although pharmacologic agents with activity against hepatitis B are in development, there has been interest in immunologic therapy of chronic hepatitis secondary to hepatitis B, potentially as an adjunct to antiviral therapy. Administration of cytokines (such as IL-12) and antibody to surface antigen are two approaches that have been studied.

Longitudinal studies of chronic carriers of hepatitis B virus (HBV) suggest a role for IL-12 in viral clearance. Not only do HBV carriers have higher levels of IL-12 than controls, but further increases above baseline are noted in HBV carriers who go on to develop anti-HBe and clear HBV compared with those who have persistent HBV replication *(23)*. Based on this observation, as well as evidence from transgenic mouse models of hepatitis B infection, it is postulated that the antiviral effect of IL-12 is mediated by interferon-γ, IL-2, and tumor necrosis factor-α (TNF-α) released by HBV-specific cytotoxic T-lymphocytes (CTLs) and that the result is suppression of HBV gene expression in infected hepatocytes by noncytolytic mechanisms *(24–27)*. A small trial of IL-12 with or without lamivudine as part of concurrent antiretroviral therapy for chronic hepatitis B infection in patients coinfected with HIV is currently accruing. It is hoped that the combination of better antiviral therapies for hepatitis B and stimulation of immune responses such as enhancement with IL-12 will be an effective strategy for chronic hepatitis.

Another approach to the treatment of chronic hepatitis B involves a human monoclonal antibody to hepatitis B surface antigen, OST-577 (Protein Design Labs). In a phase I/II trial of this antibody in patients with chronic HBV infection, subjects received either 0.5, 1.0, or 2.0 mg/kg intravenously on days 0, 1, 3, 7, 14, 21, and 35. The lower doses were well tolerated; however, two subjects in the 2.0-mg/kg cohort developed hypotension that was thought to be related to immune complex deposition. Both patients tolerated dose reduction without further hypotensive episodes. Serum animotransferase levels and serum HBV DNA were measures of efficacy; mean reductions of HBV DNA by 75% and serum SGOT by 49% were seen *(28)*. Larger studies of this antibody are needed to establish its role in the therapy of chronic HBV infection.

CYTOMEGALOVIRUS INFECTIONS

Cytomegalovirus (CMV) infections and end-organ disease following bone marrow or solid organ transplant usually represent reactivation of latent infection; more rarely, they are new infections in a seronegative host. Such infections are associated with a high degree of morbidity and mortality. Although effective antiviral therapies such as ganciclovir and foscarnet are available, they are associated with significant toxicities, and at least in the case of HIV-associated CMV infections, resistance to these agents has been demonstrated.

Enhancement of CMV-specific immune response has been another approach to the prevention and treatment of CMV disease in the period of greatest immunocompromise post transplant. The earliest approach involved restoration of humoral immunity by passive immunization with pooled anti-CMV-IgG preparations. Results of trials of such immunization are mixed; although there does not seem to be benefit in bone marrow transplant patients, there is some protection for solid organ transplant patients who receive CMV hyperimmunoglobulin, particularly following renal transplant or for patients who receive an organ from a seropositive donor *(29,30)*.

Given the partial success of pooled anti-CMV globulin, a human monclonal antibody to CMV has been developed, MSL 109, directed against the gH glycoprotein of human CMV. The antibody has been shown to have neutralizing activity against both laboratory isolates and clinical isolates of CMV, and seems to be synergistic with ganciclovir or forscarnet in inhibiting laboratory and wild-type CMV isolates in vitro *(31,32)*.

Because of this potential synergistic effect with antiviral therapy, and the antibody's long half-life after intravenous administration (approximately 14 days), several trials were conducted of the administration of MSL 109 with standard therapy (either ganciclovir or foscarnet) for the treatment of CMV retinitis in patients with the acquired immunodeficiency syndrome. The first was a phase I/II study in which patients received either 0.25, 0.5, 1.0, 2.0, or 5.0 mg/kg as an intravenous infusion every 2 weeks, begun as close as possible to the beginning of maintenance antiviral therapy of the retinitis. There were no significant adverse effects of the antibody infusions, and the median time to progression was 202 days *(33)*. Two larger trials of MSL 109 in CMV retinitis in AIDS were initiated. These parallel studies were AIDS Clinical Treatment Group (ACTG) protocol 266 (a trial of MSL 109 vs placebo with standard therapy for the treatment of newly diagnosed CMV retinitis in patients with AIDS) and the Studies of Ocular Complications of AIDS Monoclonal Antibody Cytomegalovirus Retinitis Trial (SOCA-MACRT), comparing MSL 109 versus placebo with standard therapy for the treatment of newly diagnosed or relapsed CMV retinitis. The SOCA trial showed an unanticipated difference in mortality between the treatment and placebo arms in the relapsed retinitis group, which appeared to be related to the better than expected survival outcomes in the placebo-relapsed group rather than mortality related to the monoclonal antibody itself *(34)*. Given this difference, and the apparent lack of efficacy of MSL-109 in the SOCA trial, the ACTG trial was terminated early, before adequate numbers had been accrued to be able to detect a difference between treatment and placebo groups. This monoclonal antibody is no longer being pursued as a potential therapy for CMV infections.

Another immunotherapeutic approach to CMV infections in the severely immunosuppressed is the adoptive transfer of anti-CMV cytotoxic T-cells, which has been employed in allogeneic bone marrow recipients. This population is particularly prone to CMV pneumonitis, which is associated with a mortality of 30–60% *(35,36)*. In the first 100 days following transplant, these patients are persistently deficient in class I HLA-restricted CD8+ cytotoxic lymphocytes specific for CMV; this deficiency is important in the pathogenesis of CMV disease in this population *(37)*. Given these observations, Riddell and colleagues *(38)* undertook a phase I trial of transfer of clones of CD8+ cytotoxic T-lymphocytes specific for CMV from the marrow donors to the marrow transplant recipient. Fourteen patients each received a total of four intravenous infusions of these clones from their donors; the infusions began 30–40 days after transplant and were given once a week. The infusions themselves were well tolerated. In 11 of the 14 patients, CMV cytotoxic cells could not be detected prior to the first infusion; in all 11 of these patients, CMV-specific cytotoxic cells could be detected 2 days after the first infusion, and all patients had reconstituted CMV-specific cytotoxic T-lymphocytes by days 42–49 post transplant. In a subset of these patients, this reconstitution occurred even in the absence of detectable CMV-specific CD4+ helper cells, which are required for the recovery of endogenous CMV-specific cytotoxic T-lymphocytes *(39)*. All the patients maintained cytotoxic T-lymphocyte responses specific for CMV for at least 8 weeks after completion of T-cell therapy. The magnitude of the responses decreased over time in the patients who did not recover CD4+ T-helper responses specific for CMV compared with those who did, suggesting that the recovery of a T-helper response may facilitate the maintenance of transferred CD8+ cytotoxic T-lymphocytes. None of the 14 patients treated developed CMV viremia or disease, although 2 received ganciclovir following isolation of CMV from surveillance urine cultures.

In summary, various immune-based strategies have been attempted in the treatment and prophylaxis of viral infections; some hold promise, particularly as potential adjunctive therapy to antiviral therapies. The complexity of several approaches, particularly those involving expansion and reinfusion of cell populations, has made them somewhat impractical for widespread utilization.

REFERENCES

1. McIntosh K. Respiratory syncytial virus infection in infants and children: diagnosis and treatment. Pediatr Res 1987; 9:191–196.
2. La Via WV, Marks MI, Stutman HR. Respiratory syncytial virus puzzle: clinical features, pathophysiology, treatment and prevention. J Pediatr 1992; 121:503–510.
3. Bruhn FW, Mokowsky W, Kransinski K, Lawrence R, Welliver R. Apnea associated with respiratory syncytial virus infection in young infants. J Pediatr 1977; 90:382–386.
4. Hall CB, McBride JT, Gala CL, Hildreth SW, Schnabel KC. Ribavirin treatment of respiratory syncytial virus infection in infants with underlying cardiopulmonary disease. JAMA 1985; 254:3047–3051.
5. Hall CB, Powell KR, MacDonald NE, et al. Respiratory syncytial virus infection in children with compromised immune function. N Engl J Med 1986; 315:77–81.
6. Whimbey E, Chamlin RE, Couch RB, et al. Community respiratory virus infections among hospitalized adult bone marrow transplant recipients. Clin Infect Dis 1996; 22:778–782.
7. PREVENT Study Group. Reduction of respiratory syncytial virus hospitalization among premature infants and infants with bronchopulmonary dysplasia using respiratory syncytial virus immune globulin prophylaxis. Pediatrics 1997; 99:93–99.

8. Johnson S, Griego SD, Pfarr DS, et al. A direct comparison of two humanized respiratory syncytial virus monoclonal antibodies: MEDI-493 and RSHZ19. J Infect Dis 1999; 180:35–40.

9. The Impact RSV Study Group. Palivizumab, a humanized respiratory syncytial virus monoclonal antibody, reduces hospitalization from respiratory syncytial virus infection in high-risk infants. Pediatrics 1998; 102:531–537.

10. American Academy of Pediatrics—Committee on Infectious Diseases and Committee on Fetus and Newborn. Prevention of respiratory syncytial virus infections: indications for the use of palivizumab and update on the use of RSV-IVIG. Pediatrics 1998; 102:1211–1216.

11. Randwaha PS, Yousem SA, Paradis IL, et al. The clinical spectrum, pathology, and clonal analysis of Epstein-Barr virus associated lymphoproliferative disorders in heart-lung transplant reciepients. Am J Clin Pathol. 1989; 92:177.

12. Shapiro RS, McClain K, Frizzera G, et al. Epstein-Barr virus associated B-cell lymphoproliferative disorders following bone marrow transplantation. Blood 1988; 71:1234–1243.

13. Seeley J, Svedmyr OLA, Weiland GK, et al. Epstein-Barr virus selective T cells in infectious mononucleosis are not restricted to HLA-A and B antigens. J Immunol 1981; 127:293–300.

14. Masucci MG, Bejarano MT, Masucci G, et al. Large granular lymphocytes inhibit the *in vitro* growth of autologous Epstein-Barr virus-infected cells. Cell Immunol 1981; 127:293–300.

15. Rickinson AB, Moss DJ, Wallace LE, et al. Long-term T cell-mediated immunity to Epstein Barr virus. Cancer Res 1981; 41:4216–4221.

16. O'Reilly RJ, Small TN, Papdopoulos E, Lucas K, Lacerda J, Koulova L. Adoptive immunotherapy for Epstein-Barr virus-associated lymphoproliferative disorders complicating marrow allografts. Springer Semin Immunopathol 1998; 20:455–491.

17. Rooney CM, Smith C, Ng CY, et al. Infusion of cytotoxic T cells for the prevention and treatment of Epstein-Barr virus-induced lymphoma in allogenic transplant recipients. Blood 1998; 5:1549–1555.

18. Small TN, Avigan D, Dupont B, et al. Immune reconstitution following T cell depleted bone marrow transplantation; effect of age and post-transplant graft rejection prophylaxis. Biol Blood Marrow Transplant 1997; 2:65.

19. Emanuel DJ, Lucas KG, Mallory GB, et al. Treatment of post-transplant lymphoproliferative disease in the central nervous system of a lung transplant recipient using allogenic leukocytes. Transplantation 1997; 63:1691.

20. Nalesnik MA, Rao AS, Furukawa H, et al. Autologous lymphokine-activated killer cell therapy of Epstein-Barr virus-positive and -negative lymphoproliferative disorders arising in organ transplant recipients. Transplantation 1997; 63:1200.

21. McGuirk JP, Seropian S, Howe G, Smith B, Stoddard L, Cooper DL. Use of rituximab and irradiated donor-derived lymphocytes to control Epstein-Barr virus-associated lymphoproliferation in patients undergoing related haplo-identical stem cell transplantation. Bone Marrow Transplant 1999; 24:1253–1258.

22. Cook RC, Connors JM, Gascoyne RD, Fradet G, Levy RD. Treatment of post-transplant lymphoproliferative disease with rituximab monoclonal antibody after lung transplantation. Lancet 1999; 354:1698–1699.

23. Rossol S, Marinos G, Caruscci P, Singer MV, Williams R, Naoumonv NV. Interleukin-12 induction of Th1 cytokines is important for viral clearance in chronic hepatitis B. J Clin Invest 1997; 99:3025–3033.

24. Gilles PN, Fey G, Chisari FV. Tumor necrosis factor negatively regulates hepatitis B virus gene expression in transgenic mice. J Virol 1992; 66:3955–3960.

25. Guilhot S, Guidotti LG, Chisari FV. Interleukin 2 and interferon alpha/beta downregulate hepatitis B virus gene expression in transgenic mice by a posttranscriptional mechanism. J Virol 1993; 67:7444–7449.

26. Guidotti LG, Guihlot S, Chisari FV. Interleukin 2 and interferon alpha/beta downregulate hepatitis B virus gene expression in vivo by tumor necrosis factor—dependent and independent pathways. J Virol 1994; 68:1265–1270.

27. Guidotti LG, Ando K, Hobbs MV, et al. Cytotoxic T lymphocytes inhibit hepatitis B virus gene expression by a noncytolytic mechanism in transgenic mice. Proc Natl Acad Sci USA 1994; 91:3764–3768.

28. Paar DP, Montgomerie BM, Nadler P, Schiff ER, Pollard RB. A phase I/II open-label trial to assess the safety, pharmacokinetic profile, and preliminary antiviral effects of OST-577 (a human monoclonal anti-hepatitis B surface antigen monoclonal antibody) administered to patients who are persistently hepatitis B surface antigen seropositive. In: Proceedings of the International Society for Antiviral Research, Charleston, SC, 1994 (Abstract).

29. Meyers JD. Prevention of cytomegalovirus infection after marrow transplantation. Rev Infect Dis 1989; 11:S1691–S1705.

30. Snydmena DR, Werner BG, Heinze-Lacey B, et al. Use of cytomegalovirus immune globulin to prevent cytomegalovirus disease in renal-transplant recipients. N Engl J Med 1987; 317:1049–1054.

31. Lakeman F, Blevins BS, Whitley R, Tolpin M. In vitro neutralization of CMV strains by human monoclonal antibody, MSL 109. Antiviral Res 1991; 15:77.

32. Nokta MA, Tolpin MD, Nadler PI, Pollard RB. Human monoclonal anti-CMV antibody (MSL 109): enhancement of in vitro foscarnet and ganciclovir induced inhibition of CMV replication. Antiviral Res 1994; 24:17–26.

33. Tolpin M, Pollard RB, Tierney M, Nokta MA, Wood D, Hirsch M. Combination therapy of CMV retinitis with a human monoclonal antibody (SDZ MSL 109) and either ganciclovir or foscarnet. In: Proceedings of the IX International Conference on AIDS. 1993 (Abstract).

34. The Studies of Ocular Complications of AIDS Research Group. MSL 109 adjuvant therapy for cytomegalovirus retinitis in patients with acquired immunodeficiency syndrome: the monoclonal antibody cytomegalovirus retinitis trial. Arch Ophthalmol 1997; 115:1528–1536.

35. Reed ED, Bowden RA, Dandliker PS, Lilleby KE, Myers JD. Treatment of cytomegalovirus pneumonia with ganciclovir and intravenous cytomegalovirus immunoglobulin in patients with bone marrow transplants. Ann Intern Med 1988; 109:783–788.

36. Emmanuel D, Cunningham I, Jules-Elysee K, et al. Cytomegalovirus pneumonia after bone marrow transplant successfully treated with the combination of ganciclovir and high-dose intravenous immune globulin. Ann Intern Med 1988; 109:777–782.

37. Reusser P, Riddell SR, Meyers JD, Greenberg PD. Cytotoxic lymphocyte response to cytomegalovirus after human allogenic bone marrow transplantation: patterns of recovery and correlation with cytomegalovirus infection and disease. Blood 1991; 78:1373–1380.

38. Walter EA, Greenberg PD, Gilbert MJ, et al. Reconstitution of cellular immunity against cytomegalovirus in recipients of allogenic bone marrow by transfer of T-cell clones from the donor. N Engl J Med 1995; 333:1038–1044.

39. Li CR, Greenberg PD, Gilbert MJ, Goodrich JM, Riddell SR. Recovery of HLA-restricted cytomegalovirus-specific T-cell responses after allogeneic bone marrow transplant; correlation with CMV disease and effect of ganciclovir prophylaxis. Blood 1994; 83:1971–1979.

15

Immunotherapy for Virus-Associated Malignancies

Uluhan Sili, Helen Heslop, and Cliona M. Rooney

INTRODUCTION

Estimates of the fraction of human malignancies that are associated with viral infections range from 10% to 20% *(1)*. Among viruses and their associated cancers are Epstein-Barr virus (EBV), which is associated with many different malignant diseases including lymphoproliferative disease (LPD) in immunosuppressed patients, Hodgkin's disease, Burkitt's lymphoma and nasopharyngeal carcinoma; human papillomaviruses (HPV) types 16 and 18 with cervical cancer; hepatitis B (HBV) and hepatitis C viruses with hepatocellular carcinoma; human T-cell leukemia virus-1 with adult T-cell lymphoma; and human herpes virus-8 with Kaposi's sarcoma in patients with AIDS.

Much of the evidence for the association of viruses with human cancer comes from epidemiologic data *(2)*. EBV and HPV have a high prevalence in most populations, but only a small proportion of infected persons develops a virus-associated cancer. The period of latency between primary infection and tumor outgrowth underscores the multifactorial origins of human tumors. Further evidence for the association of viruses with cancer comes from the detection of viral DNA in tumor tissue, the ability of viruses to transform cells in vitro, and the expression of viral proteins with oncogenic potential or the ability to inactivate tumor suppressor genes. Regardless of their precise role in oncogenesis, viral tumor-associated antigens can serve as targets for immunotherapy. The cytotoxic T-lymphocyte (CTL) arm of the cellular immune response is thought to be the most important defense against tumors and virus-infected cells. In this chapter, we discuss the use of EBV-specific CTLs as immunotherapy for EBV-associated malignancies. Other tumor-associated viruses are covered only briefly.

GENERATION OF CELL-MEDIATED IMMUNE RESPONSES

The design of successful immunologic strategies to treat human virus-associated malignancies requires an understanding of the effector processes that control viral infection and the mechanisms viruses use to evade such responses. Immune responses against viruses are mediated by nonspecific effector cells, such as natural killers and macrophages, and antigen-specific T- and B-lymphocytes.

Antibody-mediated humoral immunity effectively neutralizes extracellular virus. Once inside the cell, viruses are likely to be protected from antibody and therefore

From: *Immunotherapy for Infectious Diseases*
Edited by: J. M. Jacobson © Humana Press Inc., Totowa, NJ

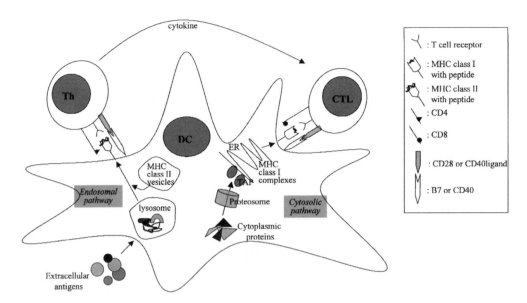

Fig. 1. Generation of cell-mediated immune response. For activation of naive T-helper (Th) and cytotoxic T-lymphocytes (CTLs), professional antigen-presenting cells (e.g., dendritic cells [DCs]) are required. DCs process the antigens and present the immunogenic peptides in an MHC context with simultaneous delivery of costimulatory signals (e.g., B7/CD28 or CD40/CD40 ligand signals) to activate T-lymphocytes. Two antigen-processing pathways are generally accepted. In the cytosolic pathway, endogenously synthesized antigens (cytoplasmic proteins) are digested in proteosomes and transported into the endoplasmic reticulum (ER) by transporters associated with antigen processing (TAPs), where they complex with MHC class I molecules for presentation to CD8+ CTLs. In the endosomal pathway, extracellular antigens are phagocytozed, digested in lysosomes, and then complexed with MHC class II molecules in vesicles for presentation to CD4+ Th-lymphocytes. See the text for more details.

become the targets of cellular immune responses, usually resulting in eradication of the infected cell by CTLs. Professional antigen-presenting cells (i.e., dendritic cells [DCs] or macrophages) and T-helper lymphocytes orchestrate the CTL response (Fig. 1).

Virus-specific CD4+ T-helper (Th) lymphocytes and CD8+ CTLs generally mediate the effector mechanisms necessary and sufficient to resolve acute infection as well as provide recall immune responses to resist reexposure to acute viruses and to control the reactivation of latent viruses. Viruses have diverse mechanisms to evade immune responses *(3)*, although in most cases the immune system prevails and controls the infection.

CD8+ CTLs recognize virus-infected cells through interaction of their T-cell receptor with peptides bound to the major histocompatibility complex (MHC) class I molecule of the infected cell. Endogenously synthesized proteins of the virus are degraded into short peptides by the antigen-processing machinery and presented in the MHC class I context *(4)*. Peptides are generally 8–10 amino acids long, are generated within cells by a cytoplasmic proteolytic complex known as the proteosome, and are then transported into the endoplasmic reticulum by transporters associated with antigen processing (TAPs), where they are complexed with MHC class I molecules for cell surface presentation *(5)*. Virtually all nucleated cells are MHC class I-positive and thus can be recognized when they are infected by a virus. For activating (priming) naive CTL precursors, the peptides must be presented by professional antigen-presenting cells (APCs), which can also provide the necessary costimulatory signals (i.e., interaction of B7 with CD28 or CD40 with CD40L on APC and T-cells, respectively) *(6)*. If the T-cell receptor is engaged without costimulatory signals, T-lymphocytes can become anergized. Activated CTLs do not need the costimulatory molecules to exert their effector functions, namely, cytolysis or induction of apoptosis of the target cell.

CD4+ Th-lymphocytes recognize exogenous antigens that are phagocytosed, processed, and presented in the context of MHC class II. Only APCs that are MHC class II-positive can activate CD4+ Th-lymphocyte precursors. Their major antiviral effect appears to be secreting cytokines and activating other effector cells, such as B-lymphocytes and CTLs. They may also have indirect antitumor activity via release of toxic cytokines (e.g., tumor necrosis factor-α [TNF-α]). CD4+ Th-lymphocyte help is crucial for the maintenance of an effective CTL response. When the infected cell is MHC class II-positive, CD4+ T-lymphocytes can also be cytolytic to the target cells *(7)*. This function has been clearly demonstrated for herpesvirus infections including cytomegalovirus, herpes simplex virus, varicella-zoster virus, and EBV *(8)*.

Endogenously synthesized antigens are generally thought to be presented as peptides on MHC class I molecules to CD8+ CTLs (i.e., the cytosolic pathway), whereas exogenous antigens are phagocytosed and presented in an MHC class II context to CD4+ Th-lymphocytes (i.e., the endosomal pathway). Alternatively, APCs can phagocytose antigens from virus-infected cells and present them on MHC class I molecules via exogenous pathways *(6)*. Viruses possess mechanisms to enter the cytosol, and virion proteins, although not endogenously synthesized, can gain access to the MHC class I pathway *(9,10)*. Thus, in some instances, the immune system might eradicate infected cells before the viral genome is expressed and progeny viruses produced.

IMMUNOTHERAPY

The goal of immunotherapy is to overcome the deficits of the host or the tumor itself and activate an effective immune response to the tumor. In the case of virus-associated malignancies, immunotherapeutic strategies can be either prophylactic (prevention of infection or prevention of tumor outgrowth in already infected individuals) or therapeutic (targeting the immune response against viral proteins expressed in tumor cells). In both applications, CTLs are regarded as the most important effector arm of the immune response against tumor or virus-infected cells, and they may be activated in vivo or ex vivo (Fig. 2). In vivo approaches such as vaccination aim to evoke an immune response by administration of an immunogen such as a peptide or DNA directly into patient. In the ex vivo approach, CTLs are activated and expanded in vitro, in a culture environment conducive to CTL growth, and then adoptively transferred into a recipient.

A tumor cell may fail to activate an effective immune response in the host for a number of reasons. First, tumor cells may fail to express an antigen that is perceived as foreign. In virus-associated malignancies, peptides derived from viral proteins can provide the target epitopes for CTLs. Second, tumor cells may fail to provide the costimulatory signals needed to activate CTLs. Optimal CTL induction can be achieved with professional APCs (e.g., DCs). Third, tumor cells may have mechanisms that inhibit the

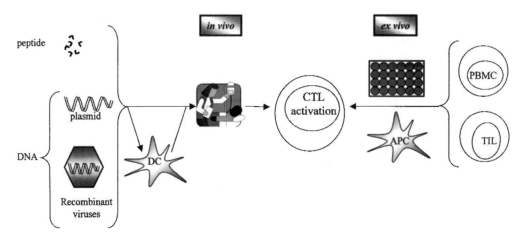

Fig. 2. Cytotoxic T-lymphocyte (CTL) activation strategies. In vivo (vaccination) strategies involve immunization with peptides (CTL-defined epitopes), naked DNA, recombinant viruses (e.g., recombinant vaccinia virus or recombinant adenovirus vectors) encoding immunogens, or antigen-loaded (peptide-pulsed or nucleic acid transfected) dendritic cells (DCs). Ex vivo (adoptive immunotherapy) strategies involve activation of antigen-specific CTLs (from peripheral blood mononuclear cells [PBMCs] or tumor-infiltrating lymphocytes [TILs]) using tumor or viral antigens expressed on antigen-presenting cells (APCs) and expanding them with T-cell growth factors in vitro with the eventual goal of infusion into patients.

generation of appropriate immune responses. For example, some tumors secrete cytokines that inhibit the activation or recruitment of professional APCs. Fourth, the host may be immunosuppressed. Ex vivo generation of CTLs may be feasible in either of the latter two contexts.

Adoptive Immunotherapy

Adoptive cellular immunotherapy is currently being used in settings in which the patient is immunosuppressed or the tumor secretes inhibitory factors. Recipients of solid organ or stem cell transplants, rendered immunodeficient by chemotherapy or radiotherapy, are at high risk for the reactivation of latent viruses, such as EBV, cytomegalovirus, and herpes zoster virus, which can produce considerable morbidity and mortality. The critical immunologic defect in these cases appears to be an inability to generate an effective CTL response; thus, in murine models, adoptive transfer of virus-specific T-cells restores protective immunity and controls established infection *(11–13)*.

In most contemporary strategies of adoptive therapy with virus-specific T-cells, antigen-specific CTL precursors are activated and expanded in vitro and then returned to the patient when sufficient numbers of cells have been obtained. The advantages of this approach are that the phenotype and function of the CTLs can be determined before treatment, antitumor activity can be ensured, and anti-host activity can be excluded. Furthermore, CTL numbers can be controlled and additional infusions given if required. Finally, the transfer of marker genes into CTL lines allows one to assess the function and persistence of the marked cells in vivo *(14)*, transfer of suicide genes may allow in vivo destruction of the CTLs should they prove toxic *(15)*, and transfer of functional genes may improve the activity of infused CTLs *(16)*. Thus, adoptive therapy with virus-specific T-lymphocytes potentially offers maximal therapeutic efficiency with minimal toxicity. We have used virus-specific CTLs for the prevention and treatment of EBV-associated malignancies in stem cell recipients, who are immunosuppressed, as well as in patients with relapsed EBV-positive Hodgkin's disease, whose tumors secrete inhibitory factors.

Vaccination

Peptides

Short, immunogenic peptides from virus-encoded proteins can be used for vaccination *(17)*. A number of naturally presented viral CTL epitopes have been identified by various techniques *(17)*. For example, a CTL response against an HPV-16-E7-encoded peptide was occasionally detected in cervical carcinoma patients *(18,19)*, suggesting the presence of a natural CTL-mediated immunity against HPV-16 in patients with cervical cancer. Similarly, T-lymphocytes from patients with HBV infection recognized the immunogenic peptides of HBV *(20)*. These specific but ineffective CTL responses might be augmented by additional in vivo stimulation with the immunogenic peptide.

Vaccination with a naturally processed and immunogenic peptide in vivo was initially tested in murine models of lymphocytic choriomeningitis virus *(21)* and Sendai virus *(22)*. An MHC class I binding peptide expressed by a recombinant vaccinia virus or injected in an adjuvant protected the mice against a challenge with a lethal dose of virus. Furthermore, vaccination with a peptide derived from HPV-16-E7 oncoprotein prevented the outgrowth of an HPV-16-induced tumor in mice *(23)*. However, the method of administration was found to be important for peptide immunotherapy *(12)*. A specific deletion of peptide-specific CTL was observed after injection of a peptide subcutaneously *(24)*. When the same peptide was loaded onto DCs or expressed as a transgene by a recombinant adenovirus vector, CTL response was detected *(12)*. Coadministration of recombinant IL-12 or addition of a helper peptide to a CTL peptide can also reverse the anergic state and help prime CTLs against the peptide *(25)*. These results indicate the importance of recruiting Th1 cells to the vaccination site. A persistent problem with single immunogenic peptides is the risk of mutations that alter the epitope, allowing the virus or tumor cell to evade the immune response. A second problem with peptides in general is that they must be tailored to suit the patient's HLA type.

Genetic Immunization

Immunotherapy by in vivo transfer of DNA encoding virus- or tumor-associated peptides or antigens is based on the rationale that qualitatively and quantitatively increased peptide presentation will lead to effective activation of both cytotoxic T-cell response and a humoral response *(26)*. DNA vaccination may be used to induce immune responses against predetermined peptides, an entire antigen, or multiple antigens. In contrast to peptide vaccination, DNA vaccination with an entire antigen results in intracellular processing and presentation of immunogenic peptides, so that the HLA type is less restrictive. The development of a protective immune response by immunization with a genetic vaccine was initially demonstrated in mice that had received intramuscular injections of naked plasmid DNA encoding the influenza virus nucleoprotein (NP). Both NP-specific antibody and CTL responses were generated, with resultant immunoprotection against intranasal challenge with influenza virus *(27)*. Since then the potential efficacy of DNA vaccination has been demonstrated in animal models infected with different pathogens. Genetic vaccines can also be administered via intravenous, intradermal, or subcutaneous routes or onto the skin by particle-mediated bombardment *(28)*.

The mechanism by which injected DNA induces immunity remains controversial *(29)*. It may be mediated by endogenous synthesis and presentation by the muscle cell, by transduction of professional APCs residing in tissue, or by crosspriming *(30)*, a process in which extracellular proteins and cellular fragments are phagocytosed and processed by professional APCs *(26,29)*.

The magnitude of the immune response to plasmid DNA vaccination appears to be determined by multiple factors. Increased immunogen expression generally augments the induction of immune responses *(31)*, and route of administration may influence the outcome of immunization. For example, epidermal delivery was reported to be quantitatively superior to intramuscular delivery in inducing immune responses *(32)*. Differences in immunization outcome owing to the route of immunogen delivery may reflect the fact that APCs are relatively more abundant in the skin, raising the possibility of direct APC transfection with cutaneous administration.

Immune responses induced by genetic immunization may be augmented by concurrent use of plasmid-encoded immunomodulatory molecules, such as cytokines, or costimulatory molecules, or by targeting the immunogenic proteins to intracellular processing organelles. An important factor in determining the outcome of immunization is the T-helper bias. The Th1-type immune response is characterized by secretion of cytokines such as interferon-γ (IFN-γ), interleukin-2 (IL-2), and IL-12, leading to the CTL response; the Th2-type response is characterized by secretion of cytokines such as IL-4 and IL-10, leading to the humoral immune response *(33)*. Thus, the pattern of cytokines expressed during initial immunization affects the character of the resultant immune response. Coinoculation of plasmids encoding granulocyte-macrophage colony-stimulating factor (GM-CSF), IL-2, IL-12, or IFN-γ was shown to augment both Th1 and CTL responses induced by DNA vaccination *(34–37)*. By contrast, coinoculation of plasmid-encoded IL-4 suppressed the CTL response generated by DNA vaccination *(34,36)*. Specific bacterial DNA sequences (unmethylated CpG dinucleotides) in noncoding regions of plasmid constructs were also identified as promoters of Th1-type immune responses culminating in CTL responses *(38,39)*.

Immune responses can be modified by directing the protein to an endogenous versus exogeneous antigen-processing pathway. Thus, expression of an adenovirus E3 leader sequence can target an epitope to the endoplasmic reticulum and result in enhancement of the CTL response generated by more efficient MHC class I-restricted presentation *(40)*. Likewise, the sorting signal from a lysosome-associated membrane protein 1 fused to an antigen can enhance both antibody and CTL responses generated by MHC class II presentation *(41,42)*.

In vivo evaluation of genetic immunization has failed to demonstrate any significant toxicity. Major concerns have included the potential induction of autoimmunity or destruction of transfected cells, but to date neither effect has been observed *(43)*. Furthermore, integration of plasmid DNA into genomic DNA with the attendant risk of insertional mutagenesis has not been detected *(44)*.

Inducing immune responses to multiple peptides is a major goal of research in genetic immunization. The string-bead approach, which links multiple different CTL or T-helper epitopes, is one of the methods proposed. Such multiepitope (polytope) vaccines might induce immunity against multiple antigenic targets, multiple strain variants, or multiple pathogens *(45)*. The polytope vaccine hypothesis was recently validated in a study in which a recombinant vaccinia virus containing 10 contiguous minimal murine CTL epitopes was used to induce primary CTL responses to all 10 epitopes in mice *(46)*.

Dendritic Cell Vaccines

DCs are the most potent antigen-presenting cells yet identified *(47)*. They are efficient in priming naive T-lymphocyte precursors, as they possess the costimulatory signals and secrete the cytokines required for this immune response. The development of techniques to generate adequate numbers of DCs from peripheral blood precursors or bone marrow progenitors has led to application of these cells in immunotherapy *(48)*. In general, peptide-pulsed DCs are more effective in eliciting immune responses than are peptides alone *(49–51)*. Introduction of antigen-coding DNA into the cytoplasm of DCs for endogenous processing and presentation allows CTL activation that is independent of HLA type. Such transduction is possible with either physical methods (e.g., liposomes) or viral vectors (e.g., adenovirus vectors) *(52–54)*. When the use of DNA vaccination against viral oncoproteins (e.g., E6 and E7 of HPV) raises safety issues, RNA-loaded APCs may offer a useful alternative *(55)*. Clinical trials of DCs loaded with tumor antigens are in progress *(48)*.

VIRUS-ASSOCIATED MALIGNANCIES

Epstein-Barr Virus

EBV, also designated human herpesvirus 4, is associated with malignancies of B-cells, epithelial cells, T-cells, natural killer cells, and muscle *(56,57)*. The development of EBV-positive tumors is associated with the latent life cycle of the virus during which it expresses up to nine viral proteins that provide targets for CTLs.

Adoptive Immunotherapy

LPDs of stem cell transplant recipients have provided an excellent system for testing the biologic efficacy of ex vivo expanded, adoptively transferred antigen-specific CTL lines. LPD represents the most immunogenic tumor (type 3 latency) among EBV-related malignancies, as all EBV latency-associated proteins are expressed by the virally transformed lymphocytes. Virus-infected B-cells expressing type 3 latency do not evade the immune response and are seen only in severely immunocompromised individuals. For example, EBV-LPD occurs in up to 20% of recipients of T-cell-depleted stem cells from HLA-mismatched or unrelated donors. No antiviral agents are reproducibly effective against EBV-LPD. Immunotherapy with unmanipulated donor leukocytes, although effective in some cases, is associated with a high incidence of disease progression, and survivors have a high incidence of graft-versus-host disease (GvHD) *(58)*. We have shown that LPD can be prevented or eradicated and GvHD avoided by using selectively expanded EBV-specific CTLs either prophylactically or as treatment for overt disease *(59)*. EBV-transformed B-cell lines are relatively easy to

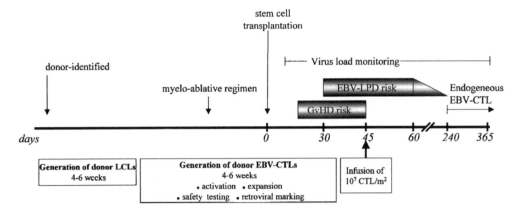

Fig. 3. Timeline for generation of Epstein-Barr virus-specific cytotoxic T-lymphocytes (EBV-CTL). To ensure that CTL lines are available by the time patients are at high risk for EBV-lymphoproliferative disease (EBV-LDP) (1–2 months after stem cell transplantation), we initiate the lines as soon as the donor is identified. The first step is the generation of the lymphoblastoid cell lines (LCLs), which takes about 4–6 weeks. Activation, expansion, and safety testing of the CTL line takes an additional 4–6 weeks. The first 26 patients received CTLs that had been genetically marked with a retrovirus vector carrying the neomycin resistance gene. Marking efficiencies of 0.5–10% allowed us to track the in vivo persistence of the CTLs and to determine their involvement in any toxicity. An initial dose escalation study revealed that low numbers of CTLs were biologically effective, and so all patients currently receive one dose of 10^7 CTL per m². The target date of infusion is day 45, at which time graft-versus-host disease (GvHD), if it is to occur, should be apparent. Endogenous EBV-specific CTLs return at about 8–9 months post transplant. Virus load monitoring is also useful for timely intervention.

establish and provide a continuous source of APCs to activate EBV-specific CTL lines from seropositive donors (Fig. 3). Since 1993, we have infused donor-derived, EBV-specific CTL lines into over 60 recipients of stem cell transplants *(60,61)*.

The most important result of the study was that none of the patients who received prophylactic CTLs developed EBV-LPD, in contrast to about 12% of controls *(61)*. Gene-marking studies showed that the infused CTL lines could expand in vivo in response to EBV reactivation and then persist for as long as 5 years. Infusion of CTLs into patients with a high virus load resulted in a dramatic drop in the virus load to low or undetectable levels. Further evidence for antitumor effects came from four patients who developed frank lymphoma before they were treated with CTLs. Subsequent infusions of the activated T-lymphocytes produced complete remissions in three of the four cases *(61)*. Marking studies showed that the EBV-specific CTLs home to tumor sites, where they accumulate or expand and ultimately cause lymphoma regression.

Experience with CTL treatment of advanced EBV-LPD has illustrated two common pitfalls of such therapy. First, if the tumor occurs in a sensitive anatomic location, the inflammatory response can be damaging. One of our patients with bulky disease in the nasopharynx showed increased swelling after the CTL infusion, requiring intubation and tracheotomy *(61)*. Second, mutation of important CTL epitopes becomes increasingly likely with tumor progression. Analysis of tumor tissue from a patient whose disease resisted CTL therapy revealed a deletion in viral DNA that removed two immunodominant epitopes against which the CTLs were specific *(59,62)*.

Recipients of solid organ transplants may be at particularly high risk for EBV-LPD if they are seronegative prior to transplantation or if they receive organs, such as gut, that carry a high B-cell load, or if they receive prolonged, intensive immunosuppressive therapy for repeat episodes of graft rejection. Surprisingly, it has been possible to generate EBV-specific CTL lines from organ recipients even after they have developed lymphoproliferative disease. This suggests that EBV-specific CTL precursors are present in the circulation but are unable to expand in vivo during treatment with immunosuppressive drugs. If such cells are moved to a supportive culture environment, they can respond to activation and proliferation signals. In the case of seronegative recipients, it may be possible to activate CTLs by using APCs such as DCs, since they are able to activate CTLs from naive precursors in vitro *(47)*. Prophylaxis with CTLs is probably not an option in these patients, since with time, in the absence of viral antigen and the presence of immunosuppressive drugs, the infused CTL may be lost. However, because regular monitoring of the virus load can permit early intervention, CTLs should be prepared in advance for patients with a high-risk status and then infused when virus DNA appears or they seroconvert.

Patients with immunodeficiency disorders are also at increased risk for EBV-LPD. As with solid organ recipients, it has been possible to generate EBV-specific CTLs from some of these patients and to use them as therapeutic agents *(63)*.

EBV-positive Hodgkin's disease is another candidate for treatment with EBV-specific CTLs. Five patients who received autologous EBV-specific CTLs in a phase I study had temporary clinical improvements, including increases in EBV-specific CTL precursor frequency, reductions in high virus loads, resolution of type B symptoms, and stabilization of disease *(64)*. Current improvements include the generation of CTL lines that are specific for the limited range of viral antigens expressed in Reed-Sternberg cells.

Vaccination

The high incidence of nasopharyngeal carcinoma (NPC) in southern China (1–2% of the general population) has been associated with early infection by EBV *(65)*. A vaccine that could prevent or delay primary infection with EBV by establishing mucosal immunity might decrease the incidence of EBV-associated NPC *(66)*. The gp340 envelope glycoprotein of EBV, the principal target for neutralizing antibodies, binds to the cellular receptor for the C3d component of complement, enabling virus to enter the B-cells. A vaccine based on purified gp340 has been shown to reduce the virus load and protect against EBV-associated LPD in cotton-top tamarins *(2)*. When tested in Chinese children, live recombinant vaccinia virus engineered to express gp340 induced EBV-specific immune responses with protection against and/or delay of EBV infection *(67)*. However, the outcome of this study may not be evident for 40 years.

Because the CTL-mediated immune response is necessary for control of EBV infection, the possibility of priming T-cells by peptide immunization, before primary infection, has been raised. One advantage of accelerating the CTL response to primary infection is that one may be able to limit subsequent colonization of the B-lymphocyte pool *(2)*. This approach would require peptides that are customized to the patients' HLA phenotype *(17)* or perhaps a polytope vaccine, as described previously *(45)*. An effective vaccine against EBV would be especially useful for seronegative recipients of solid organs from seropositive donors. Such patients are generally at greater risk of developing EBV-LPD *(68)*.

Human Papillomavirus

Infection with HPV is widespread throughout population. Over 80 strains of this virus cause a spectrum of tumors of skin and mucous membranes. HPV-1 and HPV-6 appear to be largely responsible for benign skin warts and genital warts, respectively, whereas 90% of cervical carcinomas are associated with HPV-16 and HPV-18 *(69)*. Despite the wide involvement of HPV in sexually transmitted disease and its association with malignancy, specific therapy for HPV is still not available. Surgical or chemical removal of the wart leaves the viral episome in the basal epithelium, and host cell transformation can result from random integration of oncogenic HPV DNA into the genome *(70)*.

Prophylaxis with vaccines for genital papillomaviruses might prevent infection by eliciting neutralizing antibodies *(70)*. To be effective, such vaccines must establish an immunologic barrier at the anogenital epithelium by selective stimulation of a secretory IgA-mediated anti-HPV virion response in the genital mucosa *(70)*. A phase I trial of L1 (the major capsid protein) particles to vaccinate HPV-11-naive adults is imminent. Detection of type-specific HPV DNA in the genital tract or the development of HPV-induced anogenital lesions will serve as end points of this proposed vaccination trial *(71)*.

The immunogenicity of cervical cancer is supported by the observation that it progresses rapidly in immunosuppressed patients, and spontaneous remissions are associated with lymphocyte infiltration *(73)*. Furthermore, the detection of CTL activity against HPV-16-E7-encoded immunogenic peptides in some patients with cervical intraepithelial neoplasia or cervical cancer suggested that natural immunity might be strengthened with immunotherapeutic approaches *(72)*. There is considerable interest in using HPV vaccines to eliminate residual cancer, precancerous lesions, or warts. About 60% of cervical carcinomas express the transforming proteins of HPV-16 (E6 and E7) *(49)*. Hence, these proteins are obvious targets for any immunotherapeutic approaches that successfully exploit tumor rejection antigens in murine models *(74)*. Immunization with an immunodominant peptide of HPV-16-E7 protected animals against lethal challenge with a tumor expressing this epitope, whereas immunization with peptide-pulsed DCs could eradicate established tumor *(12)*.

Vaccination with peptides has been applied in clinical trials for cervical cancer. A peptide vaccine consisting of two HPV-16-E7 HLA-A*0201-restricted CTL peptides and a helper peptide has been tested in women with end-stage cervical cancer *(73,75)*, but no correlation between vaccine dose and clinical outcome was observed. Steller et al. *(76)* also tested the effectiveness of a lipidated form of HPV-16-E7 covalently linked to a helper peptide. Activation of CTL responses, detected by IFN-γ release assay, were demonstrated in two of three evaluable patients who had been vaccinated with this peptide.

Genetic immunization with a recombinant vaccinia virus expressing the E6 and E7 epitopes of HPV-16 and HPV-18 (mutated to abrogate the transforming capacity of the virus, while retaining the predicted epitopes) was tested in eight patients with late-stage cervical cancer *(77)*. Vaccinia antibody responses were noted in all patients, with three demonstrating HPV-specific antibody responses. HPV-specific CTLs could be detected in one of three patients. Such an approach might be more effective in patients with less advanced cancers or preinvasive lesions, or perhaps even in HPV-16 or -18 carriers without detectable lesions.

To eliminate basal cells infected with HPV, some investigators have proposed E1 and E2 proteins of HPV as targets for immunotherapy, as they are required for maintenance of the episomal state *(70)*. Papilloma virus-like particles (VLPs), formed by the assembly of the major capsid protein of papillomaviruses in the absence of other viral proteins, can be engineered to carry other proteins *(78,79)*, whereas a VLP bearing an HPV-16-E7 epitope protected mice from challenge with E7-transformed tumor cells *(79)*.

Hepatitis B Virus

HBV replicates in the liver and causes hepatic dysfunction *(80)*. Most HBV infections are self-limiting and are effectively controlled by the immune system. A small fraction of HBV infections can become persistent or chronic if the immune system fails to resolve the infection completely. Persons with chronic HBV infection are at substantially increased risk of developing cirrhosis and primary hepatocellular carcinoma. Although no specific HBV sequence has been implicated in the development of hepatocellular carcinoma, the virus appears to act as a mutagenic agent, and viral gene expression may not be required for tumor growth. IFN-α treatment is helpful in some cases, but a satisfactory medical treatment for chronic HBV infection is still unavailable. Immunologic intervention with the conventional hepatitis B vaccine relies on primary prevention. The vaccine is composed of a highly purified preparation of hepatitis B surface antigen (HbsAg). Virtually 100% of persons who develop HBsAg antibody titers of > 10 mIU/mL after primary vaccination are protected against primary infection. However, the vaccine is of no benefit to individuals already infected or who have chronic disease. The ultimate goal of hepatitis B vaccination is to decrease the incidence of HBV-related chronic liver disease and hepatocellular carcinoma. Recent studies in Taiwan have demonstrated a reduction in the incidence of primary liver cancer in children born after the implementation of routine hepatitis B vaccination programs *(80)*.

From 2.5 to 5% of immunized adults with HbsAg do not develop an antibody response. This rate increases to 40% in high-risk patients, such as those on hemodialysis *(81)*. Chimpanzees that received intramuscular vaccination with plasmid DNA encoding the major and middle HBV envelope proteins developed strong group-, subtype-, and preS2-specific antibodies compared with those achieved by traditional antigen-based vaccination *(31)*. Thus, genetic immunization may lead to a lower rate of unresponsiveness.

Patients who successfully clear HBV develop a strong HLA class I-restricted CTL response, whereas in those with chronic hepatitis B, the response is weak or undetectable. Hence, a vaccine capable of inducing a CTL response to HBV may be capable of eradicating chronic infection and thereby eliminating the risk of developing cirrhosis or hepatocellular carcinoma. Twenty-six normal volunteers were immunized with an HLA-A*0201-restricted CTL epitope from the HBV core antigen linked to a tetanus toxoid-derived helper epitope with palmitic acid residues used as adjuvants *(82,83)*. This vaccination proved to be safe and generated primary HBV-specific CTL responses. This was the first demonstration that a CTL peptide can induce a primary CTL response in humans and provides the rationale for a larger clinical trial in patients chronically infected with HBV *(83)*.

CONCLUSIONS AND FUTURE PERSPECTIVES

Adoptive immunotherapy with antigen-specific CTLs has proved to be safe and effective in immunosuppressed patients. Our clinical trials have suggested that the prophylactic use of ex vivo generated CTLs is optimal and provides protection against virus-associated tumor formation. If CTLs are used therapeutically, attention must be paid to the potential of a damaging inflammatory response and the emergence of "antigen-loss variants." As with any immunotherapeutic strategy, the use of polyclonal CTL lines targeted to more than one antigen or to antigens that are essential for the transformed phenotype may preclude the outgrowth of "escape mutants." Tumors in patients who are not immunosuppressed will probably be more difficult to treat because of tumor-mediated immune evasion strategies.

Genetic immunization and vaccination with peptides have also proved to be efficacious in eliciting specific immune responses. As clinical trials progress, it will be important to identify the best method of administering these agents. Genetic immunization with entire protein sequences offers natural processing and presentation of peptides, precluding the need to determine the immunogenic peptide for the patient's HLA type. Among the advantages offered by peptide-based approaches are safety, easier clinical grade production, and specific induction of immune responses to subdominant epitopes. The uses of single peptides for vaccination will probably lead to epitope-loss mutants and should therefore be avoided. Polytope vaccines linking different CTL epitopes may offer better protection. The optimal strategy is likely to be disease-dependent. Clearly, the use of dendritic cells for both peptide vaccination and genetic immunization results in more potent responses.

REFERENCES

1. Wang FCS, Kieff ED. Medical virology. In: Fauci AS, Braunwald E, Isselbacher KJ, et al. (eds.) Harrison's Online. New York: McGraw-Hill, 2000.
2. Rickinson AB. Immune intervention against virus-associated human cancers. Ann Oncol 1995; 6(suppl 1):69–71.
3. McMichael A. T cell responses and viral escape. Cell 1998; 93:673–676.
4. Jondal M, Schirmbeck R, Reimann J. MHC class I-restricted CTL responses to exogenous antigens. Immunity 1996; 5:295–302.
5. Pamer E, Cresswell P. Mechanisms of MHC class I—restricted antigen processing. Annu Rev Immunol 1998; 16:323–358.
6. Sigal LJ, Crotty S, Andino R, Rock KL. Cytotoxic T-cell immunity to virus-infected non-haematopoietic cells requires presentation of exogenous antigen [see comments]. Nature 1999; 398:77–80.
7. Lanzavecchia A. Mechanisms of antigen uptake for presentation. Curr Opin Immunol 1996; 8:348–354.
8. Borysiewicz LK, Sissons JPG. Cytotoxic T cells and human herpes virus infections. In: Oldstone MBA (ed). Cytotoxic T-Lymphocytes in Human Viral and Malaria Infections. Berlin: Springer-Verlag, 1994, pp. 123–150.
9. Gilbert MJ, Riddell SR, Plachter B, Greenberg PD. Cytomegalovirus selectively blocks antigen processing and presentation of its immediate-early gene product. Nature 1996; 383:720–722.
10. Smith CA, Woodruff LS, Kitchingman GR, Rooney CM. Adenovirus-pulsed dendritic cells stimulate human virus-specific T-cell responses in vitro. J Virol 1996; 70:6733–6740.
11. Melief CJ, Kast WM. Efficacy of cytotoxic T lymphocytes against virus-induced tumors. Cancer Cells 1990; 2:116–120.

12. Velders MP, Schreiber H, Kast WM. Active immunization against cancer cells: impediments and advances. Semin Oncol 1998; 25:697–706.

13. Zinkernagel RM, Doherty PC. Immunological surveillance against altered self components by sensitised T lymphocytes in lymphocytic choriomeningitis. Nature 1974; 251:547–548.

14. Heslop HE, Ng CY, Li C, et al. Long-term restoration of immunity against Epstein-Barr virus infection by adoptive transfer of gene-modified virus-specific T lymphocytes. Nat Med 1996; 2:551–555.

15. Bonini C, Ferrari G, Verzeletti S, et al. HSV-TK gene transfer into donor lymphocytes for control of allogeneic graft-versus-leukemia [see comments]. Science 1997; 276:1719–1724.

16. Hwu P, Yannelli J, Kriegler M, et al. Functional and molecular characterization of tumor-infiltrating lymphocytes transduced with tumor necrosis factor-alpha cDNA for the gene therapy of cancer in humans. J Immunol 1993; 150:4104–4115.

17. Velders MP, Nieland JD, Rudolf MP, et al. Identification of peptides for immunotherapy of cancer. It is worth the effort. Crit Rev Immunol 1998; 18:7–27.

18. Ressing ME, Offringa R, Toes RE, et al. Immunotherapy of cancer by peptide-based vaccines for the induction of tumor-specific T cell immunity. Immunotechnology 1996; 2:241–251.

19. Ressing ME, van Driel WJ, Celis E, et al. Occasional memory cytotoxic T-cell responses of patients with human papillomavirus type 16-positive cervical lesions against a human leukocyte antigen-A *0201-restricted E7-encoded epitope. Cancer Res 1996; 56:582–588.

20. Sette A, Vitiello A, Reherman B, et al. The relationship between class I binding affinity and immunogenicity of potential cytotoxic T cell epitopes. J Immunol 1994; 153:5586–5592.

21. Schulz M, Zinkernagel RM, Hengartner H. Peptide-induced antiviral protection by cytotoxic T cells. Proc Natl Acad Sci USA 1991; 88:991–993.

22. Kast WM, Roux L, Curren J, et al. Protection against lethal Sendai virus infection by in vivo priming of virus-specific cytotoxic T lymphocytes with a free synthetic peptide. Proc Natl Acad Sci USA 1991; 88:2283–2287.

23. Feltkamp MC, Smits HL, Vierboom MP, et al. Vaccination with cytotoxic T lymphocyte epitope-containing peptide protects against a tumor induced by human papillomavirus type 16-transformed cells. Eur J Immunol 1993; 23:2242–2249.

24. Toes RE, Blom RJ, Offringa R, Kast WM, Melief CJ. Enhanced tumor outgrowth after peptide vaccination. Functional deletion of tumor-specific CTL induced by peptide vaccination can lead to the inability to reject tumors. J Immunol 1996; 156:3911–3918.

25. Grohmann U, Bianchi R, Ayroldi E, et al. A tumor-associated and self antigen peptide presented by dendritic cells may induce T cell anergy in vivo, but IL-12 can prevent or revert the anergic state. J Immunol 1997; 158:3593–3602.

26. White SA, Conry RM, Strong TV, Curiel DT, LoBuglio AL. Polynucleotide-mediated immunization therapy of cancer. In: Lattime EC, Gerson SL (eds). Gene Therapy of Cancer. San Diego: Academic Press, 1999, pp. 271–283.

27. Ulmer JB, Fu TM, Deck RR, et al. Protective CD4+ and CD8+ T cells against influenza virus induced by vaccination with nucleoprotein DNA. J Virol 1998; 72:5648–5653.

28. Tang DC, DeVit M, Johnston SA. Genetic immunization is a simple method for eliciting an immune response. Nature 1992; 356:152–154.

29. Butterfield LH, Ribas A, Economou JS. DNA and dendritic cell-based genetic immunization against cancer. In: Lattime EC, Gerson SL (eds). Gene Therapy of Cancer. San Diego: Academic Press, 1999, pp. 285–298.

30. Inaba K, Turley S, Yamaide F, et al. Efficient presentation of phagocytosed cellular fragments on the major histocompatibility complex class II products of dendritic cells. J Exp Med 1998; 188:2163–2173.

31. Davis HL, McCluskie MJ, Gerin JL, Purcell RH. DNA vaccine for hepatitis B: evidence for immunogenicity in chimpanzees and comparison with other vaccines. Proc Natl Acad Sci USA 1996; 93:7213–7218.

32. Barry MA, Johnston SA. Biological features of genetic immunization. Vaccine 1997; 15:788–791.

33. Constant SL, Bottomly K. Induction of Th1 and Th2 CD4+ T cell responses: the alternative approaches. Annu Rev Immunol, 1997; 15:297–322.

34. Chow YH, Chiang BL, Lee YL, et al. Development of Th1 and Th2 populations and the nature of immune responses to hepatitis B virus DNA vaccines can be modulated by code-livery of various cytokine genes. J Immunol 1998; 160:1320–1329.

35. Fallarino F, Uyttenhove C, Boon T, Gajewski TF. Improved efficacy of dendritic cell vaccines and successful immunization with tumor antigen peptide-pulsed peripheral blood mononuclear cells by coadministration of recombinant murine interleukin-12. Int J Cancer 1999; 80:324–333.

36. Geissler M, Gesien A, Tokushige K, Wands JR. Enhancement of cellular and humoral immune responses to hepatitis C virus core protein using DNA-based vaccines augmented with cytokine-expressing plasmids. J Immunol 1997; 158:1231–1237.

37. Kim JJ, Nottingham LK, Tsai A, et al. Antigen-specific humoral and cellular immune responses can be modulated in rhesus macaques through the use of IFN-gamma, IL-12, or IL-18 gene adjuvants. J Med Primatol 1999; 28:214–223.

38. Halpern MD, Kurlander RJ, Pisetsky DS. Bacterial DNA induces murine interferon-gamma production by stimulation of interleukin-12 and tumor necrosis factor-alpha. Cell Immunol 1996; 167:72–78.

39. Sato Y, Roman M, Tighe H, et al. Immunostimulatory DNA sequences necessary for effective intradermal gene immunization. Science 1996; 273:352–354.

40. Ciernik IF, Berzofsky JA, Carbone DP. Induction of cytotoxic T lymphocytes and antitumor immunity with DNA vaccines expressing single T cell epitopes. J Immunol 1996; 156:2369–2375.

41. Lin KY, Guarnieri FG, Staveley-O'Carroll KF, et al. Treatment of established tumors with a novel vaccine that enhances major histocompatibility class II presentation of tumor antigen. Cancer Res 1996; 56:21–26.

42. Wu TC, Guarnieri FG, Staveley-O'Carroll KF, et al. Engineering an intracellular pathway for major histocompatibility complex class II presentation of antigens. Proc Natl Acad Sci USA 1995; 92:11671–11675.

43. Conry RM, LoBuglio AF, Curiel DT. Polynucleotide-mediated immunization therapy of cancer. Semin Oncol 1996; 23:135–147.

44. Nichols WW, Ledwith BJ, Manam SV, Troilo PJ. Potential DNA vaccine integration into host cell genome. Ann NY Acad Sci 1995; 772:30–39.

45. Suhrbier A. Multi-epitope DNA vaccines. Immunol Cell Biol 1997; 75:402–408.

46. Thomson SA, Sherritt MA, Medveczky J, et al. Delivery of multiple CD8 cytotoxic T cell epitopes by DNA vaccination. J Immunol 1998; 160:1717–1723.

47. Banchereau J, Steinman RM. Dendritic cells and the control of immunity. Nature 1998; 392:245–252.

48. Timmerman JM, Levy R. Dendritic cell vaccines for cancer immunotherapy. Annu Rev Med 1999; 50:507–529.

49. De Bruijn ML, Schuurhuis DH, Vierboom MP, et al. Immunization with human papillomavirus type 16 (HPV16) oncoprotein-loaded dendritic cells as well as protein in adjuvant induces MHC class I-restricted protection to HPV16-induced tumor cells. Cancer Res 1998; 58:724–731.

50. Hsu FJ, Benike C, Fagnoni F, et al. Vaccination of patients with B-cell lymphoma using autologous antigen-pulsed dendritic cells. Nat Med 1996; 2:52–58.

51. Ossevoort MA, Feltkamp MC, van Veen KJ, Melief CJ, Kast WM. Dendritic cells as carriers for a cytotoxic T-lymphocyte epitope-based peptide vaccine in protection against a human papillomavirus type 16-induced tumor. J Immunother Emphasis Tumor Immunol 1995; 18:86–94.

52. Arthur JF, Butterfield LH, Roth MD, et al. A comparison of gene transfer methods in human dendritic cells. Cancer Gene Ther 1997; 4:17–25.

53. Morse MA, Lyerly HK, Gilboa E, Thomas E, Nair SK. Optimization of the sequence of antigen loading and CD40-ligand-induced maturation of dendritic cells. Cancer Res 1998; 58:2965–2968.

54. Zhong L, Granelli-Piperno A, Choi Y, Steinman RM. Recombinant adenovirus is an efficient and non-perturbing genetic vector for human dendritic cells. Eur J Immunol 1999; 29:964–972.

55. Boczkowski D, Nair SK, Snyder D, Gilboa E. Dendritic cells pulsed with RNA are potent antigen-presenting cells in vitro and in vivo. J Exp Med 1996; 184:465–472.

56. McClain KL, Leach CT, Jenson HB, et al. Association of Epstein-Barr virus with leiomyosarcomas in children with AIDS [see comments]. N Engl J Med 1995; 332:12–18.

57. Su IJ, Lin KH, Chen CJ, et al. Epstein-Barr virus-associated peripheral T-cell lymphoma of activated CD8 phenotype. Cancer 1990; 66:2557–2562.

58. Lucas KG, Burton RL, Zimmerman SE, et al. Semiquantitative Epstein-Barr virus (EBV) polymerase chain reaction for the determination of patients at risk for EBV-induced lymphoproliferative disease after stem cell transplantation. Blood 1998; 91:3654–3661.

59. Rooney CM, Smith CA, Ng CYC, et al. Infusion of cytotoxic T cells for the prevention and treatment of Epstein-Barr virus-induced lymphoma in allogeneic transplant recipients. Blood 1998; 92:1549–1555.

60. Heslop HE, Brenner MK, Rooney CM. Donor T cells to treat EBV-associated lymphoma [letter; comment]. N Engl J Med 1994; 331:679–680.

61. Rooney CM, Smith CA, Ng CY, et al. Infusion of cytotoxic T cells for the prevention and treatment of Epstein-Barr virus-induced lymphoma in allogeneic transplant recipients. Blood 1998; 92:1549–1555.

62. Gottschalk S, Ng CYC, Perez M, Brenner MK, Heslop HE, Rooney CM. Mutation in EBV produces immunoblastic lymphoma unresponsive to CTL immunotherapy. Blood 1998; 92:321a (Abstract).

63. Khanna R, Bell S, Sherritt M, et al. Activation and adoptive transfer of Epstein-Barr virus-specific cytotoxic T cells in solid organ transplant patients with posttransplant lymphoproliferative disease. Proc Natl Acad Sci USA 1999; 96:10391–10396.

64. Roskrow MA, Rooney CM, Heslop HE, et al. Administration of neomycin resistance gene marked EBV specific cytotoxic T-lymphocytes to patients with relapsed EBV-positive Hodgkin disease. Hum Gene Ther 1998; 9:1237–1250.

65. Moss DJ, Burrows SR, Suhrbier A, Khanna R. Potential antigenic targets on Epstein-Barr virus-associated tumours and the host response. In: Chadwick DJ, Marsh J (eds). Vaccines Against Virally Induced Cancers. New York: John Wiley & Sons, 1994, pp. 4–20.

66. Krause PR, Straus SE. Herpesvirus vaccines. Development, controversies, and applications. Infect Dis Clin North Am 1999; 13:61–81, vi.

67. Gu SY, Huang TM, Ruan L, et al. First EBV vaccine trial in humans using recombinant vaccinia virus expressing the major membrane antigen. Dev Biol Stand 1995; 84:171–177.

68. Rickinson AB, Moss DJ. Human cytotoxic T lymphocyte responses to Epstein-Barr virus infection. Annu Rev Immunol 1997; 15:405–431.

69. Bosch FX, Manos MM, Munoz N, et al. Prevalence of human papillomavirus in cervical cancer: a worldwide perspective. International biological study on cervical cancer (IBSCC) Study Group [see comments]. J Natl Cancer Inst 1995; 87:796–802.

70. Tindle RW. Immunomanipulative strategies for the control of human papillomavirus associated cervical disease. Immunol Res 1997; 16:387–400.

71. Galloway DA. Is vaccination against human papillomavirus a possibility? Lancet, 1998; 351(suppl 3):22–24.

72. Nimako M, Fiander AN, Wilkinson GW, Borysiewicz LK, Man S. Human papillomavirus-specific cytotoxic T lymphocytes in patients with cervical intraepithelial neoplasia grade III. Cancer Res 1997; 57:4855–4861.

73. van Driel WJ, Ressing ME, Brandt RM, et al. The current status of therapeutic HPV vaccine. Ann Med 1996; 28:471–477.

74. Chen L, Mizuno MT, Singhal MC, et al. Induction of cytotoxic T lymphocytes specific for a syngeneic tumor expressing the E6 oncoprotein of human papillomavirus type 16. J Immunol 1992; 148:2617–2621.

75. van Driel WJ, Ressing ME, Kenter GG, et al. Vaccination with HPV16 peptides of patients with advanced cervical carcinoma: clinical evaluation of a phase I-II trial. Eur J Cancer 1999; 35:946–952.

76. Steller MA, Gurski KJ, Murakami M, et al. Cell-mediated immunological responses in cervical and vaginal cancer patients immunized with a lipidated epitope of human papillomavirus type 16 E7. Clin Cancer Res 1998; 4:2103–2109.

77. Borysiewicz LK, Fiander A, Nimako M, et al. A recombinant vaccinia virus encoding human papillomavirus types 16 and 18, E6 and E7 proteins as immunotherapy for cervical cancer [see comments]. Lancet 1996; 347:1523–1527.

78. Dupuy C, Buzoni-Gatel D, Touze A, Le Cann P, Bout D, Coursaget P. Cell mediated immunity induced in mice by HPV 16 L1 virus-like particles. Microbiol Pathogen 1997; 22:219–225.

79. Peng S, Frazer IH, Fernando GJ, Zhou J. Papillomavirus virus-like particles can deliver defined CTL epitopes to the MHC class I pathway. Virology 1998; 240:147–157.

80. Mahoney FJ. Update on diagnosis, management, and prevention of hepatitis B virus infection. Clin Microbiol Rev 1999; 12:351–366.

81. Waters JA, Foster GR, Thursz MR, Thomas HC. Hepatitis B virus infection and immunity. In: McCance DJ (ed). Human Tumor Viruses. Washington, DC: ASM, 1998, pp. 283–299.

82. Bertoni R, Sidney J, Fowler P, Chesnut RW, Chisari FV, Sette A. Human histocompatibility leukocyte antigen-binding supermotifs predict broadly cross-reactive cytotoxic T lymphocyte responses in patients with acute hepatitis. J Clin Invest 1997; 100:503–513.

83. Vitiello A, Ishioka G, Grey HM, et al. Development of a lipopeptide-based therapeutic vaccine to treat chronic HBV infection. I. Induction of a primary cytotoxic T lymphocyte response in humans. J Clin Invest 1995; 95:341–349.

16

Immunotherapy of Bacterial Infections and Sepsis

Sam T. Donta

INTRODUCTION

The use of immunoglobulins for the prevention and treatment of bacterial infections has been an important principle and component of antibacterial therapies over the past 70 years. From its origins in the preantibiotic era as treatment for pneumococcal infections (using serotype-specific antisera) to its use as adjunctive therapy in sepsis, the concept of immunotherapy of bacterial infections has been very attractive and popular. A number of issues, however (often practical as well as controversial) have hindered even greater progress in this field.

Conceptually, immunoglobulins directed against surface products of bacteria (such as polysaccharides, lipopolysaccharides, and proteins) or against soluble products such as toxins released by bacteria should provide one means of hindering, if not stopping, the progression of the infectious process. Immunotherapy would not be expected to impact on pathogenetic events that take place on an intracellular level.

The timing of any immunotherapy would appear to play a key role in its effectiveness. Immunoprophylaxis should be the most effective means of preventing the establishment of the infectious process. Also, the earlier immunoglobulins are administered once infection has been initiated, the greater is the impact of immunotherapy.

IMMUNOTHERAPY OF SPECIFIC BACTERIAL INFECTIONS

Staphylococcus aureus

There have been a number of attempts to develop type-specific antibodies for use in the treatment of staphyloccal infections (1–4). Most of them have focused on the development of vaccines to induce immunity against staphylococci (1,2) or the use of non-virulent staphylococci to colonize individuals and prevent colonization by virulent staphylococci (3,4). None of these strategies has been shown to be effective to date, although it should be possible eventually to develop a vaccine against staphylococcal antigens that could induce protective immunity against invasive disease. One such antigen would be the toxic shock syndrome toxin (TSST).

Pooled immunoglobulins have been used in the treatment of staphylococcal-associated toxic shock syndrome (5,6). This appears to be a successful strategy in some cases, but

From: *Immunotherapy for Infectious Diseases*
Edited by: J. M. Jacobson © Humana Press Inc., Totowa, NJ

no controlled clinical trials have been conducted to evaluate its potential fully, and no TSST-specific, hyperimmune, sera have been developed to further evaluate their potential efficacy in reducing the morbidity and mortality of this disease.

Because staphylococci, especially *S. aureus,* have become increasingly resistant to antibiotics currently in use, emphasis should be placed on the development of both active vaccines and hyperimmune sera directed against specific antigens to prevent and treat invasive disease.

Streptococci

Prior to the advent of antimicrobials, antisera were developed to combat pneumococcal infections, especially pneumonia *(7).* The use of these preparations became standard practice and did lead to a significant reduction in the mortality of the disease. As effective antibiotics were developed, the use of antipneumococcal sera was abandoned. Now that strains of pneumococci have become resistant to β-lactams, it may become necessary to reconsider the use of antisera as adjunctive, if not primary, therapy of serious pneumococcal infections. It should not be difficult to prepare hyperimmune sera from individuals immunized with polyvalent preparations of pneumococcal polysaccharides who have high titers against the prevalent serotypes of pneumococci.

No antisera directed against the polysaccharides or proteins of any of the hemolytic streptococci have been developed to date. In studies of the use of various intravenous immunoglobulin (IVIG) preparations in the prevention and treatment of sepsis in low-birth-weight and other neonates, there appeared to be a small, but significant effect on decreasing the mortality rate associated with sepsis *(8,9).* Group B streptococci are an important cause of neonatal sepsis, but these studies did not specifically address these organisms, and it is as yet unclear whether the use of standard IVIG preparations would prevent or augment the treatment of serious group B streptococcal infections. Group B streptococci can also cause serious disease in adults, especially those with underlying diabetes, cirrhosis, and malignancy, but these infections have not posed a threat in terms of antibiotic resistance, and it would seem unlikely that hyperimmune antisera to group B streptococcal antigens would significantly facilitate the resolution of the disease, compared with the use of antibiotics alone. It would seem important, however, to develop vaccines against specific group B streptococcal antigens for use in susceptible adults, if not in neonates.

Group A streptococcal infections remain an important cause of morbidity and mortality in most human populations. Attempts to develop vaccines that induce protective immunity have faltered because of potential cross-reactions with normal human tissues *(10).* Nonetheless, these attempts should continue, as should the development of specific, hyperimmune sera, to augment the treatment of serious infections such as necrotizing fasciitis, septicemia, and complicated cellulitis. Streptococcal toxins, especially TSST, appear to be important virulence factors in the pathogenesis of systemic infection *(11),* and the early use of IVIG, similar to that in staphylococcal infections, appears to ameliorate the effects of TSST-associated streptococcal infections *(12).* Ideally, controlled clinical studies should be conducted to prove that this approach would work. In this regard, hyperimmune sera directed against TSST should be developed for use in such studies, and for use in selected clinical situations.

Other Gram-Positive Organisms

The use of specific hyperimmune globulins in the treatment of diseases associated with toxins produced by corynebacteria and clostridia is now well established *(13–15)*. Diphtheria antitoxin, when administered early in the disease, appears to prevent a number of complications associated with diphtheria *(13)*. Similarly, the use of tetanus and botulinum antitoxins is critical to the recovery of patients with tetanus and botulism *(14,15)*. One anecdotal study suggested that the use of IVIG facilitated the resolution of *Clostridium difficile* enterocolitis *(16)*.

Gram-Negative Cocci and Coccobacilli

Hemophilus influenzae is an important cause of invasive disease, especially meningitis, in infants and young children. An effective vaccine directed against a major outer membrane protein, as well as a vaccine directed against the specific polysaccharide, has now been in routine use *(17)*. Currently available antibiotics are still very effective against disease caused by *H. influenzae* in children and adults; thus, it would not appear necessary to try to develop hyperimmune antisera for adjunctive use in the treatment of serious infections caused by this organism.

Neisserial infections, especially those caused by *Neisseria meningitidis* and *Neisseria gonorrhea,* remain worldwide problems. Vaccines have been developed for Groups A and C meningococci, and work is proceeding on developing a vaccine for group B as well *(18,19)*. Work is also proceeding on the development of a gonococcal-specific vaccine *(20)*. As for the potential use of hyperimmune IVIG preparations directed against meningococci or gonococci, there would not seem to be any compelling need for the development of such sera.

Gram-Negative Bacilli

Much attention has been paid to the prevention and treatment of infections caused by enteric Gram-negative bacilli and *Pseudomonas aeruginosa*. Infections caused by these organisms have been of increasing importance as pathogens, especially in hospitals, causing significant morbidity and mortality *(21)*. As more immunosuppressive treatments are used to control malignancies and other disorders, the incidence of secondary infections caused by Gram-negative bacilli increases. The ability of these organisms to become resistant to antibiotics over relatively short periods also presents a compelling argument for the development of effective prophylactic and therapeutic strategies to combat the frequently life-threatening infections associated with them. It would appear at times that significant progress has been made in this area, only to find evidence to the contrary. Nonetheless, the bulk of the evidence supports the idea that successful immunization against these organisms is possible and that immunotherapy of infection in progress is also possible.

Braude et al. *(22)* and McCabe *(23)* made the initial observations that the core glycolipids of the endotoxin molecule, common to all Enterobacteriaceae, could be used to prevent infection from both homologous and heterologous enteric bacteria and that antisera directed against this endotoxin core could both prevent and treat infections caused by different enteric bacteria. Clinical trials initially using human antiserum to the core of the endotoxin molecule of a mutant *E. coli,* and subsequently a monoclonal antibody preparation (HA-1A) against the same J5 mutant, showed that both mortality and morbidity (i.e., shock) could be prevented in patients with documented Gram-negative bacteremia *(24,25).* A number of other clinical trials also showed therapeutic or prophylactic benefit of immunoglobulin preparations *(26–28),* although other trials did not show any benefit of core-endotoxin hyperimmune globulin over that of standard IVIG preparations *(29,30).* Because overall mortality of patients was not reduced in control patients in the HA-1A trial, implying an adverse effect of the antibody preparation in patients with Gram-positive bacteremia or with no defined etiology, because two other trials failed to show a beneficial effect against Gram-negative sepsis, and because of a number of other issues, including the use of subanalyses, and the potential costs of this therapy, the HA-1A preparation did not receive U.S. Food and Drug Administration approval for use in patients with suspected Gram-negative sepsis. The various issues, however, remain unresolved, as argued by Cross et al *(31),* and it is hoped that this approach will be re-examined and refined, not abandoned.

Another series of trials directed against infections caused by *Klebsiella* species and *Pseudomonas aeruginosa* ended without definitive conclusions. In these trials, patients in intensive care units in Department of Veterans Affairs hospitals in the United States were given hyperimmune sera derived from immunized human volunteers to determine whether these preparations were more effective than an albumin placebo in preventing infection, mortality, and morbidity caused by these important pathogens. In the first trial, it appeared that *Klebsiella* infections were being prevented and modified, but because there was no effect against *Pseudomonas* infections, that trial was stopped by the Data Monitoring Board (DMB) and a new trial begun using greater concentrations of hyperimmune sera *(32).* The second trial was never completed, however, because of the many adverse effects (e.g., hypotension, fever) of the hyperimmune IVIG preparation and because the DMB was not convinced that the trial would yield significant differences when and if sufficient patient enrollment could be achieved. Subsequent analyses suggested that the hyperimmune preparation had a therapeutic effect on patients who were already infected at the time of patient entry into the study, but the numbers did not achieve statistical significance. No subsequent studies were considered by the manufacturer or by the Department of Veterans Affairs, leaving the possibility of therapeutic and/or prophylactic benefit unresolved.

Miscellaneous Observations

Limited, anecdotal, studies in various other settings have suggested some therapeutic and prophylactic benefit of standard IVIG preparations. These include sepsis following cardiac surgery in high-risk patients *(33),* patients with cerebrospinal fluid shunt infections *(34),* and patients with multiple myeloma *(35).* No effect was found in preventing infections in pediatric head trauma patients *(36).* One report suggested that early treatment with IVIG prevented polyneuropathy following multiple organ failure and Gram-negative sepsis *(37).* Another report suggested that IVIG facilitated the recovery of lymphocytic meningoradiculitis associated with Lyme disease *(38).* Experimentally, the use of human IVIG protected rabbits from diarrhea and death associated with *E. coli* shiga-like toxin *(39).*

CONCLUSIONS

The immunotherapy of bacterial infections, including sepsis, remains an important issue and consideration as adjunctive treatment of various infections. Experimental evidence strongly supports the concept, but implementation has continued to encounter numerous hurdles. The bulk of the clinical experience also supports the use of specific immunotherapies in a number of clinical settings, but more research is needed to provide statistical proof of its efficacy. As these trials are very expensive ventures, it is difficult for manufacturers to have the incentive to develop specific preparations and to support clinical trials. As the occurrence of infections and sepsis exacts a very high toll, however, it would seem important for federal funding agencies to support the development of such products and the clinical trials to prove their efficacy. Ultimately, it is hoped that vaccines will prevent many specific infections, but there will always be a need for adjunctive immunotherapy directed against specific bacterial products.

REFERENCES

1. Lee JC, Perez NE, Hoplins CA, Pier GB. Purified capsular polysaccharide-induced immunity to Staphylococcus aureus infection. J Infect Dis 1998; 157:723–730.
2. Fattom A, Schneerson R, Szu SC, Vann WF, Shiloach J, Karakawa WW, Robbins JB. Synthesis and immunologic properties in mice of vaccines composed of Staphylococcus aureus type 5 and type 8 capsular polysaccharides conjugated to Pseudomonas aeruginosa exotoxin A. Infect Immunity 1990; 58:2367–2374.
3. Shinefield HR, Sutherland JM, Ribble JC, Eichenwald HF. Bacterial interference: its effect on nursery-acquired infection with Staphylococcus aureus. Am J Dis Child 1963; 105:655–662.
4. Drutz DJ, Van Way MH, Schaffner W, and Koenig MG. Bacterial interference in the therapy of recurrent staphylococcal infections. N Engl J Med 1996; 275:1161–1165.
5. Barry W, Hudgins L, Donta ST, Pesanti EL. Intravenous immunoglobulin therapy for toxic shock syndrome. JAMA 1992; 267:3315–3316.
6. Scott DF, Best GK, King JM, Thompson MR, Adinolfi LE, Bonventre PF. Passive protection of rabbits infected with toxic shock syndrome-associated strains of *Staphylococcus aureus* by monoclonal antibody to toxic shock syndrome toxin 1. Rev Infect Dis 1989; 11:S214–S218.
7. Austrian R, and Gold J. Pneumococcal bacteremia with especial reference to bacteremic pneumococcal pneumonia. Ann Intern Med 1964; 60:759–776.
8. Jenson HG, Pollock BH. The role of intravenous immunoglobulin for the prevention and treatment of neonatal sepsis. Semin Perinatol 1998; 22:50–63.
9. Lassiter HA. Intravenous immunoglobulin in the prevention and treatment of neonatal bacterial sepsis. Adv Pediatr 1992; 39:71–99.
10. Beachey EH, Stollerman GH, Bisno AL. A strep vaccine: how close? Hospital Practice 1979; 11:49–57.
11. Stevens DL. Invasive group A streptococcal infections. Clin Infect Dis 1992; 14:2–13.
12. Lamothe F, D'Amico P, Ghosn P, Tremblay C, Braidy J, Patenaude J-V. Clinical usefulness of intravenous human immunoglobulins in invasive group A streptococcal infections: case report and review. Clin Infect Dis 1995; 21:1469–1470.
13. Hoeprich PD. Diphtheria, in Infectious Disease, 3rd eds, Harper & Row, 1983, 25:300–307
14. Donta ST. Tetanus, in Intensive Care Medicine, 3rd eds, Little Brown & Co, 1996 97:1227–1230
15. Merson MH, Hughes JM, Dowell VR, Taylor A, Barker WH, Gangarosa Ej. Current trends in Botulism in the United States. JAMA 1974; 229:1305–1308.

16. Salcedo J, Keates S, Pothoulakis D, et al. Intravenous immunoglobulin therapy for severe *Clostridium difficile* colitis. Gut 1997; 41:366–370.

17. Santosham M, Rivin B, Wolff M, Reid R, Newcomer W, Letson GW, Alemeido-Hill J, Thompson C, Siber GR. Prevention of Haemophilus influenzae type b infections in Apache and Navajo children. J Infect Dis 1992; 165:S144–S151.

18. Gold R, Lepow ML, Goldschneider I, Draper TF, Gotschlich EC. Kinetics of antibody production to group A and group C meningococcal polysaccharide vaccines administered during the first six years of life: prospects for routine immunization of infants and children. J Infect Dis 1979; 140:690–697.

19. Frasch CE, Peppler MS. Protection against group B Neisseria meningitidis disease: preparation of soluble protein and protein-polysaccharide immunogens. Infect Immunity 1982; 37:271–280.

20. Virji M, Heckels JE, Watt PJ. Monoclonal antibodies to gonococcal pili: studies on antigenic determinants on pili from variants of strain P9. J Gen Micriobiol 1983; 129:1965–1973.

21. Cryz SJ Jr, Sadoff JC, Cross AS, Furer E. Safety and immunogenicity of a polyvalent *Pseudomonas aeruginosa* O-polysaccharide-toxin A vaccine in humans. Antibiot Chemother 1989; 42:177–183.

22. Braude AI, Ziegler EJ, McCutchan JA, Douglas, H. Immunization against nosocomial infection. Am J Med 1981; 70:463–466.

23. McCabe WR. Immunization with R mutants of *S. minnesota*. Part I. Protection against challenge with heterologous gram-negative bacilli. J Immunol 1972; 108:601–610.

24. Ziegler EJ, McCutchan JA, Fierer J, et al. Treatment of gram-negative bacteremia and shock with human antiserum to a mutant *Escherichia coli*. N Engl J Med 1982; 307:1225–1230.

25. Ziegler EJ, Fisher CJ Jr, Sprung CL, et al. Treatment of gram-negative bacteremia and septic shock with HA-1A human monoclonal antibody against endotoxin. N Engl J Med 1991; 324:429–436.

26. Baumgartner JD, McCutchan JA, van Melle G, et al. Prevention of gram-negative shock and death in surgical patients by antibody to endotoxin core glycolipid. Lancet 1985; 8446:59–63.

27. Schedel I, Dreikhausen U, Nentwig B, et al. Treatment of gram-negative septic shock with an immunoglobulin preparation: a prospective, randomized clinical trial. Crit Care Med 1991; 19:1104–1113.

28. Greenman RL, Schein RMH, Martin MA, et al. A controlled clinical trial of E5 murine monoclonal IgM antibody to endotoxin in the treatment of gram-negative sepsis. JAMA 1991; 266:1097–1102.

29. Calandra T, Glauser MP, Schellekens J, Verhoef J, and the Swiss-Dutch J5 Immunoglobulin Study Group. Treatment of gram-negative septic shock with human IgG antibody to *Escherichia coli* J5: a prospective, double-blind, randomized trial. J Infect Dis 1988; 158:312–319.

30. Cometta A, Baumgartner JD, Lee ML, Hanique G, Glauser MP. Prophylactic intravenous administration of standard immune globulin as compared with core-lipopolysaccharide immune globulin in patients at high risk of postsurgical infection. N Engl J Med 1992; 327:234–240.

31. Cross AS, Opal SM, Bhattacharjee AK, et al. Immunotherapy of sepsis: flawed concept of faulty implementation. Vaccine 1999; 17:S13–S21.

32. Donta ST, Peduzzi P, Cross AS, Sadoff J, Haakenson C, Cryz SJ Jr, for the Federal Hyperimmme Immunoglobulin Trial Study Group: Immunoprophylaxis against *Klebsiella* and *Pseudomonas* infections. J Infect Dis 1996; 174:537–543.

33. Pilz G, Kreuzer E, Kaab S, Appel R, Werdan K. Early sepsis treatment with immunoglobulins after cardiac surgery in score-identified high-risk patients. Chest 1994; 105:76–82.

34. Ersahin Y, Mutluer S, Kocaman S. Immunoglobulin prophylaxis in shunt infections: a prospective randomized study. Childs Nerv Syst 1997; 13:546–549.

35. Chapel HM, Lee M, Hargreaves R, Pamphilon DH, Prentice AG. Randomized trial of intravenous immunoglobulin as prophylaxis against infection in plateau-phase multiple myeloma. Lancet 1994; 343:1059–1063.
36. Gooding AM, Bastian JF, Peterson BM, Wilson NW. Safety and efficacy of intravenous immunoglobulin prophylaxis in pediatric head trauma patients: a double-blind controlled trial. J Crit Care 1993; 8: 212–216.
37. Mohr M, Englisch L, Roth A, Burchardi H, Zielmann S. Effects of early treatment with immunoglobulin on critical illness polyneuropathy following multiple organ failure and gram-negative sepsis. Intensive Care Med 1997; 23:1144–1149.
38. Crisp D, Ashby P. Lyme radiculoneuritis treated with intravenous immunoglobulin. Neurology 1996; 46:1174–1175.
39. Havens PL, Dunne WM, Burd EM. Effects of human intravenous immune globulin on diarrhea caused by shiga-like toxin I and shiga-like toxin II in infant rabbits. Microbiol Immunol 1992; 36:1077–1083.

17

Immunotherapy for Tuberculosis and Other Mycobacterial Infections

Robert S. Wallis and John L. Johnson

INTRODUCTION

At least one-fourth of the world's population is infected with *Mycobacterium tuberculosis,* resulting in nearly 4 million deaths worldwide each year, more than any other single pathogen. In some areas, such as southern Africa and southeast Asia, tuberculosis case rates have approached 200 cases per 100,000 persons/year, or nearly 0.2% annually *(1),* despite vaccination with *M. bovis* bacille Calmette-Guérin (BCG) and increased access to chemotherapy. In other regions, including eastern Europe and Russia, multidrug-resistant (MDR) infection has emerged as a major threat to public health *(2).* As a consequence, there is greater urgency to define the factors involved in host resistance to mycobacterial infection and to evaluate their potential therapeutic application in clinical trials.

Basic clinical observations have shaped our understanding of mycobacterial immunity. The initial infection with *M. tuberculosis* is usually inapparent. It is followed by acquisition of delayed-type hypersensitivity and partial immunity to exogenous reinfection. Although active TB can arise shortly after exposure, most TB cases represent reactivation disease, which is separated in both time and distance from the initial infection. In a normal host, the risk of TB is approximately 5% during the first year after initial infection, and 5% subsequently, distributed over as much as decades. The risk of TB is increased in the very young and the elderly, owing to impaired cellular immune function. The risk is greatest in individuals with advanced HIV-1 infection, in whom the likelihood of progression to active TB may be increased by as much as 170-fold *(3–6).* These observations underscore the critical role of cell-mediated immunity and, in particular, the importance of antigen-specific CD4+ T-cells in mycobacterial immunity.

CYTOKINE REGULATION OF MACROPHAGE ACTIVATION

As intracellular pathogens, mycobacteria possess the capacity to replicate within the phagocytic cells that comprise the major effector arm of the cellular immune system. Resting human monocytes and macrophages are relatively permissive of intracellular

From: *Immunotherapy for Infectious Diseases*
Edited by: J. M. Jacobson © Humana Press Inc., Totowa, NJ

replication of *M. tuberculosis,* with doubling times of 16–26 hours in vitro *(7).* At this stage, the infection can be affected by factors reflecting natural immunity. In mice, resistance of resting macrophages to infection with most intracellular pathogens is controlled by the products of a gene on chromosome 1 identified as the *bcg* locus *(8,9).* Macrophages of BCG-resistant strains demonstrate increased respiratory burst activity as assessed by peroxide production and enhanced capacity for inhibition of replication of *M. bovis* BCG and *M. intracellulare (10,11).* Recent studies suggest that the human correlate of this gene may also play a role in determining TB susceptibility *(12).* Natural killer (NK) cells may also play a role in mycobacterial resistance *(13).* Natural resistance may be most important late in HIV disease, when acquired, antigen-driven CD4 responses have substantially declined.

The formation of granulomas at the site of initial infection is a critical early event in mycobacterial immunity. The capacity to produce interleukin-1 (IL-1) and tumor necrosis factor-α (TNF-α) is increased in monocytes from patients with active TB *(14,15).* IL-1β, TNF-α, and IL-12 are produced within tuberculous granulomas *(16),* in response to intact mycobacteria as well as specific polysaccharides and proteins *(17–22).* These cytokines are essential and sufficient to induce formation of granulomas when coupled to inert particles *(23).* TNF-α and (to a lesser extent) granulocyte/macrophage colony-stimulating factor (GM-CSF) appear to act in an autocrine fashion to limit intracellular mycobacterial growth *(24–29).* Granuloma formation is absent in mice lacking the gene for TNF-α or treated with neutralizing TNF-α antibody, which results in progressive, lethal mycobacterial infection *(30,31).* IL-12 may act at this stage of infection, by activating NK cells *(13).* Other products of activated macrophages, including IL-6 and calcitriol (1,25 dihydroxy vitamin D_3), also restrict intracellular mycobacterial growth *(7,32–36).* Sufficient concentrations of vitamin D $(10^{-7}–10^{-9}$ M) may be produced within granulomas for growth inhibition to occur. (For a summary of effects, see Table 1.)

In most cases, however, this level of macrophage activation is not sufficient to contain mycobacterial replication, especially in human hosts. Control of most intracellular pathogens (including *Toxoplasma, Legionella,* and *Leishmania* organisms as well as mycobacteria) requires factors produced by antigen-specific lymphocytes, including CD4+, CD8+, and γδ T-cells *(37–41).* The critical role of interferon-γ (IFN-γ) produced by these cells can be readily demonstrated in murine models of TB *(42,43).* Mice with targeted disruption of the IFN-γ gene or the gene for the IFN-γ receptor show increased susceptibility to *M. tuberculosis* and *M. bovis* BCG *(44–47).* In such animals, intravenous or aerogenic challenge with a normally sublethal number of *M. tuberculosis* bacilli leads to death, with extensive tissue necrosis and increased numbers of acid-fast bacilli. Defects that prevent the clonal expansion and activation of IFN-γ-producing T-cells, such as deficiencies in IL-12 or IL-18, have similar effects *(48,49).* Mutations affecting the IFN-γ or IL-12 receptors in humans also result in increased mycobacterial susceptibility *(50–53).*

Cytotoxic T-cells also appear to contribute toward control of intracellular mycobacterial by a granule-dependent mechanism. Granulysin, a protein found in granules of cytotoxic T-lymphocytes (CTLs), reduced the viability of a broad spectrum of pathogenic bacteria, fungi, and parasites in vitro. Granulysin directly killed extracellular

Table 1
Effect of Cytokines and Other Mononuclear Cell Products on Macrophage Activation for Inhibition of Intracellular Mycobacterial Growth

Activating	Deactivating
IL-2	IL-1α
IL-4	IL-3
1,25(OH)$_2$-D$_3$	IL-6
GM-CSF	IL-10
TNF-α	TGF-β
IFN-γ	PGE$_2$
IL-12	
IL-15	

Abbreviations: GM-CSF, granulocyte/macrophage colony-stimulating factor; IFN-γ, interferon-γ; IL, interleukin; 1,25(OH)$_2$-D$_3$, 1,25 dihydroxy vitamin D$_3$; PGE$_2$, prostaglandin E$_2$; TGF-β, transforming growth factor-β; TNF-α, tumor necrosis factor-α.

mycobacteria and, in combination with perforin, decreased the viability of intracellular *M. tuberculosis (54,55)*. However, cytotoxicity *per se* does not appear to be a major factor in control of intracellular bacilli *(56,57)*.

IMMUNOPATHOGENESIS OF TUBERCULOSIS

The specific genetic defects described above appear to account for only a small fraction of human TB cases. Nonetheless, there is substantial evidence of immune dysregulation in patients with active disease. Up to 25% have a negative tuberculin skin test on initial evaluation *(58)*; this percentage is increased in those with disseminated or miliary disease *(59)*. Up to 60% of patients demonstrate reduced responses to *M. tuberculosis* purified protein derivative (PPD) in vitro in terms of T-cell blastogenesis, production of IL-2 and IFN-γ, and surface expression of IL-2 receptors *(60,61)*. These abnormalities are accompanied by increased levels of *M. tuberculosis*-reactive antibody and increased capacity for production of the cytokines IL-1 and TNF-α by monocytes *(14,15)*.

Several studies indicate that activation of suppressive mechanisms in blood monocytes contributes to this process. Depletion of monocytes partially restores T-cell responses and IL-2 production, although not completely so. Blood monocytes in TB show increased expression of HLA-DR, IL-2 and TNF receptors, B$_7$, and FcγRI and RIII *(62,63)*. When stimulated in vitro, they produce increased quantities of IL-10, transforming growth factor-β (TGF-β) and prostaglandin E$_2$ (PGE$_2$) *(22,64–69)*. This altered macrophage cytokine profile may be a consequence of intracellular infection. Mycobacterial lipoarabinomannan, for example, blocks activation of macrophages by IFN-γ via production of PGE$_2$ and TGF-β and also inhibits mitogen-induced T-cell activation in a dose-dependent fashion *(70–74)*. This hypothesis is supported by the observation that the immunologic abnormalities are most pronounced in patients with far advanced disease. The immunologic defects may thus be a consequence of the advanced disease stage and high bacillary burden in these patients.

Mechanisms other than the production of immunosuppressive factors by monocytes may also be involved in the reduced T-cell responses in peripheral blood in TB.

Several studies have indicated compartmentalization of T-cell responses at the site of disease *(75–78)*. In addition, intrinsic T-cell refractoriness, possibly associated with a tendency toward apoptosis (programmed cell death), may be present in the peripheral blood *(79)*.

Immunologically mediated tissue damage and other toxicities also appear to be responsible for many of the clinical manifestations of TB. TNF-α appears to be the cause of much of the fever, wasting, inflammation, and tissue necrosis characteristic of the disease.

HIV AND TUBERCULOSIS

Coinfection with HIV is the most potent risk factor for active TB in a person latently infected with *M. tuberculosis.* TB typically is an early complication of HIV infection, occurring prior to an AIDS-defining illness in 50–67% of HIV-infected patients *(80)*. Before the introduction of protease inhibitors, the diagnosis carried an expected mortality of 21% at 9 months, even in those subjects presenting without other AIDS-defining conditions *(81)*. Death was infrequently (13%) due to active TB, however. More often, it resulted from other AIDS-related causes (particularly *Pneumocystis carinii* or bacterial pneumonia, or wasting syndrome), which may occur shortly after the diagnosis of tuberculosis.

Several studies indicate that the adverse interactions of *M. tuberculosis* and HIV are bidirectional, i.e., that TB affects HIV disease in addition to the better recognized converse interaction. TB is characterized by prolonged antigenic stimulation and immune activation, even in HIV-positive subjects *(79,82)*. Antigen-induced T-cell activation and expression of the proinflammatory cytokines TNF-α and other inflammatory cytokines in turn promote HIV expression by latently infected cells *(83–89)*. *M. tuberculosis* and its proteins and glycolipids directly stimulate HIV replication by mechanisms involving monocyte production of TNF-α *(90–93)*. In the lung, TNF-α and HIV-1 RNA are both increased in bronchoalveolar lavage fluid of involved segments of lungs of patients with pulmonary TB and HIV-1 infection *(94)*. Phylogenetic analysis of V3 sequences demonstrated that HIV-1 RNA present in bronchoalveolar fluid had diverged from plasma, indicating that pulmonary TB enhances local HIV-1 replication in vivo. In this context, IL-10 and TGF-β expression may be of benefit to the host, in that they inhibit antigen-induced HIV expression, via inhibitory effects on lymphocyte activation *(88)*.

These interactions appear to have significant clinical consequences. Plasma HIV viral load increases 5- to 160-fold in HIV-infected persons during the acute phase of TB *(95)*. Subsequently, new AIDS-defining opportunistic infections occur at a rate 1.4 times that of CD4-matched HIV-infected control subjects without a history of TB (95% confidence interval: 0.94–2.11) *(96)*. Cases also had a shorter overall survival than did controls ($p = 0.001$), as well as an increased risk for death (odds ratio = 2.17). The adverse effect on survival is most pronounced in those individuals with the greatest evidence for macrophage activation (neopterin $\geq$ 14 ng/mL, or soluble type II TNF-α receptor $\geq$ 6.5 ng/mL, or negative tuberculin skin tests; $p < 0.01$) *(97)*. Thus, although active TB may be an independent marker of advanced immunosuppression in HIV-infected patients, it may also act as a cofactor to accelerate the clinical course of HIV infection.

CLINICAL TRIALS

As summarized above, current evidence suggests that protective host responses against *M. tuberculosis* are dependent on Th1 responses mediated by interactions of CD4 T-lymphocytes and macrophages. IL-2 and IFN-γ are crucial cytokines produced by antigen-responsive T-cells that activate macrophages to inhibit intracellular mycobacterial growth and may also act indirectly to enhance specific cytotoxic T-cell and NK cell responses. Other cytokines such as TGF-β enhance fibrosis and scarring near tuberculous lesions and result in loss of functional pulmonary parenchyma.

These observations have led to the hypothesis that administration of endogenous IFN-γ or IL-2 and other agents might augment host cell-mediated immune responses in active TB, improve or accelerate clearance of tubercle bacilli, and improve clinical outcomes. The availability of highly purified recombinant cytokines, the increasing rates of MDR tuberculosis, and successful experience with adjunctive therapy using human cytokines in cancer therapy and the treatment of other infectious diseases have led to strong interest in their possible role in the therapy of human mycobacterial diseases.

The general goals of immunotherapy in TB treatment are to shorten the duration of therapy for drug-susceptible disease or improve cure rates in drug-resistant disease. Current approaches to the immunotherapy of tuberculosis center on promoting Th1 responses by administration of Th1 cytokines or immunomodulators, inhibition of macrophage-deactivating toxic cytokines such as TGF-β, and inhibition of proinflammatory cytokines by specific or general cytokine inhibitors such as corticosteroids, thalidomide, or pentoxifylline. IL-2, IFN-α, IFN-γ, IL-12, and a heat-killed *M. vaccae* immunotherapeutic agent are being evaluated in controlled clinical trials *(98–101)*. Other potential interventions include administering IL-18 or blocking immunosuppressive cytokines such as TGF-β and IL-10 *(102)*.

Interleukin-2

Data from animal studies, in vitro studies using human cells, and clinical trials in other mycobacterial infections suggest that IL-2 may play a central role in controlling murine TB infection. Murine models of *M. lepraemurium, M. avium,* and *M. bovis* BCG infection have shown that IL-2 can be useful in limiting infection, possibly by activating macrophages through an interferon-mediated mechanism or directly via the development of cytotoxic T-lymphocytes specific for mycobacterial antigens *(103–105)*. Humans infected with *M. tuberculosis* often have absent or weak PPD skin test response and decreased in vitro proliferative responses to PPD. These abnormalities are associated with deficient IL-2-induced cell proliferation and decreased IL-2R generation *(61)*. These observations form the basis for studies of recombinant IL-2 as adjunctive immunotherapy against mycobacterial disease in humans.

Early clinical trials with IL-2 in patients with leprosy and leishmaniasis, as well as other serious infections caused by intracellular pathogens, demonstrated that IL-2 immunotherapy may be useful in controlling these infections *(106–108)*. In leprosy patients, IL-2 administration led to enhanced local cell-mediated immune responses and resulted in more rapid and extensive reduction in *M. leprae* bacilli compared with multidrug chemotherapy alone. The administration of IL-2 at low doses of 10 μg (180,000 IU) twice a day for 8 days led to body-wide infiltration of CD4+ T-cells, monocytes, and Langerhans cells in the skin and a decline in the total body burden of *M. leprae (109)*. IL-2 appeared to facilitate the destruction of leprosy bacilli in these patients. The presumed mechanism of this antibacterial effect is via the destruction of oxidatively incompetent dermal macrophages and the extracellular liberation of bacilli and their subsequent uptake and destruction by newly emigrated and oxidatively competent monocytes from the circulation.

Two clinical trials have examined IL-2 as an adjunct to TB treatment in humans. A pilot study of IL-2 was performed in 20 TB patients in Bangladesh and South Africa to evaluate its safety and microbiologic and immunologic activities *(100)*. The patient population was diverse and included new, partially treated, and chronic MDR cases. Patients received 30 days of twice daily intradermal injections of 12.5 µg (225,000 IU) of IL-2 in addition to combination chemotherapy. Patients in all three groups showed improvement of clinical symptoms during the 30-day treatment period. Results of direct sputum smears for acid-fast bacilli (AFB) demonstrated conversion to negative following IL-2 and chemotherapy in all the newly diagnosed patients and in five of seven patients with MDR TB. Patients receiving IL-2 did not experience clinical deterioration or any significant side effects.

A recent randomized clinical trial of 35 patients with MDR TB in South Africa compared daily or pulsed IL-2 therapy with placebo *(101)*. Patients received the best available combination chemotherapy based on individual drug susceptibility testing results. Twelve patients received 12.5 µg (225,000 IU) IL-2 intradermally twice daily. Nine patients received pulsed IL-2 therapy (twice daily intradermal injection of 25 µg [450,000 IU] IL-2 daily for 5 days, followed by 9 days off IL-2 treatment, for three cycles), and 14 subjects received placebo. Immunotherapy or placebo was given in conjunction with combination chemotherapy during the first 30 days of the study. The total dose of IL-2 in both active treatment groups was identical. Patients receiving pulsed IL-2 therapy did not respond to treatment, whereas the patients receiving daily therapy did respond. Among patients who were sputum AFB smear-positive at the time of study entry, five of eight patients receiving daily IL-2 treatment had reduced or cleared sputum mycobacterial load compared with two of seven subjects receiving pulsed IL-2 and three of nine subjects in the placebo group. Chest X-ray improvement after 6 weeks of anti-TB treatment was present in 7 of 12 patients receiving daily IL-2 compared with 2 of 9 patients on pulsed IL-2 treatment and 5 of 12 patients receiving placebo. The number of circulating CD25+ (low-affinity IL-2 receptor-bearing T-cells) and CD56+ (NK) cells was significantly increased in patients receiving daily IL-2 but not in the pulsed IL-2 or placebo arms.

No significant side effects related to IL-2 treatment were observed. One patient developed mild flu-like symptoms during two cycles of pulsed IL-2 treatment. Patients receiving IL-2 developed mild self-limited local induration and pruritus at injection sites. All patients receiving IL-2 treatment completed the study. The results of these studies suggest that IL-2 administration in combination with conventional combination chemotherapy is safe in patients with TB and may potentiate the antimicrobial cellular immune response to TB. Additional studies are needed to confirm these initial findings and assess long-term clinical benefits. Another randomized placebo-controlled trial of daily IL-2 (450,000 IU daily) in HIV-noninfected patients with smear-positive, drug-susceptible pulmonary TB is currently ongoing in Uganda.

Interferon-γ

Because of its critical role in macrophage activation and host defenses against mycobacterial diseases, adjunctive treatment with IFN-γ has been studied in several small trials. In lepromatous leprosy, intradermal therapy with low-dose IFN-γ resulted in increased local T-cell and monocyte infiltration, HLA-DR (Ia) antigen expression, and decreased bacillary load *(110)*. In another study, twice or thrice weekly therapy with 25–50 μg/m^2 of subcutaneous IFN-γ was administered to seven HIV-noninfected patients with disseminated *M. avium* complex infection who had failed to respond to antibiotic therapy *(111)*. Within 8 weeks of beginning IFN treatment, all seven patients had significant and sustained clinical improvement. In contrast, IFN-γ therapy was not found to be beneficial in patients with advanced AIDS and disseminated *M. avium* complex infection *(112)*.

IFN-γ immunotherapy also has been studied in MDR TB, for which drug treatment options are limited. In a case report, adjunctive treatment with IFN-γ and GCSF was successful in the treatment of a leukemic patient with intracerebral and spinal cord MDR TB *(113)*. High-dose systemic therapy with IFN-γ has, however, been associated with frequent side effects including fatigue, myalgias, and malaise. Treatment with aerosolized IFN-γ has been studied in an attempt to decrease these systemic side effects and deliver therapy directly to the site of disease in the lung. In an open-label study in five patients with MDR TB, aerosolized IFN-γ 500 μg three times weekly for 1 month was well tolerated and resulted in decreased sputum bacillary burden and stable or improved body weight *(114)*. Further studies of aerosolized IFN-γ are warranted to determine the optimal dose and duration of therapy.

Interferon-α

Interferon-α is another immunomodulatory cytokine produced by mononuclear phagocytes stimulated by bacteria and viruses. IFN-α modulates differentiation of T-cells toward the Th1 phenotype, induces production of IFN-γ and IL-2, and inhibits proliferation of Th2 cells. Two small studies have examined a possible role for IFN-α in TB treatment. A randomized open-label trial in 20 HIV-seronegative TB patients in Italy studied the effects of aerosolized IFN-α 3 million units thrice weekly during the first 2 months of TB treatment *(115)*. Patients treated with IFN-α had significantly earlier improvement in fever, sputum bacillary burden by quantitative microscopy after 1 week of treatment, and pulmonary consolidation after 2 months than patients receiving placebo. No adverse effects were noted in the IFN-α treatment group. In another pilot study, IFN-α2b (3 million units weekly) was administered subcutaneously for 3 months as an adjunct to chemotherapy for five patients with chronic MDR TB *(116)*. Two of the five patients became consistently sputum culture-negative over a 30-month follow-up period.

Interleukin-12

IL-12 is a pivotal cytokine that enhances host responses to intracellular pathogens by inducing IFN-γ production and Th1 responses at sites of disease. Patients with congenital abnormalities of IL-12 receptors are highly susceptible to serious mycobacterial and salmonella infections *(52,53)*. Administration of IL-12 to severe combined immunodeficient (SCID) or CD4+ T-cell-depleted mice infected with *M. avium* enhances IFN-γ production and had modest activity against *M. avium (117)*. Recombinant IL-12 also has been shown to upregulate *M. tuberculosis*-induced IFN-γ responses in human peripheral blood mononuclear cells (PBMCs) and alveolar macrophages *(118,119)*. Because of these properties, there has been considerable interest in exploring a possible role for IL-12 immunotherapy in TB, balanced by concerns about its nonspecific mechanism of action and potential toxicity. An early phase I trial of IL-12 immunotherapy in TB is currently under way in the Gambia.

Thalidomide

Thalidomide, or α-*N*-phthalimidoglutarimide, is a synthetic derivative of glutamic acid that was initially released as a sedative in Europe in 1957 but was withdrawn from most countries 4 years later after recognition of its serious teratogenic effects, particularly limb-shortening defects and phocomelia. The use of thalidomide as adjunctive therapy in inflammatory and mycobacterial diseases has an interesting history. In 1965 an Israeli dermatologist prescribed thalidomide as a sedative for six patients with lepromatous leprosy and erythema nodosum leprosum (ENL) *(120)*. ENL is a serious reaction characterized by painful nodules, fever, malaise, wasting, vasculitis, and peripheral neuritis that develops in 10–50% of patients treated for lepromatous leprosy. All six patients treated with thalidomide improved within hours. This clinical observation spurred a series of studies by other researchers to investigate its underlying mechanisms.

It is now recognized that thalidomide has complex antiinflammatory, immunologic, and metabolic effects. Its activity has been attributed, at least in part, to its demonstrated ability to inhibit TNF-α synthesis in vitro and in vivo *(121,122)*. Thalidomide also inhibits neutrophil phagocytosis, monocyte chemotaxis, and angiogenesis and, to a lesser degree, inhibits lymphocyte proliferation to antigenic and mitogenic stimuli *(123–125)*. Thalidomide inhibits HIV-1 replication in the U-1 monocytoid cells and PBMC from patients with advanced AIDS, primarily by inhibition of TNF-α *(126,127)*. These studies indicate potential clinical roles of thalidomide to limit TNF-related clinical toxicities and to reduce cytokine-related HIV expression.

Thalidomide has subsequently been studied in several diseases in which immunologically mediated mechanisms cause pathology. Thalidomide is effective for recurrent oral, esophageal, and rectal apthous ulcers in patients with AIDS *(128)*. It is also beneficial in chronic graft-versus-host disease after bone marrow transplantation, discoid lupus erythematosus, Behçet's disease, and pyoderma gangrenosum and other inflammatory skin diseases. Thalidomide also has modest activity in HIV wasting syndrome, severe ulcerative colitis, microsporidial diarrhea, wasting in HIV-infected patients with TB, and refractory *M. avium* complex infection in HIV-noninfected persons. Adjunctive immunotherapy with thalidomide was studied in a double-blind placebo-controlled trial of 39 HIV-infected adults with and without active TB *(129)*. Patients with active TB treated with thalidomide had decreased plasma TNF-α and HIV-1 viral levels and greater weight gain than patients in the placebo group.

Thalidomide has also been evaluated as adjunctive therapy for TB meningitis, a relatively common form of TB that often has serious sequelae. The severe inflammation in the subarachnoid space is believed to play a central pathophysiologic role in the cerebral edema, vasculitis, and infarction typically seen in this form of TB. Levels of TNF-α and other inflammatory cytokines are increased in the cerebrospinal fluid in patients with tuberculous meningitis and are correlated with disease progression and brain injury in an animal model of tuberculous meningitis *(130)*. Rabbits treated with the combination of thalidomide and anti-TB drugs are protected from death compared with animals treated only with anti-TB drugs *(131)*. Based on these promising pre-clinical data, a randomized, placebo-controlled trial of adjunctive thalidomide in HIV-noninfected children with tuberculous meningitis is currently under way in South Africa comparing treatment with thalidomide or placebo in addition to standard anti-TB drugs and corticosteroids during the first month of TB treatment.

The side effect profile of thalidomide varies considerably among different patient groups. Aside from its teratogenic effects, the major toxicity of thalidomide is a peripheral polyneuropathy that occurs in 20–50% of patients. It is predominantly sensory and can be irreversible. Other side effects include sedation, orthostatic hypotension, xerostomia, and rash. Thalidomide was approved in 1998 for use in the United States for the treatment of severe erythema nodosum leprosum and is under active investigation in other immunologically mediated conditions such as HIV wasting syndrome. Because of its teratogenicity and neurologic toxicity, its use has been reserved for conditions refractory to other medical therapy and is strictly regulated in women of child-bearing age. Patients on chronic therapy must be followed closely for neurologic toxicities.

Other Inhibitors of TNF-α

Pentoxifylline is a phosphodiesterase inhibitor used for treatment of intermittent claudication, in which it acts to increase the deformability of the red blood cell membrane. Pentoxifylline also inhibits the production of TNF-α at the transcriptional level, as well as the effects of the cytokine on target tissues *(132–134)*. It reduces the pulmonary toxicity of TNF-α in animal models of sepsis *(135)*. Pentoxifylline inhibits HIV-1 expression by monocytes and lymphocytes in acute and chronic in vitro expression models *(136,137)*. Oral administration of 1200–2400 mg daily to AIDS patients without TB or other active opportunistic infections results in reduced TNF-α mRNA in circulating mononuclear cells, reduced capacity to produce TNF-α following stimulation in cell culture, and reduced serum triglyceride, but it has no effect on plasma HIV RNA *(138,139)*.

A double-blind, placebo-controlled study of adjunctive therapy with pentoxifylline (1800 mg/day) as a timed-release formulation was performed in Ugandan HIV-infected patients with pulmonary TB. Subjects had early HIV disease (mean CD4 cell count, 380/μL) and did not receive other antiretroviral drugs. They were treated for the first 4 months with standard TB therapy. Pentoxifylline resulted in decreased plasma HIV RNA and serum $β_2$-microglobulin and, in a subset of moderately anemic patients, improved blood hemoglobin levels. Trends were noted toward reduced TNF-α production in vitro and improved performance scores, but these did not reach statistical significance. No effect was noted on body mass, CD4 cell count, TB relapse, or survival *(140,141)*.

Several studies of prednisolone or other corticosteroids as adjunctive therapy for HIV plus TB are currently under way. Like pentoxifylline and thalidomide, prednisolone inhibits TNF-α expression but also affects many other cellular processes. An uncontrolled trial of prednisolone 0.5 mg/kg for 6 months and then 0.3 mg/kg daily in AIDS patients without TB found increased numbers of circulating CD4 cells (Δ119/μL from baseline) but no effect on plasma HIV RNA *(142)*. A pilot study of prednisolone in HIV plus TB, administered during the second month of TB therapy, found that a daily dose of 2 mg/kg was required to decrease expresson of TNF-α and HIV RNA

(A. Hise and R.S. Wallis, unpublished observations). The high dose requirement may be a consequence of induction of hepatic enzymes by rifampin. Prednisolone is inexpensive and readily available worldwide and has the potential for wide clinical use should these studies show it to be beneficial.

Therapeutic Vaccines

In 1890 Koch demonstrated that intradermal injection of tuberculous guinea pigs with old tuberculin led to rapid necrosis and sloughing of tuberculous lesions—the Koch phenomenon. Nonetheless, immunotherapy with tuberculin was subsequently administered to TB patients with mixed and generally unimpressive results. Other immunotherapeutic preparations were also tried without substantial results. Interest in therapeutic vaccines declined following the development of modern anti-TB chemotherapy; however, recognition of the limitations of current combination chemotherapy such as its relatively long 6-month duration and increasing rates of MDR TB, led to renewed work in this area. Stanford and colleagues *(143)* postulated that immunotherapy with environmental mycobacteria may activate protective immune responses, but not tissue-destructive Koch reactivity, and may hasten the clearance of persisting tubercle bacilli, potentially shortening the duration of therapy. Rapidly growing environmental mycobacteria that may have been responsible for modulating the protective responses of BCG vaccine against leprosy in some areas were studied as potential immunotherapeutic agents. Mycobacteria that were capable of inducing in vitro responses to common mycobacterial antigens but not delayed-type hypersensitivity responses (a surrogate for tissue-destructive Koch responses) were sought.

M. vaccae is a rapidly growing environmental mycobacterium that has low pathogenicity for humans *(144)*. *M. vaccae* was originally isolated from the soil in an area of Uganda where BCG vaccination had been shown to be protective against leprosy. Heat-killed preparations of *M. vaccae* have been studied as an adjunct to standard anti-TB drug therapy for over a decade. *M. vaccae* expresses antigens common to many mycobacteria *(145)*, and earlier studies suggested that it may favorably modify host immune responses in TB and leprosy *(146)*. Heat-killed *M. vaccae* preparations have been hypothesized to work in two ways: (i) by restoring host recognition of shared mycobacterial antigens; and (2) by promoting Th1 responses important to host defenses against intracellular pathogens. Because heat-killed *M. vaccae* is inexpensive, simple to administer, and could potentially be implemented by TB control programs in developing countries, there has been great interest in performing controlled trials to evaluate its potential role in TB treatment.

M. vaccae has usually been administered as an intradermal injection of an autoclaved preparation of the organism given within the first few days to first month after the initiation of standard chemotherapy. The heat-killed vaccine has been demonstrated to be safe in HIV-infected and HIV-noninfected adults. Side effects owing to *M. vaccae* have been mild and infrequent. Forty percent of subjects in an earlier trial developed a local scar similar to a BCG vaccination scar *(147)*.

In early studies, heat-killed preparations of *M. vaccae* showed activity as an adjunct to anti-TB chemotherapy. In studies from the Gambia and Vietnam, the proportion of TB cases cured was increased and mortality decreased among those treated with a heat-killed *M. vaccae* immunotherapeutic agent *(148)*. Other studies in Nigeria, Romania, and Iran also suggested activity in TB patients with drug-susceptible and drug-resistant tuberculosis *(149–152)*. These studies suffered from methodologic problems including insufficient sample sizes, nonrandom treatment allocation, high losses to follow-up, and the use of various TB drug treatment regimens *(153)*.

Three recent clinical trials have examined the role of immunotherapy with heat-killed *M. vaccae* in a more rigorous fashion. In Romania, 206 previously untreated patients with pulmonary TB were randomized to receive *M. vaccae* immunotherapeutic agent or placebo 1 month after the beginning of anti-TB treatment *(151)*. In this trial, which included patients with both drug-susceptible and drug-resistant TB, sputum cultures 1 month after the administration of *M. vaccae* (i.e., 2 months after the onset of anti-TB chemotherapy) were negative in 86% of patients in the immunotherapy group compared with 76% of the placebo arm ($p = 0.08$). Patients who received *M. vaccae* had significantly greater weight gain after 2 and 6 months of TB treatment and decrement in cavitary disease at 6 months. In a companion study of 102 patients with chronic or relapsed TB, 60% of whom were infected with bacilli resistant to at least one first-line drug, 77% patients treated with *M. vaccae* had successful treatment outcomes at 1 year compared with 52% of patients treated with chemotherapy only ($p < 0.02$) *(150)*. Sputum culture negativity at 2 months was significantly higher in *M. vaccae* than placebo recipients.

In contrast, a randomized clinical trial from South Africa found no difference in the rate of sputum culture conversion, weight gain, radiographic improvement, survival, or decrease in erythrocyte sedimentation rate after 2 months of TB treatment *(154)*. This study included 374 HIV-infected and HIV-noninfected patients with pulmonary TB, treated with standard short-course chemotherapy and a single intradermal injection of heat-killed *M. vaccae* or placebo 1 week after the onset of anti-TB treatment. In a similar clinical trial done in HIV-noninfected TB patients in Uganda, the rate of sputum culture conversion after 1 month of TB treatment was twofold higher in the *M. vaccae* group compared with the placebo arm after 1 month of TB treatment ($p = 0.01$) and was comparable between the groups thereafter *(155)*. Weight gain and improvement in cough and chest pain did not differ between treatment groups. Treatment with *M. vaccae* was also associated with greater improvement in radiographic extent of disease at the end of anti-TB treatment and at 1-year follow-up.

The reasons underlying the disparate results of these studies are unclear but may reflect differences in exposure and sensitization to environmental mycobacteria between the trial sites that might obscure any potential benefit from the immunotherapeutic agent *(148)*. At the present time, immunotherapy with *M. vaccae* should continue to be regarded as experimental therapy. The promising results in several studies suggest that further research with *M. vaccae* is warranted. Another large study of *M. vaccae* immunotherapy is currently under way in Zambia.

CONCLUSIONS

The evolution of *Mycobacterium tuberculosis* as an intracellular pathogen has led to a complex relationship between the organism and its host, the human mononuclear phagocyte. The products of *M. tuberculosis*-specific T-lymphocytes, particularly IFN-γ, are essential for macrophage activation for intracellular mycobacterial killing. However, some cytokines, including products of both lymphocytes and phagocytic cells, may contribute to disease pathogenesis, by enhancing mycobacterial survival and by causing many of the pathologic features of the disease. In HIV-associated mycobacterial infections, cytokines may mediate accelerated progression of HIV disease. The objectives of adjunctive immunotherapy for tuberculosis are also complex. In some situations, such as MDR disease, clearance of bacilli may be enhanced by administration of IL-2, IL-12, or IFN-γ, or possibly by using inhibitors of the deactivating cytokines TGF-β and IL-10. In other circumstances, such as in HIV coinfection, it may be desirable to reduce the nonspecific inflammatory response—and thereby reduce HIV expression—using inhibitors of TNF-α such as pentoxifylline, prednisone, or soluble TNF receptor. Further clinical trials are needed to define the clinical role for immunotherapy of tuberculosis and other mycobacterial infections.

REFERENCES

1. Global Tuberculosis Programme. Global Tuberculosis Control WHO Report 1999. Geneva: WHO, 1999.
2. Global Tuberculosis Programme. Anti-tuberculosis drug resistance in the world. 1998.
3. Villarino ME, Dooley SW, Geiter LJ, Castro KG, Snider DE Jr. Management of persons exposed to multidrug-resistant tuberculosis. MMWR 1992; 41:61–71.
4. Selwyn PA, Alcabes P, Hartel D, et al. Clinical manifestations and predictors of disease progression in drug users with human immunodeficiency virus infection. N Engl J Med 1992; 327:1697–1703.
5. Di Perri G, Cruciani M, Danzi MC, et al. Nosocomial epidemic of active tuberculosis among HIV-infected patients. Lancet 1989; 2:1502–1504.
6. Daley CL, Small PM, Schecter GF, et al. An outbreak of tuberculosis with accelerated progression among persons infected with the human immunodeficiency virus. An analysis using restriction-fragment-length polymorphisms. N Engl J Med 1992; 326:231–235.
7. Crowle AJ, Elkins N. Relative permissiveness of macrophages from black and white people for virulent tubercle bacilli. Infect Immun 1990; 58:632–638.
8. Skamene E, Forget A. Genetic basis of host resistance and susceptibility to intracellular pathogens. Adv Exp Med Biol 1988; 239:23–37.
9. Radzioch D, Hudson T, Boule M, Barrera L, Urbance JW, Varesio L, Skamene E. Genetic resistance/susceptibility to mycobacteria: phenotypic expression in bone marrow derived macrophage lines. J Leukoc Biol 1991; 50:263–272.
10. Stach JL, Gros P, Forget A, Skamene E. Phenotypic expression of genetically-controlled natural resistance to *Mycobacterium bovis* (BCG). J Immunol 1984; 132:888–892.
11. Goto Y, Buschman E, Skamene E. Regulation of host resistance to *Mycobacterium intracellulare* in vivo and in vitro by the *bcg* gene. Immunogenetics 1989; 30:218–221.
12. Bellamy R, Ruwende C, Corrah T, McAdam KP, Whittle HC, Hill AV. Variations in the NRAMP1 gene and susceptibility to tuberculosis in West Africans [see comments]. N Engl J Med 1998; 338:640–644.
13. Bermudez LE, Wu M, Young LS. Interleukin-12-stimulated natural killer cells can activate human macrophages to inhibit growth of *M. avium.* Infect Immun 1995; 63:4099–4104.
14. Fujiwara H, Kleinhenz ME, Wallis RS, Ellner JJ. Increased interleukin-1 production and monocyte suppressor cell activity associated with human tuberculosis. Am Rev Respir Dis 1986; 133:73–77.
15. Takashima T, Ueta C, Tsuyuguchi I, Kishimoto S. Production of tumor necrosis factor alpha by monocytes from patients with pulmonary tuberculosis. Infect Immun 1990; 58:3286–3292.
16. Chensue SW, Warmington KS, Berger AE, Tracey DE. Immunohistochemical demonstration of interleukin-1 receptor antagonist protein and interleukin-1 in human lymphoid tissue and granulomas. Am J Pathol 1992; 140:269–275.
17. Kindler V, Sappino AP. The beneficial effects of localized tumor necrosis factor production in BCG infection. Behring Inst Mitt 1991; 88:120–124.

18. Wallis RS, Paranjape R, Phillips M. Identification by two-dimensional gel electrophoresis of a 58-kilodalton tumor necrosis factor-inducing protein of *M. tuberculosis.* Infect Immun 1993; 61:627–632.
19. Moreno C, Taverne J, Mehlert A, Bate CA, Brealey RJ, Meager A, Rook GA, Playfair JH. Lipoarabinomannan from *M. tuberculosis* induces the production of tumour necrosis factor from human and murine macrophages. Clin Exp Immunol 1989; 76:240–245.
20. Wallis RS, Fujiwara H, Ellner JJ. Direct stimulation of monocyte release of interleukin 1 by mycobacterial protein antigens. J Immunol 1986; 136:193–196.
21. Valone SE, Rich EA, Wallis RS, Ellner JJ. Expression of tumor necrosis factor in vitro by human mononuclear phagocytes stimulated with whole *Mycobacterium bovis* BCG and mycobacterial antigens. Infect Immun 1988; 56:3313–3315.
22. Bermudez LE. Production of transforming growth factor-beta by *M. avium*-infected human macrophages is associated with unresponsiveness to IFN-gamma. J Immunol 1993; 150:1838–1845.
23. Kasahara K, Kobayashi K, Shikama Y, et al. The role of monokines in granuloma formation in mice: the ability of interleukin 1 and tumor necrosis factor-alpha to induce lung granulomas. Clin Immunol Immunopathol 1989; 51:419–425.
24. Denis M, Gregg EO, Ghandirian E. Cytokine modulation of *M. tuberculosis* growth in human macrophages. Int J Immunopharmacol 1990; 12:721–727.
25. Bermudez LE, Young LS. Tumor necrosis factor, alone or in combination with IL-2, but not IFN-gamma, is associated with macrophage killing of *M. avium* complex. J Immunol 1988; 140:3006–3013.
26. Rose RM, Fuglestad JM, Remington L. Growth inhibition of *M. avium* complex in human alveolar macrophages by the combination of recombinant macrophage colony-stimulating factor and interferon-gamma. Am J Respir Cell Mol Biol 1991; 4:248–254.
27. Denis M. Tumor necrosis factor and granulocyte macrophage-colony stimulating factor stimulate human macrophages to restrict growth of virulent *M. avium* and to kill avirulent *M. avium:* killing effector mechanism depends on the generation of reactive nitrogen intermediates. J Leukoc Biol 1991; 49:380–387.
28. Bermudez LE, Young LS. Recombinant granulocyte-macrophage colony-stimulating factor activates human macrophages to inhibit growth or kill *M. avium* complex. J Leukoc Biol 1990; 48:67–73.
29. Denis M, Gregg EO. Recombinant tumour necrosis factor-alpha decreases whereas recombinant interleukin-6 increases growth of a virulent strain of *M. avium* in human macrophages. Immunology 1990; 71:139–141.
30. Kaneko H, Yamada H, Mizuno S, et al. Role of tumor necrosis factor-alpha in *Mycobacterium*-induced granuloma formation in tumor necrosis factor-alpha-deficient mice. Lab Invest 1999; 79:379–386.
31. Kindler V, Sappino AP, Grau GE, Piguet PF, Vassalli P. The inducing role of tumor necrosis factor in the development of bactericidal granulomas during BCG infection. Cell 1989; 56:731–740.
32. Ladel CH, Blum C, Dreher A, Reifenberg K, Kopf M, Kaufmann SH. Lethal tuberculosis in interleukin-6-deficient mutant mice. Infect Immun 1997; 65:4843–4849.
33. Bellamy R, Ruwende C, Corrah T, et al. Tuberculosis and chronic hepatitis B virus infection in Africans and variation in the vitamin D receptor gene. J Infect Dis 1999; 179:721–724.
34. Roy S, Frodsham A, Saha B, Hazra SK, Mascie-Taylor CG, Hill AV. Association of vitamin D receptor genotype with leprosy type. J Infect Dis 1999; 179:187–191.
35. Denis M. Killing of *M. tuberculosis* within human monocytes: activation by cytokines and calcitriol. Clin Exp Immunol 1991; 84:200–206.
36. Rook GA, Taverne J, Leveton C, Steele J. The role of gamma-interferon, vitamin D3 metabolites and tumour necrosis factor in the pathogenesis of tuberculosis. Immunology 1987; 62:229–234.

37. Boom WH. The role of T-cell subsets in *M. tuberculosis* infection. Infect Agents Dis 1996; 5:73–81.

38. Tsukaguchi K, Balaji KN, Boom WH. CD4+ alpha beta T cell and gamma delta T cell responses to *M. tuberculosis.* Similarities and differences in Ag recognition, cytotoxic effector function, and cytokine production. J Immunol 1995; 154:1786–1796.

39. Nacy CA, Meltzer MS, Leonard EJ, Wyler DJ. Intracellular replication and lymphokine-induced destruction of *Leishmania tropica* in C3H/HeN mouse macrophages. J Immunol 1981; 127:2381–2386.

40. Murray HW, Spitalny GL, Nathan CF. Activation of mouse peritoneal macrophages in vitro and in vivo by interferon-gamma. J Immunol 1985; 134:1619–1622.

41. Bhardwaj N, Nash TW, Horwitz MA. Interferon-gamma-activated human monocytes inhibit the intracellular multiplication of *Legionella pneumophila.* J Immunol 1986; 137:2662–2669.

42. Rook GA, Champion BR, Steele J, Varey AM, Stanford JL. I-A restricted activation by T cell lines of anti-tuberculosis activity in murine macrophages. Clin Exp Immunol 1985; 59:414–420.

43. Flesch I, Kaufmann SH. Mycobacterial growth inhibition by interferon-gamma-activated bone marrow macrophages and differential susceptibility among strains of *M. tuberculosis.* J Immunol 1987; 138:4408–4413.

44. Cooper AM, Dalton DK, Stewart TA, Griffin JP, Russell DG, Orme, IM. Disseminated tuberculosis in interferon gamma gene-disrupted mice. J Exp Med 1993; 178:2243–2247.

45. Flynn JL, Chan J, Triebold KJ, Dalton DK, Stewart TA, Bloom BR. An essential role for interferon gamma in resistance to *M. tuberculosis* infection. J Exp Med 1993; 178:2249–2254.

46. Kamijo R, Le J, Shapiro D, et al. Mice that lack the interferon-gamma receptor have profoundly altered responses to infection with bacillus Calmette-Guérin and subsequent challenge with lipopolysaccharide. J Exp Med 1993; 178:1435–1440.

47. Dalton DK, Pitts-Meek S, Keshav S, Figari IS, Bradley A, Stewart TA. Multiple defects of immune cell function in mice with disrupted interferon-gamma genes. Science 1993; 259:1739–1742.

48. Kobayashi K, Yamazaki J, Kasama T, et al. Interleukin (IL)-12 deficiency in susceptible mice infected with *M. avium* and amelioration of established infection by IL-12 replacement therapy. J Infect Dis 1996; 174:564–573.

49. Sugawara I, Yamada H, Kaneko H, Mizuno S, Takeda K, Akira S. Role of interleukin-18 (IL-18) in mycobacterial infection in IL-18-gene-disrupted mice. Infect Immun 1999; 67:2585–2589.

50. Holland SM, Dorman SE, Kwon A, et al. Abnormal regulation of interferon-gamma, interleukin-12, and tumor necrosis factor-alpha in human interferon-gamma receptor 1 deficiency. J Infect Dis 1998; 178:1095–1104.

51. Frucht DM, Holland SM. Defective monocyte costimulation for IFN-gamma production in familial disseminated *M. avium* complex infection: abnormal IL-12 regulation. J Immunol 1996; 157:411–416.

52. de Jong R, Altare F, Haagen IA, et al. Severe mycobacterial and *Salmonella* infections in interleukin-12 receptor-deficient patients. Science 1998; 280:1435–1438.

53. Altare F, Durandy A, Lammas D, et al. Impairment of mycobacterial immunity in human interleukin-12 receptor deficiency. Science 1998; 280:1432–1435.

54. Kaufmann SH. Cell-mediated immunity: dealing a direct blow to pathogens. Curr Biol 1999; 9:R97–R99.

55. Stenger S, Hanson DA, Teitelbaum R, et al. An antimicrobial activity of cytolytic T cells mediated by granulysin. Science 1998; 282:121–125.

56. Cooper AM, D'Souza C, Frank AA, Orme IM. The course of *M. tuberculosis* infection in the lungs of mice lacking expression of either perforin- or granzyme-mediated cytolytic mechanisms. Infect Immun 1997; 65:1317–1320.

57. Stenger S, Mazzaccaro RJ, Uyemura K, et al. Differential effects of cytolytic T cell subsets on intracellular infection. Science 1997; 276:1684–1687.

58. Nash DR, Douglass JE. Anergy in active pulmonary tuberculosis. A comparison between positive and negative reactors and an evaluation of 5 TU and 250 TU skin test doses. Chest 1980; 77:32–37.

59. Daniel TM, Oxtoby MJ, Pinto E, Moreno E. The immune spectrum in patients with pulmonary tuberculosis. Am Rev Respir Dis 1981; 123:556–559.

60. Onwubalili JK, Scott GM, Robinson JA. Deficient immune interferon production in tuberculosis. Clin Exp Immunol 1985; 59:405–413.

61. Toossi Z, Kleinhenz ME, Ellner JJ. Defective interleukin 2 production and responsiveness in human pulmonary tuberculosis. J Exp Med 1986; 163:1162–1172.

62. Toossi Z, Sedor JR, Lapurga JP, Ondash RJ, Ellner JJ. Expression of functional interleukin 2 receptors by peripheral blood monocytes from patients with active pulmonary tuberculosis. J Clin Invest 1990; 85:1777–1784.

63. Tweardy DJ, Schacter BZ, Ellner JJ. Association of altered dynamics of monocyte surface expression of human leukocyte antigen DR with immunosuppression in tuberculosis. J Infect Dis 1984; 149:31–37.

64. Ellner JJ. Regulation of the human cellular immune response to *M. tuberculosis*. The mechanism of selective depression of the response to PPD. Bull Int Union Tuberc Lung Dis 1991; 66:129–132.

65. Toossi Z, Ellner JJ. The role of TGF beta in the pathogenesis of human tuberculosis. Clin Immunol Immunopathol 1998; 87:107–114.

66. Bermudez LE, Champsi J. Infection with *M. avium* induces production of interleukin-10 (IL-10), and administration of anti-IL-10 antibody is associated with enhanced resistance to infection in mice. Infect Immun 1993; 61:3093–3097.

67. Shiratsuchi H, Johnson JL, Ellner JJ. Bidirectional effects of cytokines on the growth of *M. avium* within human monocytes. J Immunol 1991; 146:3165–3170.

68. Rastogi N, Bachelet M, Carvalho de Sousa JP. Intracellular growth of *M. avium* in human macrophages is linked to the increased synthesis of prostaglandin E2 and inhibition of the phagosome-lysosome fusions. FEMS Microbiol Immunol 1992; 4:273–279.

69. Kleinhenz ME, Ellner JJ, Spagnuolo PJ, Daniel TM. Suppression of lymphocyte responses by tuberculous plasma and mycobacterial arabinogalactan. Monocyte dependence and indomethacin reversibility. J Clin Invest 1981; 68:153–162.

70. Dahl KE, Shiratsuchi H, Hamilton BD, Ellner JJ, Toossi Z. Selective induction of TGFβ in human monocytes by LAM of *M. tuberculosis*. Infect Immun 1996; 64:399–405.

71. Sibley LD, Adams LB, Krahenbuhl JL. Inhibition of interferon-gamma-mediated activation in mouse macrophages treated with lipoarabinomannan. Clin Exp Immunol 1990; 80:141–148.

72. Sibley LD, Hunter SW, Brennan PJ, Krahenbuhl JL. Mycobacterial lipoarabinomannan inhibits gamma interferon-mediated activation of macrophages. Infect Immun 1988; 56:1232–1236.

73. Chan J, Fan XD, Hunter SW, Brennan PJ, Bloom BR. Lipoarabinomannan, a possible virulence factor involved in persistence of *M. tuberculosis* within macrophages. Infect Immun 1991; 59:1755–1761.

74. Chujor CS, Kuhn B, Schwerer B, Bernheimer H, Levis WR, Bevec D. Specific inhibition of mRNA accumulation for lymphokines in human T cell line Jurkat by mycobacterial lipoarabinomannan antigen. Clin Exp Immunol 1992; 87:398–403.

75. Schwander SK, Torres M, Sada E, et al. Enhanced responses to *M. tuberculosis* antigens by human alveolar lymphocytes during active pulmonary tuberculosis. J Infect Dis 1998; 178:1434–1445.

76. Barnes PF, Mistry SD, Cooper CL, Pirmez C, Rea TH, Modlin RL. Compartmentalization of a CD4+ T lymphocyte subpopulation in tuberculous pleuritis. J Immunol 1989; 142:1114–1119.

77. Ellner JJ. Pleural fluid and peripheral blood lymphocyte function in tuberculosis. Ann Intern Med 1978; 89:932–933.
78. Rossi GA, Balbi B, Manca F. Tuberculous pleural effusions. Evidence for selective presence of PPD-specific T-lymphocytes at site of inflammation in the early phase of the infection. Am Rev Respir Dis 1987; 136:575–579.
79. Vanham G, Toossi Z, Hirsch CS, et al. Examining a paradox in the pathogenesis of human pulmonary tuberculosis: immune activation and suppression/anergy. Tuber Lung Dis 1997; 78:145–158.
80. Ellner JJ. Tuberculosis in the time of AIDS. The facts and the message. Chest 1990; 98:1051–1052.
81. Small PM, Schecter GF, Goodman PC, Sande MA, Chaisson RE, Hopewell PC. Treatment of tuberculosis in patients with advanced human immunodeficiency virus infection. N Engl J Med 1991; 324:289–294.
82. Wallis RS, Vjecha M, Amir Tahmasseb M, et al. Influence of tuberculosis on human immunodeficiency virus (HIV-1): enhanced cytokine expression and elevated beta 2-microglobulin in HIV-1-associated tuberculosis. J Infect Dis 1993; 167:43–48.
83. Folks TM, Justement J, Kinter A, et al. Characterization of a promonocyte clone chronically infected with HIV and inducible by 13-phorbol-12-myristate acetate. J Immunol 1988; 140:1117–1122.
84. Chun TW, Engel D, Mizell SB, Ehler LA, Fauci AS. Induction of HIV-1 replication in latently infected CD4+ T cells using a combination of cytokines [published erratum appears in J Exp Med 1998 188:following 614]. J Exp Med 1998; 188:83–91.
85. Griffin GE, Leung K, Folks TM, Kunkel S, Nabel GJ. Induction of NF-kappa B during monocyte differentiation is associated with activation of HIV-gene expression. Res Virol 1991; 142:233–238.
86. Potts BJ, Maury W, Martin MA. Replication of HIV-1 in primary monocyte cultures. Virology 1990; 175:465–476.
87. Latham PS, Lewis AM, Varesio L, et al. Expression of human immunodeficiency virus long terminal repeat in the human promonocyte cell line U937: effect of endotoxin and cytokines. Cell Immunol 1990; 129:513–518.
88. Goletti D, Weissman D, Jackson RW, Collins F, Kinter A, Fauci AS. The in vitro induction of human immunodeficiency virus (HIV) replication in purified protein derivative-positive HIV-infected persons by recall antigen response to *M. tuberculosis* is the result of a balance of the effects of endogenous interleukin-2 and proinflammatory and antiinflammatory cytokines. J Infect Dis 1998; 177:1332–1338.
89. Kinter AL, Ostrowski M, Goletti D, et al. HIV replication in CD4+ T cells of HIV-infected individuals is regulated by a balance between the viral suppressive effects of endogenous beta-chemokines and the viral inductive effects of other endogenous cytokines. Proc Natl Acad Sci USA 1996; 93:14076–14081.
90. Zhang Y, Doerfler M, Lee TC, Guillemin B, Rom WN. Mechanisms of stimulation of interleukin-1 beta and tumor necrosis factor-alpha by *M. tuberculosis* components. J Clin Invest 1993; 91:2076–2083.
91. Zhang Y, Nakata K, Weiden M, Rom WN. *M. tuberculosis* enhances human immunodeficiency virus-1 replication by transcriptional activation at the long terminal repeat. J Clin Invest 1995; 95:2324–2331.
92. Lederman MM, Georges DL, Kusner DJ, Mudido P, Giam CZ, Toossi Z. *M. tuberculosis* and its purified protein derivative activate expression of the human immunodeficiency virus. J Acquir Immune Defic Syndr Hum Retrovirol 1994; 7:727–733.
93. Mudido P, Georges D, Jacobs G, Toossi Z, Ellner JJ, Lederman MM. Mycobacteria and their products activate HIV expression. Int Conf AIDS. 1993; 9:325 (Abstract).
94. Nakata K, Rom WN, Honda Y, et al. *M. tuberculosis* enhances human immunodeficiency virus-1 replication in the lung. Am J Respir Crit Care Med 1997; 155:996–1003.

95. Goletti D, Weissman D, Jackson RW, et al. Effect of *M. tuberculosis* on HIV replication. Role of immune activation. J Immunol 1996; 157:1271–1278.
96. Whalen C, Horsburgh CR, Hom D, Lahart C, Simberkoff M, Ellner J. Accelerated course of human immunodeficiency virus infection after tuberculosis. Am J Respir Crit Care Med 1995; 151:129–135.
97. Wallis RS, Helfand MS, Whalen C, et al. Immune activation, allergic drug toxicity, and mortality in HIV-positive tuberculosis. Tuber Lung Dis 1996; 77:516–523.
98. Cooper AM, Roberts AD, Rhoades ER, Callahan JE, Getzy DM, Orme IM. The role of interleukin-12 in acquired immunity to *M. tuberculosis* infection. Immunology 1995; 84:423–432.
99. Flynn JL, Goldstein MM, Triebold KJ, Sypek J, Wolf S, Bloom BR. IL-12 increases resistance of BALB/c mice to *M. tuberculosis* infection. J Immunol 1995; 155:2515–2524.
100. Johnson BJ, Ress SR, Willcox P, et al. Clinical and immune responses of tuberculosis patients treated with low-dose IL-2 and multidrug therapy. Cytokines Mol Ther 1995; 1:185–196.
101. Johnson BJ, Bekker LG, Rickman R, et al. rhuIL-2 adjunctive therapy in multidrug resistant tuberculosis: a comparison of two treatment regimens and placebo. Tuber Lung Dis 1997; 78:195–203.
102. Hirsch CS, Ellner JJ, Blinkhorn R, Toossi Z. In vitro restoration of T cell responses in tuberculosis and augmentation of monocyte effector function against *M. tuberculosis* by natural inhibitors of transforming growth factor beta. Proc Natl Acad Sci USA 1997; 94:3926–3931.
103. Bermudez LE, Young LS. Tumor necrosis factor, alone or in combination with IL-2, but not IFN-gamma, is associated with macrophage killing of *M. avium* complex. J Immunol 1988; 140:3006–3013.
104. Bermudez LE, Stevens P, Kolonoski P, Wu M, Young LS. Treatment of experimental disseminated *M. avium* complex infection in mice with recombinant IL-2 and tumor necrosis factor. J Immunol 1989; 143:2996–3000.
105. Jeevan A, Asherson GL. Recombinant interleukin-2 limits the replication of *Mycobacterium lepraemurium* and *Mycobacterium bovis* BCG in mice. Infect Immun 1988; 56:660–664.
106. Akuffo H, Kaplan G, Kiessling R, et al. Administration of recombinant interleukin-2 reduces the local parasite load of patients with disseminated cutaneous leishmaniasis. J Infect Dis 1990; 161:775–780.
107. Hancock GE, Cohn ZA, Kaplan G. (1989) The generation of antigen-specific, major histocompatibility complex-restricted cytotoxic T lymphocytes of the CD4+ phenotype. Enhancement by the cutaneous administration of interleukin 2. J Exp Med 169:909–919.
108. Kaplan G, Kiessling R, Teklemariam S., et al. The reconstitution of cell-mediated immunity in the cutaneous lesions of lepromatous leprosy by recombinant interleukin 2. J Exp Med 1989; 169:893–907.
109. Kaplan G, Britton WJ, Hancock GE, et al. The systemic influence of recombinant interleukin 2 on the manifestations of lepromatous leprosy. J Exp Med 1991; 173:993–1006.
110. Nathan CF, Kaplan G, Levis WR, et al. Local and systemic effects of intradermal recombinant interferon-gamma in patients with lepromatous leprosy. N Engl J Med 1986; 315:6–15.
111. Holland SM, Eisenstein EM, Kuhns DB, et al. Treatment of refractory disseminated nontuberculous mycobacterial infection with interferon gamma. A preliminary report. N Engl J Med 1994; 330:1348–1355.
112. Squires KE, Brown ST, Armstrong D, Murphy WF, Murray HW. Interferon-gamma treatment for *M. avium*-intracellular complex bacillemia in patients with AIDS [letter]. J Infect Dis 1992; 166:686–687.

113. Raad I, Hachem R, Leeds N, Sawaya R, Salem Z, Atweh S. Use of adjunctive treatment with interferon-gamma in an immunocompromised patient who had refractory multidrug-resistant tuberculosis of the brain. Clin Infect Dis 1996; 22:572–574.

114. Condos R, Rom WN, Schluger NW. Treatment of multidrug-resistant pulmonary tuberculosis with interferon-gamma via aerosol. Lancet 1997; 349:1513–1515.

115. Giosue S, Casarini M, Alemanno L, et al. Effects of aerosolized interferon-alpha in patients with pulmonary tuberculosis. Am J Respir Crit Care Med 1998; 158:1156–1162.

116. Palmero D, Eiguchi K, Rendo P, Castro ZL, Abbate E, Gonzalez ML. Phase II trial of recombinant interferon-alpha2b in patients with advanced intractable multidrug-resistant pulmonary tuberculosis: long-term follow-up. Int J Tuberc Lung Dis 1999; 3:214–218.

117. Silva RA, Pais TF, Appelberg R. Evaluation of IL-12 in immunotherapy and vaccine design in experimental *M. avium* infections. J Immunol 1998; 161:5578–5585.

118. Barnes P, Zhang M, Jones B. Modulation of Th1 responses in HIV infection and tuberculosis (TB). Int Conf AIDS. 1994 Aug 7–12; 10:126 (Abstract).

119. Fenton MJ, Vermeulen MW, Kim S, Burdick M, Strieter RM, Kornfeld H. Induction of gamma interferon production in human alveolar macrophages by *M. tuberculosis*. Infect Immun 1997; 65:149–156.

120. Sheskin J. Thalidomide in the treatment of lepra reactions. Clin Pharmacol Ther 1965; 6:303

121. Sampaio EP, Sarno EN, Galilly R, Cohn ZA, Kaplan G. Thalidomide selectively inhibits tumor necrosis factor alpha production by stimulated human monocytes. J Exp Med 1991; 173:699–703.

122. Tramontana JM, Utaipat U, Molloy A, et al. Thalidomide treatment reduces tumor necrosis factor production and enhances weight gain in patients with pulmonary tuberculosis. Mol Med 1995; 1:384–397.

123. Barnhill RL, Doll NJ, Millikan LE, Hastings RC. Studies on the anti-inflammatory properties of thalidomide: effects on polymorphonuclear leukocytes and monocytes. J Am Acad Dermatol 1984; 11:814–819.

124. Keenan RJ, Eiras G, Burckart GJ, et al. Immunosuppressive properties of thalidomide. Inhibition of in vitro lymphocyte proliferation alone and in combination with cyclosporine or FK506. Transplantation 1991; 52:908–910.

125. D'Amato RJ, Loughnan MS, Flynn E, Folkman J. Thalidomide is an inhibitor of angiogenesis. Proc Natl Acad Sci USA 1994; 91:4082–4085.

126. Makonkawkeyoon S, Limson Pobre RN, Moreira AL, Schauf V, Kaplan G. Thalidomide inhibits the replication of human immunodeficiency virus type 1. Proc Natl Acad Sci USA 1993; 90:5974–5978.

127. Peterson PK, Gekker G, Bornemann M, Chatterjee D, Chao CC. Thalidomide inhibits lipoarabinomannan-induced upregulation of human immunodeficiency virus expression. Antimicrob Agents Chemother 1995; 39:2807–2809.

128. Jacobson JM, Greenspan JS, Spritzler J, et al. Thalidomide for the treatment of oral aphthous ulcers in patients with human immunodeficiency virus infection. National Institute of Allergy and Infectious Diseases AIDS Clinical Trials Group. N Engl J Med 1997; 336:1487–1493.

129. Klausner JD, Makonkawkeyoon S, Akarasewi P, et al. The effect of thalidomide on the pathogenesis of human immunodeficiency virus type 1 and *M. tuberculosis* infection. J Acquir Immune Defic Syndr Hum Retrovirol 1996; 11:247–257.

130. Tsenova L, Bergtold A, Freedman VH, Young RA, Kaplan G. Tumor necrosis factor alpha is a determinant of pathogenesis and disease progression in mycobacterial infection in the central nervous system [In Process Citation]. Proc Natl Acad Sci USA 1999; 96:5657–5662.

131. Tsenova L, Sokol K, Freedman VH, Kaplan G. A combination of thalidomide plus antibiotics protects rabbits from mycobacterial meningitis-associated death. J Infect Dis 1998; 177:1563–1572.

132. Doherty GM, Jensen JC, Alexander HR, Buresh CM, Norton JA. Pentoxifylline suppression of tumor necrosis factor gene transcription. Surgery 1991; 110:192–198.

133. Tilg H, Eibl B, Pichl M, et al. Immune response modulation by pentoxifylline in vitro. Transplantation 1993; 56:196–201.

134. Zabel P, Schade FU, Schlaak M. Inhibition of endogenous TNF formation by pentoxifylline. Immunobiology 1993; 187:447–463.

135. Lilly CM, Sandhu JS, Ishizaka A, et al. Pentoxifylline prevents tumor necrosis factor-induced lung injury. Am Rev Respir Dis 1989; 139:1361–1368.

136. Fazely F, Dezube BJ, Allen-Ryan J, Pardee AB, Ruprecht RM. Pentoxifylline (Trental) decreases the replication of the human immunodeficiency virus type 1 in human peripheral blood mononuclear cells and in cultured T cells. Blood 1991; 77:1653–1656.

137. Steigbigel RT, Craddock B. Effect of pentoxifylline on HIV-1 replication in human lymphocytes and macrophages. Int Conf AIDS. 1992 July 19–24; 8:A56 (Abstract).

138. Dezube BJ, Pardee AB, Chapman B, et al. Pentoxifylline decreases tumor necrosis factor expression and serum triglycerides in people with AIDS. NIAID AIDS Clinical Trials Group. J Acquir Immune Defic Syndr Hum Retrovirol 1993; 6:787–794.

139. Dezube BJ, Lederman MM, Spritzler JG, et al. High-dose pentoxifylline in patients with AIDS: inhibition of tumor necrosis factor production. National Institute of Allergy and Infectious Diseases AIDS Clinical Trials Group. J Infect Dis 1995; 171:1628–1632.

140. Wallis RS, Nsubuga P, Okwera A, et al. Pentoxifylline in human immunodeficiency virus-seropositive tuberculosis: a randomized, controlled trial. J Infect Dis 1996; 174:727–733.

141. Wallis RS, Johnson JL, Okwera A, et al. Pentoxifylline in human immunodeficiency virus-positive tuberculosis: safety at 4 years [letter]. J Infect Dis 1998; 178:1861

142. Andrieu JM, Lu W, Levy R. Sustained increases in CD4 cell counts in asymptomatic human immunodeficiency virus type 1-seropositive patients treated with prednisolone for 1 year. J Infect Dis 1995; 171:523–530.

143. Stanford JL, Rook GA, Bahr G, et al. *M. vaccae* in immunoprophylaxis and immunotherapy of leprosy and tuberculosis. Vaccine 1990; 8:525–530.

144. Hachem R, Raad I, Rolston KV, et al. Cutaneous and pulmonary infections caused by *M. vaccae*. Clin Infect Dis 1996; 23:173–175.

145. Stanford JL, Paul RC. A preliminary report on some studies of environmental mycobacteria. Ann Soc Belg Med Trop 1973; 53:389–393.

146. Stanford JL. Immunotherapy for leprosy and tuberculosis. Prog Drug Res 1989; 33: 415–448, 415–448.

147. Stanford JL, Bahr GM, Rook GA, et al. Immunotherapy with *M. vaccae* as an adjunct to chemotherapy in the treatment of pulmonary tuberculosis. Tubercle 1990; 71:87–93.

148. Stanford JL, Grange JM. New concepts for the control of tuberculosis in the twenty first century. J R Coll Physicians Lond 1993; 27:218–223.

149. Etemadi A, Farid R, Stanford JL. Immunotherapy for drug-resistant tuberculosis [letter]. Lancet 1992; 340:1360–1361.

150. Corlan E, Marica C, Macavei C, Stanford JL, Stanford CA. Immunotherapy with *M. vaccae* in the treatment of tuberculosis in Romania. 2. Chronic or relapsed disease. Respir Med 1997; 91:21–29.

151. Corlan E, Marica C, Macavei C, Stanford JL, Stanford CA. Immunotherapy with *M. vaccae* in the treatment of tuberculosis in Romania. 1. Newly-diagnosed pulmonary disease. Respir Med 1997; 91:13–19.

152. Onyebujoh PC, Abdulmumini T, Robinson S, Rook GA, Stanford JL. Immunotherapy with *M. vaccae* as an addition to chemotherapy for the treatment of pulmonary tuberculosis under difficult conditions in Africa. Respir Med 1995; 89:199–207.

153. de Bruyn G, Garner P. *M. vaccae* immunotherapy for treating tuberculosis (Cochrane Review). In: The Cochrane Library, no.1. Oxford: Update Software, 1999.

154. Anonymous. Immunotherapy with *M. vaccae* in patients with newly diagnosed pulmonary tuberculosis: a randomised controlled trial. Durban Immunotherapy Trial Group. Lancet 1999; 354:116–119.

155. Johnson JL, Kamya RM, Okwera A, et al. Randomized controlled trial of Mycobacterium vaccae immunotherapy in non-human immunodeficiency virus-infected Ugandan adults with newly diagnosed pulmonary tuberculosis. The Uganda-Case Western Reserve University Research Collaboration. J Infect Dis 2000; 181:1304–1312.

18

Immunotherapy for Fungal Infections

Arturo Casadevall

INTRODUCTION

Most fungal pathogens are low-virulence organisms that seldom cause serious infections in individuals with intact immune function. However, fungal infections have emerged as a major medical problem in the second half of the 20th century. Factors that have contributed to this phenomenon are: (1) the development of therapies for cancer and autoimmune disorders that produce immune suppression as a consequence of their therapeutic effects; (2) increased use of indwelling vascular devices and invasive surgical techniques that compromise the integrity of the skin; (3) the use of broad spectrum antibacterial drugs that disrupt the host microbial flora and predispose to fungal superinfection; and (4) the epidemic of HIV infection that has resulted in many individuals with impaired immunologic function at risk for fungal infection. Fungi are notorious for producing chronic infections requiring prolonged therapy. The problems posed by fungal infections are compounded by the availability of only a few antifungal drugs that are relatively ineffective in patients with impaired immunity. In fact, many types of fungal infections in patients with impaired immune function cannot be eradicated with antifungal therapy. For example, cryptococcosis, coccidioidomycosis, and histoplasmosis are generally considered to be incurable in patients with advanced HIV infection. The major fungal infections and the conditions that predispose to them are listed in Table 1.

Since most life-threatening fungal infections occur in patients with impaired immunity, therapies designed to reconstitute or activate the immune system are logical adjuncts to antifungal chemotherapy. Immunotherapy can be used to correct the underlying immunologic defect or to recruit additional resources of the immune system to fight the infection. Examples of immunotherapies designed to correct or compensate for immunologic defects are neutrophil transfusions and immunoglobulin administration in patients with neutropenia and hypogammaglobulinemia, respectively. Examples of immunotherapies designed to provide additional immunologic resources include the administration of cytokines to stimulate immune function or passive antibody therapy.

Immunotherapy can be nonspecific or pathogen-specific. Nonspecific immunotherapy is designed to enhance general immune function by administration of immune modulators such as cytokines and growth factors. Pathogen-specific immunotherapy is designed to

From: *Immunotherapy for Infectious Diseases*
Edited by: J. M. Jacobson © Humana Press Inc., Totowa, NJ

Table 1
Major Fungal Infections and Risk Factors

Infection	Pathogen	Major predisposing immunologic deficit	Major risk factors
Aspergillosis	*Aspergillus* sp.	Neutropenia	Antineoplastic chemotherapy, late stage HIV infection
Blastomycosis	*Blastomyces dermatitides*	Defects in cell-mediated immunity	Immunosuppressive therapy, late stage HIV infection; can occur in normal individuals
Candidiasis	*Candida* sp.	Neutropenia	Immunosuppressive therapy, HIV infection, antibiotic use, surgical procedures, indwelling catheters
Coccidioidomycosis	*Coccidioides immitis*	Defects in cell-mediated immunity	Late stage HIV infection, pregnancy, certain ethnic groups; may occur in normal individuals
Cryptococcosis	*Cryptococcus neoformans*	Defects in cell-mediated immunity	Late stage HIV infection, corticosteroid use, lymphoproliferative malignancies; may occur in normal individuals
Histoplasmosis	*Histoplasma capsulatum*	Defects in cell-mediated immunity	Late stage HIV infection, corticosteroid therapy; may occur in normal individuals
Mucormycosis	*Rhizopus* sp.	Diabetic ketoacidosis, neutropenia	Diabetes mellitus, antineoplastic chemotherapy
Paracoccidioidomycosis	*Paracoccidioides brasiliensis*	Defects in cell-mediated immunity	Late stage HIV infection; may occur in normal individuals
Penicilliosis	*Penicillium marneffei*	Defects in cell-mediated immunity	Late stage HIV infection, immunosuppressive therapy
Sporotrichosis	*Sporothrix schenckii*	Defects in cell-mediated immunity	Late stage HIV infection; may occur in normal individuals

Table 2
Categories of Immunotherapies under Development or in Current Use

Replacement
  Granulocyte transfusions
  IVIG
Nonspecific augmentative
  Granulocyte transfusions from CSF-stimulated donors
  G-CSF
  GM-CSF
  M-CSF
  IFN-γ
Specific augmentative
  Vaccines
  Specific antibody
  Fungal extract
  Transfer factor

Abbreviations: CSF, colony-stimulating factor; G, granulocyte; IFN-γ, interferon-γ; IVIG, intravenous immunoglobulin; M, macrophage.

stimulate immune function against specific pathogens by eliciting new immune responses or augmenting existing responses. The different types of immune therapies described in this chapter are listed in Table 2. However, the distinctions between the various forms of immune therapy are blurred by the complexity and redundancy of the immune system. For example, replacement immune therapies can augment the immune system, whereas specific immunotherapy can have nonspecific effects. Administration of colony-stimulating factors (CSFs) to neutropenic patients for the purpose of stimulating bone marrow recovery may also enhance the function of host effector cells, and such therapy has both replacement and augmentative qualities. Hence, categorization of immune therapies as replacement, augmentative, specific, and nonspecific is done with the knowledge that these labels may need revision as we learn more about the complex interrelationships between the components of the immune system.

At this time there are no immunotherapies for fungal infections that are part of standard antifungal therapeutic protocols. Most, if not all, immunotherapies for fungal infections can be characterized under the label of experimental therapy. Nevertheless, this is an area of intense interest, and the field is evolving rapidly. For other recent reviews on the subject of immunotherapy for fungal infections see refs. 1–7.

IMMUNOCOMPROMISED HOSTS AND FUNGAL INFECTIONS

When evaluating therapies, it is important to consider two features of fungal infections: (1) fungal pathogens are highly diverse organisms; and (2) susceptibility to individual fungal infections usually depends on the type of immune defect present. Fungal pathogens are free-living organisms that are acquired from either the environment or the endogenous flora. The mechanisms of pathogenesis differ for the various fungal pathogens. For example, *Aspergillus* sp. produce powerful hydrolytic enzymes that destroy tissue, whereas *Cryptococcus neoformans* cells classically elicit a weak inflammatory response. Differences in pathogenic strategies used by the different fungal species suggest that optimal immunotherapy may require an individualized approach to each type of fungal infection. Susceptibility to a particular fungal infection is, in turn, a function of the specific immunological deficit of the host. Patients with neutropenia are at high risk for *Candida* and *Aspergillus* infections, whereas those with impaired cellular immunity are at high risk for the endemic mycosis (i.e., histoplasmosis, coccidioidomycosis, blastomycosis, penicilliosis). Each fungal infection must be considered in the context of the immunologic deficit of the host, and therapy should be targeted at restoring or compensating for that particular immunologic impairment. An important concept is that it may be possible to use immune therapy to compensate for immunologic deficits by taking advantage of the many defense functions that comprise the immune system. For example, neutropenic mice can be protected against experimental candidiasis by administration of specific antibody, even though the role of natural antibody-mediated immunity in candidiasis is uncertain *(8)*. Hence, it may be possible to design effective immune therapies that promote eradication of fungal infections without the vastly more complicated task of having to reverse the underlying immunologic deficit.

APPROACH TO THE LITERATURE
ON IMMUNOTHERAPY FOR FUNGAL INFECTIONS

The literature on immunotherapies for fungal infections consists of animal studies and human clinical data. In general, animal studies are usually well controlled and rigorously performed. In contrast, most of the information available about immunotherapy in humans comes from case reports and small studies. Hence, the reader must exercise caution when interpreting the human data and making inferences that are applicable to specific clinical situations. It is important to consider that the literature may be biased toward favorable outcomes since these are more likely to be reported than negative experiences. Firm conclusions about the value of specific types of immunotherapy for specific fungal infections must await the completion of well-controlled studies. Nevertheless, case reports and small studies provide important clinical information that can be used to design larger trials or guide heroic therapies in desperately ill patients with fungal infections refractory to standard therapy.

NONSPECIFIC REPLACEMENT IMMUNE THERAPIES

Granulocyte Transfusions

Granulocyte transfusions were first used in the 1960s for the treatment and prevention of infection in patients with severe polymorphonuclear (PMN) leukocyte deficiency (neutropenia) resulting from cancer therapy. Granulocyte transfusions provide mature PMNs to serve an antimicrobial role. Leukocyte preparations containing primarily PMNs can be isolated from the blood of healthy donors by centrifugation or leukopharesis. Although granulocyte transfusions may help neutropenic patients survive a bout of infection, their use has been controversial because of high cost, significant toxicity, and lack of evidence that they affect long-term survival (for review, see ref. *9*).

The popularity of granulocyte transfusions diminished significantly in the 1980s because of several developments (reviewed in refs. *10* and *11*). First, alternatives to granulocyte transfusions became available in the form of CSFs that promoted more rapid bone marrow recovery and shortened the duration of chemotherapy-associated neutropenia. Second, highly effective antibiotics were introduced that reduced the incidence and mortality of serious bacterial infections in neutropenic hosts. Third, a variety of problems were associated with granulocyte transfusions, including concerns about transmission of viral infection, toxic reactions, and alloimmunization. Fourth, the logistics of collecting leukocytes and separating granulocytes were complex and often resulted in inadequate numbers of cells for granulocyte transfusions.

In the past decade, interest in granulocyte transfusions was rekindled by several factors. Granulocyte (G)-CSF was found to be useful in mobilizing large numbers of PMNs from donors with normal antimicrobial function *(12)*. In addition to increasing quantity, G-CSF administration to donors also activates PMNs and produces a qualitative improvement in their antimicrobial efficacy. Furthermore, G-CSF and interferon-γ (IFN-γ) can be used to preserve leukocyte function after isolation from donors, irradiation, and storage *(13)*. The availability of G-CSF provided a solution to the problems of PMN quantity and quality that were serious obstacles for granulocyte transfusion therapy in the past. Another factor stimulating interest in granulocyte transfusion was the realization that antimicrobial chemotherapy was not sufficient to treat infections in some neutropenic patients. The increasing prevalence of antimicrobial-resistant organisms diminished the efficacy of many empiric antibiotic regimens in patients with prolonged neutropenia. The fact that some infections do not respond to antimicrobial therapy unless PMNs are present has led several authorities to propose wider use of granulocyte transfusions *(10)*. However, many questions remain regarding the appropriate use of granulocyte transfusions, including the selection of patients, the quality and safety of G-CSF-stimulated leukocytes, the indications for therapy, and the cost benefit of this intervention *(10,14)*.

The effectiveness of granulocyte transfusions against invasive fungal infections may be lower than that against bacterial infections *(10)*. At this time, there are not sufficient data to recommend routine granulocyte transfusions for neutropenic patients with invasive fungal infections *(10)*. Nevertheless, several reports suggest that granulocyte transfusions can be useful for the therapy of some types of fungal infection in patients with prolonged neutropenia *(15–18)*. *Fusarium* infections in neutropenic patients respond poorly to antifungal therapy, and resolution usually requires recovery of bone marrow function *(16)*. Some patients with *Fusarium* infection and neutropenia have responded favorably to CSF-elicited granulocyte transfusions, and it has been suggested that this modality can "buy time" until recovery from myelosuppression *(16)*. There is one report of a successful therapy of disseminated *Fusarium* infection using a combination of amphotericin B, granulocyte/macrophage (GM)-CSF, and granulocyte transfusions (see Table 4). A man with invasive *Aspergillus* sinusitis was successfully managed with amphotericin B colloidal dispersion and granulocyte transfusions from G-CSF-stimulated donors during the neutropenic period following bone marrow transplant *(17)*. Another man with disseminated *Aspergillus* infection in the setting of aplastic anemia was cured by combination therapy with amphotericin B, itraconazole, granulocyte transfusions from G-CSF-stimulated donors, GM-CSF, and G-CSF *(19)*. An 8-year-old boy with chronic granulomatous disease and *Aspergillus* infection was cured by bone marrow transplantation, CSF-mobilized granulocyte transfusions, and amphotericin B *(20)*. Two individuals with *Candida tropicalis* fungemia following bone marrow transplantation were cured by combination-therapy amphotericin B and granulocyte transfusions from G-CSF-stimulated donors *(18)*. These cases are noteworthy because systemic fungal infections in patients with prolonged neutropenia seldom respond to antifungal chemotherapy.

A complication particular to the use of neutrophil transfusions for the therapy of fungal infections is lethal pulmonary reactions following the combined use of amphotericin B and leukocyte infusions *(21)*. The mechanism for this toxic reaction is thought to be increased PMN capillary plugging because of amphotericin B-mediated pulmonary toxicity *(21)*. Amphotericin B promotes leukocyte aggregation in vitro *(22)*. Pulmonary toxicity has also been observed in rabbits given PMN and amphotericin B infusion. However, another study found no significant toxicity for combination therapy of amphotericin B and granulocyte transfusions and suggested that concomitant administration of both agents could be done safely *(23)*. Nevertheless, if amphotericin B and granulocyte transfusions are to be given to the same patient, it has been recommended that the infusions be separated by at least 4–6 hours *(10)*.

In summary, granulocyte transfusions represent a replacement form of immunotherapy for neutropenic patients that was once in vogue and is now experiencing a renaissance. The evidence that granulocyte transfusions are useful for the treatment of infection is limited largely to bacterial infections. There are no prospective randomized trials demonstrating a survival benefit from granulocyte transfusions in patients with invasive fungal infections. However, occasional patients with transient neutropenia and fungal infection may benefit from granulocyte transfusions, and each case must be evaluated on individual basis.

Other Agents

Dinitrochlorobenzene was successfully used in one patient for topical treatment of a nasal cutaneous lesion of *Coccidioides immitis* refractory to amphotericin B *(24)*. The rationale for dinitrochlorobenzene application was to sensitize the skin for delayed cutaneous hypersensitivity, thereby eliciting a local immune response that would eradicate the fungal infection *(24)*. Dinitrochlorobenzene in acetone was applied to the lesion of this individual and elicited an intense local inflammatory response followed by resolution of the lesion with reversal of anergy to *C. immitis* antigens *(24)*. This well-documented report suggests that a chronic fungal dermatitis may respond to immunotherapy that elicits inflammatory responses.

Chloroquine is an antimalarial drug that has recently been shown to have antifungal properties in vitro and in experimental animal infection. Unlike classical antifungal agents, chloroquine appears to function primarily as an immune modulator by enhancing macrophage antifungal function. For *Histoplasma capsulatum,* chloroquine enhances human macrophage killing by limiting the availability of intracellular iron *(25)*. For *Cryptococcus neoformans,* chloroquine enhances the activity of macrophages through an iron-independent effect that involves raising of phagolysosomal pH *(26)*. Chloroquine therapy has prolonged survival in mice infected with *H. capsulatum (25)* and *C. neoformans (26,27)*. Although there is no information available for the efficacy of chloroquine in human fungal infections, the finding of antifungal efficacy in vitro and in mice suggests potential usefulness in human infection.

Another agent with potential antifungal efficacy is diethylcarbamazine, an immune-modulating compound used for the therapy of lymphatic filariasis. Diethylcarbamazine has activity against *C. neoformans* in experimental murine infection *(28–30)*. Like chloroquine, there is no information about its efficacy as an antifungal agent in humans, but its activity in mice suggests possible usefulness against human infection.

NONSPECIFIC AUGMENTATIVE IMMUNE THERAPIES

Colony-Stimulating Factors

CSFs are natural proteins that stimulate the differentiation of bone marrow progenitor cells to mature effector cells. Three types of CSFs have been identified, cloned, and produced in forms suitable for clinical use: granulocyte, granulocyte/macrophage, and macrophage (for reviews, see refs. *31–33*). G-CSF and GM-CSF are licensed for use in the United States, whereas M-CSF is available in Japan *(31)*. These factors are produced for clinical use in bacterial, yeast, or mammalian expression systems *(32)*.

The availability of CSFs has improved the management of neutropenia associated with chemotherapy and bone marrow transplantation by shortening the length of neutropenic episodes. Since the major fungal infections in patients with cancer and/or bone marrow transplantation are associated with neutropenic episodes, CSF administration is, in theory, an important form of prophylactic antifungal immunotherapy. There is considerable evidence from laboratory studies that CSFs can augment host immune function and the efficacy of antifungal agents against a variety of fungal pathogens and these compounds may have clinical use in a direct antifungal mode. G-CSF, GM-CSF, and M-CSF have all been shown to have powerful in vitro and in vivo effects in potentiating effector cell function against many fungal pathogens (Table 3). However, most studies to date have produced no conclusive evidence that use of G-CSF or GM-CSF reduces the incidence of fungal infections or improves survival in neutropenic patients *(34)*.

G-CSF

G-CSF promotes proliferation and differentiation of PMN progenitor cells (reviewed in refs. *31* and *32*). Administration of G-CSF results in an increased number of peripheral blood PMNs, including band forms (left shift). Neutrophils from individuals given G-CSF have enhanced superoxide production. Neutrophils from patients with AIDS have impaired activity against *Candida albicans,* which can be restored by incubation in G-CSF *(35)*. G-CSF is used clinically to promote bone marrow recovery after chemotherapy and bone marrow transplantation and to treat chronic neutropenia, myelodysplastic syndrome, and aplastic anemia *(31)*. G-CSF administration is also useful for treating AIDS-associated neutropenia and may reduce the incidence of infections in patients with advanced HIV infection *(36)*. G-CSF enhances PMN antifungal activity against a variety of fungal pathogens (Table 3).

Administration of G-CSF to human volunteers results in significant augmentation of PMN activity against *C. albicans, Aspergillus fumigatus,* and *Rhizopus arrhizus (37)*. The enhanced killing power of PMNs from G-CSF-treated individuals is attributed to enhanced respiratory bursts and suggests that G-CSF administration produces qualitative improvements in granulocyte function *(37)*. Several anecdotal case reports suggest that G-CSF is beneficial as an adjunct to other therapeutic modalities for fungal infections, which are notoriously difficult to treat (Table 4). Furthermore, a randomized trial of therapy with ceftazidime and amikacin alone versus the same antibiotics plus G-CSF in neutropenic patients with presumed infection revealed a significant trend toward

Table 3
Augmentation of Antifungal Efficacy of Host Effector Cells Against Specific Fungi by Growth Factors[1]

Factor	Fungus	Effect	Ref. no.
G-CSF	*Aspergillus fumigatus*	Prevents PMN and monocyte suppression by corticosteroids	(80)
	Aspergillus fumigatus	↑ PMN-induced damage to hyphae	(81)
	Candida sp.	↑ PMN-induced damage to pseudohyphae	(82)
	Candida albicans	↑ PMN oxidative burst	(83)
	Candida albicans	↑ PMN fungicidal activity	(84)
	Candida albicans	Enhances efficacy of azole drugs in mice	(85)
	Cryptococcus neoformans	↑ PMN fungicidal activity	(35)
	Cryptococcus neoformans	Reversal of HIV-associated PMN dysfunction	(86)
GM-CSF	*Aspergillus fumigatus*	Prevents monocyte suppression by corticosteroids	(87)
	Candida albicans	↑ Macrophage antifungal activity	(88,89)
	Cryptococcus neoformans	↑ Monocyte fungistatic activity	(90)
	Torulopsis glabrata	↑ PMN killing and oxidative burst	(91)
M-CSF	*Candida albicans*	Enhances fluconazole efficacy	(92)
	Candida albicans	Prolongs survival and reduces organ fungal burden	(93)
	Cryptococcus neoformans	↑ Macrophage antifungal activity	(94)
	Cryptococcus neoformans	Synergy with fluconazole in vitro	(94,95)
	Cryptococcus neoformans	↑ Monocyte fungistatic activity	(95)

Abbreviations: CSF, colony-stimulating factor; G, granulocyte; M, macrophage; PMN, polymorphonuclear leukocyte.
[1]This is not a complete list.

fewer bloodstream bacterial infections and no fungal superinfections in patients receiving G-CSF *(38)*. However, Amphotericin B and G-CSF is not sufficient therapy for *Aspergillus* in many patients: Dornbusch et al. *(39)* reported the cases of five children treated with combination therapy of whom one was cured, two died, and two required surgery for removal of pulmonary lesions.

GM-CSF

The effects of GM-CSF are similar to those of G-CSF except that it acts on cells at an earlier progenitor stage in which cells are capable of differentiating into either granulocyte or monocyte lineages. Consequently, GM-CSF administration increases not only PMNs but also eosinophils and monocytes. The increased number of PMNs in patients given GM-CSF is also a consequence of significantly increased circulating half-life, which is prolonged from 8 to 48 hours (reviewed in ref. *32*). GM-CSF is used clinically to promote bone marrow recovery after chemotherapy for solid tumors, to promote engraftment of bone marrow cells, and for treatment of graft failure, aplastic anemia, and myelodysplastic syndromes. GM-CSF has been shown to enhance phagocytic cell function against several fungal pathogens (Table 3).

Table 4
Case Reports of Unusual Fungal Infections Treated with Growth Factors or Cytokines as Adjunctive Therapy

Infection	Predisposing conditions	Therapy	Outcome	Ref. no.
Blastoschizomyces capitis	Neutropenia, myelosuppressive therapy for leukemia	AmB and GM-CSF	Cured	*(60)*
Disseminated *Fusarium*	Neutropenia, myelosuppressive therapy for leukemia	AmB, 5-FC, GM-CSF	Remission	*(96)*
Cutaneous mucormycosis (*Absidia corymbifera*)	Neutropenia, aplastic anemia, bone marrow transplantation	AmB, surgical debridement, G-CSF	Cured	*(97)*
Pulmonary mucormycosis	Neutropenia, myelosuppressive therapy for leukemia	AmB, 5-FC, miconazole, pneumonectomy, G-CSF	Cured	*(98)*
Sinonasal mucormycosis (*Scopulariopsis candida*)	Neutropenia, myelosuppressive therapy for lymphoma	AmB, itraconazole, surgical debridement, G-CSF	Cured	*(99)*
Paecilomyces varioti	Chronic granulomatous disease	AmB, itraconazole, IFN-γ	Cured	*(100,101)*
Pseudallescheria boydii	Chronic granulomatous disease	Miconazole, IFN-γ	Cured	*(53)*
Trichosporonosis (*Trichosporon beigelii*)	Neutropenia, myelosuppressive therapy for leukemia	AmB, G-CSF	Cured	*(102)*
Trichosporonosis (*Trichosporon beigelii*)	Neutropenia, myelosuppressive therapy for multiple myeloma	AmB, G-CSF	Died	*(103)*
Disseminated zygomycosis (*Rhizomucor pusillus*)	Aplastic anemia, cyclosporin, antithymocyte globulin	AmB, G-CSF	Remission	*(104)*

Abbreviations: AmB, amphotericin B; 5-FC, 5-fluorocytosine; CSF, colony-stimulating factor; G, granulocyte; M, macrophage; IFN-γ, interferon-γ.

There has been some concern that GM-CSF administration may impair PMN migration to sites of infection because of GM-CSF-mediated effects on neutrophil adhesion. However, clinical experience suggests that this concern may be unfounded. One case report measured migration of labeled white blood cells in a patient with fungal infection treated with GM-CSF and pentoxifylline and demonstrated their localization to the site of infection *(40)*. A small retrospective study that analyzed the incidence of fungal infections in patients who had received GM-CSF and other cytokines suggested that GM-CSF had a protective role in bone marrow transplant patients *(41)*. Another retrospective study of infectious disease complications in autologous bone marrow transplant patients suggested no deleterious effects of GM-CSF on host immune function *(42)*. In fact, there was a significant reduction in the incidence of total infectious complications and days of amphotericin B therapy as well as a trend toward fewer fungal infections *(42)*. Since the time to resolution of neutropenia did not differ in patients with and without GM-CSF therapy, these results were interpreted as suggesting that GM-CSF enhanced monocyte-macrophage function and that this reduced infections *(42)*.

GM-CSF has been used as an adjunct to amphotericin B therapy in a few patients. Bodey et al. *(43)* reported a pilot study in which GM-CSF was administered to eight patients with malignancy, severe neutropenia, and proven systemic fungal infection in doses ranging from 100 to 750 $\mu g/m^2/day$. Of the eight patients, four were cured, two had a partial response, and two failed therapy *(43)*. A capillary leak syndrome developed as an adverse effect in three of the eight patients, contributing to one death and resulting in renal failure in another patient, presumably because the dose of GM-CSF was excessive *(43)*. In a small study conducted by the Eastern Cooperative Oncology Group, the overall mortality of patients with acute myeloid leukemia and fungal infection was 13% in the group receiving GM-CSF and 75% in the control group *(44)*. Whether this reduction in mortality was a result of earlier bone marrow recovery or enhanced effector cell function is unclear *(44)*. Although encouraging, such data are preliminary, derived from a relatively few patients, and must be interpreted with caution.

M-CSF

The effects of this growth factor are limited to monocytic cell populations. M-CSF promotes proliferation, activation, and differentiation of monocytes and macrophages. M-CSF stimulates macrophages to produce higher levels of oxidants and enhances their ability to kill intracellular bacteria and fungi. Because the macrophage is a central host effector cell for defense against most, if not all, fungal infections, M-CSF is of particular interest as an immunotherapeutic agent in fungal infections. Several studies have shown that M-CSF can enhance macrophage function against fungi (Table 3).

Nemunaitis and collaborators *(45,46)* used M-CSF in doses ranging from 100 to 2000 $\mu g/m^2/day$ as an adjunct to antifungal therapy in 24 patients with bone marrow transplants complicated by invasive fungal infections. Of these patients, 25% resolved their infection, 50% could not be evaluated for judging the efficacy of the intervention, and 25% did not respond *(45)*. In a larger follow-up study, bone marrow transplant patients with fungal infections treated with M-CSF and antifungal therapy had significantly improved long-term survival compared with historical controls treated with antifungal therapy alone *(46)*. The results suggest that benefits of adjunctive M-CSF therapy occur primarily in the subset of patients with *Candida* infections *(46)*. This encouraging study suggests the need for randomized controlled trials to evaluate the efficacy of M-CSF as adjunctive therapy for invasive fungal infections *(47)*. M-CSF administration is well tolerated. The major side effects are a transient dose-related thrombocytopenia that may be caused by enhanced function of splenic phagocytic cells *(45)*.

Interferon-γ

IFN-γ is a T-cell-derived cytokine that has powerful effects on macrophage cell activation *(48)*. Since macrophages are critically important for the control of many fungal infections, there has been considerable interest in the potential usefulness of INF-γ for therapy of fungal infections. IFN-γ has been used with some success in combination with conventional therapy for patients with mycobacterial infections *(49)*. Studies in animals provide encouragement for the use of IFN-γ as an adjunct to antifungal therapy (reviewed in refs. *1* and *5*). For example, a single dose of IFN-γ enhanced the efficacy of amphotericin B against *Cryptococcus neoformans* in mice *(50)*. However, at this time there is relatively little clinical information available regarding the usefulness of IFN-γ in the treatment of fungal infections. IFN-γ administration has been used successfully as adjunctive therapy for infection in a few patients with unusual fungal infections in the setting of chronic granulomatous disease (CGD) (reviewed in ref. *51*) (Table 3). CGD is an inherited immunodeficiency that results from a diminished ability of PMNs to produce the microbicidal respiratory burst. Patients with CGD are susceptible to a variety of pathogens including fungi, and IFN-γ can reduce the frequency of fungal infections, including *Aspergillus (52)*. The cases of *Paecilomyces varioti* infection in patients with CGD were cured with a combination of IFN-γ and amphotericin B (Table 4). A 10-year-old boy with CGD and disseminated *Pseudallescheria boydii* infection was cured with combination of miconazole and IFN-γ *(53)*. Administration of IFN-γ is generally well tolerated. Most of the clinical adverse reactions consist of fever, chills, headache, and injection site erythema *(49,52)*.

INTRAVENOUS IMMUNE GLOBULIN

Passive antibody administration modifies the course of several fungal infections *(54)*. The only antibody preparation available for clinical use is immunoglobulin. Since antibodies to fungal antigens are sometimes found in normal human sera, the administration of immunoglobulin could, in theory, be useful in therapy. However, there are very few data to support the routine use of intravenous immunoglobulin (IVIG) for treatment or prevention of fungal infections. Combination therapy of amphotericin B and IVIG for experimental *C. albicans* in mice resulted in a modest improvement in survival *(55)*. Prophylactic IVIG administration was associated with a reduction in fungal infections in liver transplant recipients *(56)* but not in bone marrow recipients *(57)*.

PATHOGEN-SPECIFIC IMMUNE THERAPY

Therapeutic Vaccine for Pythium insidisum

Pythiosis insidiosi is a rare human fungal infection caused by *Pythium insidisum*. In horses, pythiosis is a relatively common infection that is treated with surgery, antifungal agents, and a therapeutic vaccine composed of *Pythium* antigens. Mendoza et al. have described Two vaccines for pythiosis have been described made from either *P. insidiosum* whole cells or soluble concentrated antigens *(59)*. Both vaccines are effective in achieving cures in horses with recent infection *(58)*. This therapeutic vaccine apparently mediates its effects by eliciting strong inflammatory responses that result in eradication of infection *(58)*. There is one case report of the use of this vaccine in humans that describes the case of a 14-year-old Thai boy with *P. insidiosum* arteritis who was apparently cured by vaccine therapy *(59)*. The efficacy of this vaccine in horses suggests that for some fungal infections, it may be possible to develop vaccine therapy with specific antigen preparations that stimulate the immune system to control infection.

Transfer Factor

Transfer factor is an extract from lymphoid cells sensitized with antigen that can transfer cell-mediated reactivity in the form of delayed cutaneous hypersensitivity response (reviewed in ref. *60*). Although many aspects of this phenomenon remain controversial, transfer factor has been used for the treatment of refractory fungal infections *(60–62)*. Chronic mucocutaneous candidiasis in patients without HIV infection is a rare disease characterized by chronic *C. albicans* infections of the nails, skin, and mucous membranes *(63)*. Several remarkable remissions of candidal infection have been reported in some patients with chronic mucocutaneous candidiasis treated with transfer factor *(60)*. Graybill et al. *(64)* reported three patients with disseminated coccidioidomycosis who were treated with transfer factor and amphotericin B. All three patients displayed increased cellular responses to *C. immitis* antigens after receiving transfer factor, and two manifested significant improvement with prolonged remissions *(64)*. Transfer factor was also used successfully in patients with histoplasmosis *(65)* and cryptococcosis *(66)* in conjunction with amphotericin B.

For these case reports, it is difficult to separate the potential therapeutic contribution of transfer factor from that of standard antifungal therapy. The use of transfer factor has been plagued by inconsistent results in clinical trials, and its use remains experimental. In fact, interest in transfer factor therapy has waned in recent years, as indicated by the relative paucity of new studies in the literature. Guidelines for the preparation of dialyzable leukocyte extracts containing transfer factor have been proposed *(62)*.

Fungal Antigens

Although not a classic fungal infection, brief mention will be made of the use of fungal antigens to treat allergic fungal sinusitis. Allergic fungal sinusitis has histologic features resembling those of allergic bronchopulmonary aspergillosis and is characterized by association with asthma, nasal polyps, and allergic mucin, a viscous secretion that contains degenerating eosinophils and Charcot-Leyden crystals *(67,68)*. *Aspergillus* species are frequently cultured from mucin, but a variety of other fungal species have been cultured from patients with allergic fungal sinusitis including *Bipolaris, Curvelaria, Alternaria,* and *Cladosporium (69)*. The standard therapy for allergic fungal sinusitis is surgical drainage and corticosteroid administration, but relapses are common *(67)*. Because of the immunologic nature of this disease, immunotherapy has been suggested to be potentially beneficial *(69)*. Immunotherapy for allergic fungal sinusitis involves the injection of fungal antigens to which an individual shows a positive reaction to intradermal testing *(69)*. Although there have been concerns about whether the administration of fungal antigens to individuals with allergic sinusitis would be harmful, a 2-year uncontrolled study revealed that it is safe and possibly beneficial *(20)*. A recent prospective study suggests that postoperative immunotherapy with specific antigens to which the patient manifests sensitivity was beneficial in patients with allergic fungal sinusitis *(68)*.

Specific Antibody Therapy

In contrast to immunoglobulin preparations prepared from donor sera, specific antibody therapy refers to the use of antibody preparations with high activity against specific fungal pathogens. Examples include monoclonal antibodies (MAbs) to fungal antigens and antibodies obtained from immunized hosts. Passive antibody therapy was widely used in the preantibiotic era for the treatment of many bacterial and viral infections *(70,71)*. In recent years, there has been new interest in reintroducing passive antibody therapy for the treatment of infectious diseases *(71)*. Although the role of humoral immunity in protection against fungi has been a controversial subject, it is now clear that certain MAbs to fungal antigens can protect against experimental infection *(54)*. In the past, several patients with *C. neoformans* infections have been treated with specific antibody (reviewed in ref. *72*). Administration of specific rabbit antibodies to patients with *C. neoformans* infection was well tolerated and resulted in clearance of serum cryptococcal antigens *(72)*. A MAb to *C. neoformans* capsular polysaccharide is in advanced preclinical development, and clinical trials in patients with cryptococcosis are expected shortly *(73)*. For cryptococcosis, antibody therapy is envisioned as an adjunct to antifungal therapy with the goals of reducing mortality and improving cure rates. Protective MAbs to *C. albicans* have also been identified that are candidates for clinical use *(74)*.

ADVERSE OUTCOMES

As noted already, much of the clinical experience with immune therapy for fungal infections consists of anecdotal case reports and small studies that usually describe some beneficial effect. Importantly, there are also a few case reports of adverse outcomes associated with the use of some types of immune therapy. A 10-year-old girl developed massive fatal hemoptysis after treatment with amphotericin B and GM-CSF for pulmonary aspergillosis *(75)*. Given that cavitation and hemoptysis in pulmonary aspergillosis are associated with resolution of neutropenia, this raised concern that these complications may become more frequent as CSFs are increasingly used to reduce neutropenia *(75)*. Another small study reported that 2 of 12 patients who received autologous bone marrow transplants and were treated with experimental interleukin-12 (IL-12) immunotherapy developed fatal fungal infections, one with *Aspergillus* and the other with mucor *(76)*. Since this rate of infection was higher than expected for autologous bone marrow recipients, the authors speculated that IL-12 therapy may have had unintended consequences on immune function *(76)*. In this regard, it is noteworthy that IL-2 therapy has been associated with a fivefold increased risk of bacteremia and *Staphylococcus aureus* infections, possibly because of an IL-2-mediated defect in neutrophil chemotactic function *(77,78)*. These reports highlight the need for controlled studies to determine the benefits and risks of immune therapy.

CONCLUSION AND FUTURE PROSPECTS

The development of various types of immunotherapy is potentially the most important advance in the therapy of human fungal infections since the introduction of amphotericin B in the late 1950s. The impetus for developing immunotherapy comes from the fact that fungal infections carry very high mortality and morbidity in patients with impaired immunity despite aggressive antifungal chemotherapy. Many fungal infections cannot be cured in severely immunocompromised patients with existing antifungal therapy. The limitations of antimicrobial chemotherapy in patients with impaired immune function combined with major advances in the field of clinical immunology provide a fertile environment for the development of immune therapies against fungal infections.

There is clear evidence that CSFs can shorten the period of myelosuppression and neutropenia associated with vulnerability to many fungal infections. There are also many encouraging reports of the use of granulocyte transfusions, CSFs, and IFN-γ in combination with antifungal agents for the treatment of fungal infections. The anecdotal reports of cures in infections due to mucor, *Fusarium,* and other rare fungal pathogens in patients with neutropenia are noteworthy, given the dismal historical experience in the treatment of these infections. However, most clinical information regarding the use of immunotherapy in severe fungal infections is anecdotal, fragmentary, and not controlled for variables that can affect the outcome. Since we do not know the number of patients treated with immunotherapy unsuccessfully, the literature may be biased toward case reports of successful outcomes. Until prospective controlled studies are completed, the efficacy of such measures must be considered uncertain.

Although there is a clear need for controlled trials of immunotherapy against fungal infections, such trials are likely to be very difficult because of several factors. First, many fungal infections are relatively rare, and only multicenter studies can accumulate enough patients for meaningful studies. Second, the increasing number of reports of successful outcomes after immune therapy raises difficult ethical questions of whether such studies should be done given that conventional antifungal therapy has such a poor historical record. Third, large sample sizes may be needed since biologic differences in the patients and in the type of fungal infection could result in significant patient-to-patient variability in response and outcome. For example, the risk of fungal infection in patients with neutropenia depends on many variables, including underlying illness, antibiotic use, type of chemotherapy, and so on (reviewed in ref. *79*). In addition, there is uncertainty in the classification of some fungal pathogens. Fungal infections categorized as *Mucormycosis* or *Fusarium* are caused by any of many species of fungi, which may exhibit biologic differences in pathogenesis and response to therapy. Even the most common type of fungal infection, candidiasis, can be caused by any of several *Candida* species. Hence, the successful development of immune therapies may be critically dependent on parallel advances in mycologic taxonomy, human genetics, diagnostic techniques, and immunology.

The dawn of immune therapy for fungal infections is now, and one can anticipate that some types of immunotherapies will become routine in the future. The initial experience with the use of immunotherapy provides encouragement for the study, development, and use of immune modulators as adjuncts of standard antifungal therapy. Several promising agents are already available, and the major challenge is to learn how to use those modalities in patients with fungal infection. In the next few years, one can anticipate that dozens of compounds in the form of cytokines, interleukins, growth factors, vaccines, and antibodies may become available, providing physicians with powerful options for enhancing immune function. In fact, the biologic revolution may deliver potential immune therapeutic agents to the bedside at a rate faster than the medical mycology community can evaluate them. Biologic response modifiers and immune therapies are complex modalities that require a sophisticated understanding of immune function and microbial pathogenesis for optimal use. Considering the diversity of fungal pathogens, the complexity of the immune system, the variety of immune modulators available, and the heterogeneity of patients with immune deficiencies at risk for fungal infection, the current challenge is to design systems for the expedient testing of immune therapy.

REFERENCES

1. Kullberg BJ. Trends in immunotherapy of fungal infections. Eur J Clin Microbiol Infect Dis 1997; 16:51–55.
2. Wingard JR, Elfenbein GJ. Host immunologic augmentation for the control of infection. Infect Dis Clin North Am 1996; 10:345–364.
3. Anaissie EJ. Immunomodulation in the treatment of invasive fungal infections: present and future directions. Clin Infect Dis 1998; 26:1264–1265.
4. Walsh TJ, Hiemenz J, Anaissie EJ. Recent progress and current problems in treatment of invasive fungal infections in neutropenic patients. Infect Dis Clin North Am 1996; 10:365–400.
5. Stevens DA. Combination immunotherapy and antifungal therapy. Clin Infect Dis 1998; 26:1266–1269.
6. Rodriguez-Adrian LJ, Grazziutti ML, Rex JH, Anaissie EJ. The potential role of cytokine therapy for fungal infections in patients with cancer: is recovery from neutropenia all that is needed? Clin Infect Dis 1998; 26:1270–1278.
7. Roilides E, Dignani MC, Anaissie EJ, Rex JH. The role of immunoreconstitution in the management of refractory opportunistic fungal infections. Med Mycol 1998; 36(suppl 1):12–25.
8. Han Y, Cutler JE. Assessment of a mouse model of neutropenia and the effect of an anti-candidiasis monoclonal antibody in these animals. J Infect Dis 1997; 175:1169–1175.
9. DiNubile MJ. Therapeutic role of granulocyte transfusions. Rev Infect Dis 1985; 7:232–243.
10. Chanock SJ, Gorlin JB. Granulocyte transfusions. Time for a second look. Infect Dis Clin North Am 1996; 10:327–343.
11. Wright DG. Leukocyte transfusions: thinking twice. Am J Med 1984; 76:637–644.
12. Dale DC, Liles WC, Llewellyn C, Rodger E, Price TH. Neutrophil transfusions: kinetics and functions of neutrophils mobilized with granulocyte-colony-stimulating factor and dexamethasone. Transfusion 1998; 38:713–721.
13. Rex JH, Bhalla SC, Cohen DM, Hester JP, Vartivarian SE, Anaissie EJ. Protection of human polymorphonuclear leukocyte function from the deleterious effects of isolation, irradiation, and storage by interferon-γ and granulocyte-colony-stimulating factor. Transfusion 1995; 35:605–611.
14. Strauss RG. Neutrophil (granulocyte) transfusions in the new millennium. Transfusion 1998; 38:710–712.
15. Clarke K, Szer J, Shelton M, Coghlan D, Grigg A. Multiple granulocyte transfusions facilitating successful unrelated bone marrow transplantation in a patient with very severe aplastic anemia complicated by suspected fungal infection. Bone Marrow Transplant 1995; 16:723–726.

16. Boutati EI, Anaissie EJ. *Fusarium,* a significant emerging pathogen in patients with hematologic malignancy: ten years' experience at a cancer center and implications for management. Blood 1998; 90:999–1008.

17. Verschraegen CF, Van Besiern KW, Dignani C, Hester JP, Anderson BS, Anaissie EJ. Invasive aspergillus sinusitis during bone marrow transplantation. Scand J Infect Dis 1997; 29:436–438.

18. Di Mario A, Sica S, Salutari P, Ortu-La Barbera E, Marra R, Leone G. Granulocyte colony-stimulating factor-primed leukocyte transfusions in *Candida tropicalis* fungemia in neutropenic patients. Haematologica 1997; 82:362–363.

19. Catalano M, Fontana R, Scarpato N, Picardi M, Rocco S, Rotoli B. Combined treatment with amphotericin-B and granulocyte transfusion from G-CSF-stimulated donors in an aplastic patient with invasive aspergillosis undergoing bone marrow transplantation. Haematologica 1997; 82:71–72.

20. Mabry RL, Mabry CS. Immunotherapy for allergic fungal sinusitis: the second year. Otolaryngol Head Neck Surg 1997; 117:367–371.

21. Wright DG, Robichaud KJ, Pizzo PA, Deisseroth AB. Lethal pulmonary reactions associated with the combined use of amphotericin B and leukocyte transfusions. N Engl J Med 1981; 304:1185–1189.

22. Boxer LA, Ingraham LM, Allen J, Oseas RS, Baehner RL. Amphotericin-B promotes leukocyte aggregation of nylon-wool-fiber-treated polymophonuclear leukocytes. Blood 1981; 58:518–523.

23. Dana BW, Durie BGM, White RF, Huestis DW. Concomitant administration of granulocyte transfusions and amphotericin B in neutropenic patients: absence of significant pulmonary toxicity. Blood 1998; 57:90–93.

24. Burch WM, Snyderman R. Induction of cellular immunity to *Coccidioides immitis* after sensitization with dinitrochlorobenzene. Ann Intern Med 1992; 96:329–331.

25. Newman SL, Gootee L, Brunner G, Deepe GS Jr. Chloroquine induces human macrophage killing of *Histoplasma capsulatum* by limiting the availability of intracellular iron and is therapeutic in a murine model of histoplasmosis. J Clin Invest 1994; 93:1422–1429.

26. Levitz SM, Harrison TS, Tabuni A, Liu X. Chloroquine induces human mononuclear phagocytes to inhibit and kill *Cryptococcus neoformans* by a mechanism independent of iron deprivation. J Clin Invest 1997; 100:1640–1646.

27. Mazzola R, Barluzzi R, Brozzetti A, et al. Enhanced resistance to *Cryptococcus neoformans* infection induced by chloroquine in a murine model of meningoencephalitis. Antimicrob Agents Chemother. 1997; 41:802–807.

28. Kitchen LW. Adjunctive immunologic therapy for *Cryptococcus neoformans* infections. Clin Infect Dis 1996; 23:209–210.

29. Kitchen LW, Ross JA, Turner BS, Hernandez JE, Mather FJ. Diethylcarbamazine enhances blood microbicidal activity. Adv Ther 1995; 12:22–29.

30. Kitchen LW, Ross JA, Hernandez JE, Zarraga AL, Mather FJ. Effect of administration of diethylcarbamazine on experimental bacterial and fungal infections in mice. Int J Antimicrob Agents 1992; 1:259–268.

31. Nemunitis J. A comparative review of colonly-stimulating factors. Drugs 1997; 54:709–729.

32. Lieschke GJ, Burgess AW. Granulocyte colony-stimulating factor and granulocyte-macrophage colony-stimulating factor. N Engl J Med 1992; 327:28–35.

33. Enelow RI, Sullivan GW, Carper HT, Mandell GL. Cytokine-induced human multinucleated giant cells have enhanced candidacidal activity and oxidative capacity compared with macrophages. J Infect Dis 1992; 166:664–668.

34. Offner F. Hematopoietic growth factors in cancer patients with invasive fungal infections. Eur J Clin Microbiol Infect Dis 1997; 16:50–63.

35. Vecchiarelli A, Monari C, Baldelli F, et al. Beneficial effects of recombinant human granulocyte colony-stimulating factor on fungicidal activity of polymorphonuclear leukocytes from patients with AIDS. J Infect Dis 1995; 171:1448–1454.

36. Kuritzkes DR, Parenti D, Ward DJ, et al. Filgastrim prevents severe neutropenia and reduces infective morbidity in patients with advanced HIV infection: results of a randomized, multicenter, controlled trial. AIDS 1998; 12:65–74.

37. Liles WC, Huang JE, van Burik JH, Bowden RA, Dale DC. Granulocyte colony-stimulating factor administered in vivo augments neutrophil-mediated activity against opportunistic fungal pathogens. J Infect Dis 1997; 175:1012–1015.

38. Avilés A, Guzmán R, García EL, Talavera A, Díaz-Maqueo JC. Results of a randomized trial of granulocyte colony-stimulating factor in patients with infection and severe neutropenia. Anti-Cancer Drugs 1996; 7:392–397.

39. Dornbusch HJ, Urban CE, Pinter H, et al. Treatment of invasive pulmonary aspergillosis in severely neutropenic children with malignant disorders using liposomal amphotericin B (Ambisome), granulocyte colony stimulating factor, and surgery: report of five cases. Pediatr Hematol Oncol 1995; 12:577–586.

40. Montgomery B, Bianco JA, Jacobsen A, Singer JW. Localization of transfused neutrophils to site of infection during treatment with recombinant human granulocyte-macrophage colony-stimulating factor and pentoxifylline. Blood 1991; 78:533–541.

41. Peters BG, Adkins DR, Harrison BR, et al. Antifungal effects of yeast-derived rhu-GM-CSF in patients receiving high-dose chemotherapy given with or without autologous stem cell transplantation: a retrospective analysis. Bone Marrow Transplant 1996; 18:93–102.

42. Nemunaitis J, Buckner CD, Dorsey KS, Willis D, Meyer W, Appelbaum FR. Retrospective analysis of infectious disease in patients who received recombinant human granulocyte-macrophage colony-stimulating factor versus patients not receiving a cytokine who underwent autologous bone marrow transplantation for treatment of lymphoid cancer. Am J Clin Oncol 1998; 21:341–346.

43. Bodey GP, Anaissie EJ, Gutterman J, Vadhan-Raj S. Role of granulocyte-macrophage colony-stimulating factor as adjuvant therapy for fungal infection in patients with cancer. Clin Infect Dis 1993; 17:705–707.

44. Rowe JM. Treatment of acute myeloid leukemia with cytokines: effect on duration of neutropenia and response to infection. Clin Infect Dis 1998; 26:1290–1294.

45. Nemunaitis J, Meyers JD, Buckner CD, et al. Phase I trial of recombinant human macrophage colony-stimulating factor in patients with invasive fungal infections. Blood 1991; 78:907–913.

46. Nemunaitis J, Shannon-Dorcy K, Appelbaum FR, et al. Long-term follow-up of patients with invasive fungal disease who received adjunctive therapy with recombinant human macrophage colony-stimulating factor. Blood 1993; 82:1422–1427.

47. Nemunaitis J. Use of macrophage colony-stimulating factor in the treatment of fungal infections. Clin Infect Dis 1998; 26:1279–1281.

48. Murray HW. Interferon-gamma and host antimicrobial defense: current and future clinical applications. Am J Med 1998; 97:459–467.

49. Holland SM, Eisenstein EM, Kuhns DB, et al. Treatment of refractory disseminated nontuberculous mycobacterial infection with interferon gamma. N Engl J Med 1999; 330:1348–1355.

50. Joly V, Saint-Julien L, Carbon C, Yeni P. In vivo activity of interferon-gamma in combination with amphotericin B in the treatment of experimental cryptococcosis. J Infect Dis 1994; 170:1331–1334.

51. Roilides E, Sigler L, Bibashi E, Katsifa H, Flaris N, Panteliadis, C. Disseminated infection due to *Chrysosporium zonatum* in a patient with chronic granulomatous disease and review of non-*Aspergillus* fungal infections in patients with this disease. J Clin Microbiol 1998; 37:18–25.

52. Gallin JI, Malech HL, Weening RS, et al. A controlled trial of interferon gamma to prevent infection in chronic granulomatous disease. N Engl J Med 1991; 324:509–516.

53. Phillips P, Forbes JC, Speert DP. Disseminated infection with *Pseudallescheria boydii* in a patient with chronic granulomatous disease: response to gamma-interferon plus antifungal therapy. Pediatr Infect Dis J 1991; 10:536–539.

54. Casadevall A. Antibody immunity and invasive fungal infections. Infect Immun 1995; 63:4211–4218.

55. Neely AN, Holder IA. Effects of immunoglobulin G and low-dose amphotericin B on *Candida albicans* infections in burned mice. Antimicrob Agents Chemother 1992; 36:643–646.

56. Stratta RJ, Schaefer MS, Cushing KA, et al. A randomized prospective trial of acyclovir and immune globulin prophylaxis in liver transplant recipients receiving OKT3 therapy. Arch Surg 1992; 127:55–64.

57. Klaesson S, Ringden O, Ljungman P, Aschan J, Hagglung H, Winiarski J. Does high-dose intravenous immune globulin treatment after bone marrow transplantation increase mortality in veno-occlusive disease of the liver? Transplantation 1995; 60:1225–1230.

58. Gudding R, Lund A. Immunoprophylaxis of bovine dermatophytosis. Can J Vet 1996; 36:302–306.

59. Thitithanyanont A, Mendoza L, Chuansumrit A, et al. Use of an immunotherapeutic vaccine to treat a life-threatening human arteritic infection caused by *Pythium insidiosum*. Clin Infect Dis 1998; 27:1394–1400.

60. Kirkpatrick CH. Transfer factor. J Allergy Clin Immunol 1988; 81:803–813.

61. Kauffman CA, Shea MJ, Frame PT. Invasive fungal infections in patients with chronic mucocutaneous candidiasis. Arch Intern Med 1981; 141:1076–1078.

62. Wilson GB, Fudenberg HH, Keller RH. Guidelines for immunotherapy of antigen-specific defects with transfer factor. J Clin Lab Immunol 1984; 13:51–58.

63. Kirkpatrick CH, Rich RR, Bennett JE. Chronic mucocutaneous candidiasis: model-building in cellular immunity. Ann Intern Med 1971; 74:955–978.

64. Graybill JR, Silva J Jr, Alford RH, Thor DE. Immunologic and clinical improvement of progressive coccidioidomycosis following administration of transfer factor. Cell Immunol 1973; 8:120–135.

65. Smith GR, Griffin DE, Graybill JR. Chronic pulmonary histoplasmosis: improved lymphocyte response with transfer factor. Ann Intern Med 1976; 84:708–710.

66. Allen R, Barter CE, Chachoua LL, Cleeve L, O'Connell JM, Daniel FJ. Disseminated cryptococcosis after transurethral resection of the prostate. Aust NZ J Med 1982; 12:296–299.

67. Allphin AL, Strauss M, Abdul-Karim FW. Allergic fungal sinusitis: problems in diagnosis and treatment. Laryngoscope 1991; 101:815–820.

68. Folker RJ, Marple BF, Mabry RL, Mabry CS. Treatment of allergic fungal sinusitis: a comparison trial of postoperative immunotherapy with specific fungal antigens. Laryngoscope 1998; 108:1623–1627.

69. Mabry RL, Manning SC, Mabry CS. Immunotherapy in the treatment of allergic fungal sinusitis. Otolaryngol Head Neck Surg 1997; 116:31–35.

70. Casadevall A, Scharff MD. "Serum therapy" revisited: animal models of infection and the development of passive antibody therapy. Antimicrob Agents Chemother 1994; 38:1695–1702.

71. Casadevall A, Scharff MD. Return to the past: the case for antibody-based therapies in infectious diseases. Clin Infect Dis 1995; 21:150–161.

72. Gordon MA, Casadevall A. Serum therapy of cryptococcal meningitis. Clin Infect Dis 1995; 21:1477–1479.

73. Casadevall A, Cleare W, Feldmesser M, et al. Characterization of a murine monoclonal antibody to *Cryptococcus neoformans* polysaccharide that is a candidate for human therapeutic studies. Antimicrob Agents Chemother 1998; 42:1437–1446.

74. Han Y, Cutler JE. Antibody response that protects against disseminated candidiasis. Infect Immun 1995; 63:2714–2719.

75. Groll A, Renz S, Gerein V, et al. Fatal haemoptysis associated with invasive pulmonary aspergillosis treated with high-dose amphotericin B and granulocyte-macrophage colony stimulating factor (GM-CSF). Mycoses 1992; 35:67–75.

76. Toren A, Or R, Ackerstein A, Nagler A. Invasive fungal infections in lymphoma patients receiving immunotherapy following autologous bone marrow transplantation (ABMT). Bone Marrow Transplant 1997; 20:67–69.

77. Snydman DR, Sullivan B, Gill M, Gould JA, Parkinson DR, Atkins MB. Nosocomial sepsis associated with interleukin-2. Ann Intern Med 1990; 112:102–107.

78. Richards JM, Gilewski TA, Vogelzang NJ. Association of interleukin-2 therapy with staphylococcal bacteremia. Cancer 1991; 67:1570–1575.

79. Walsh TJ, Hiemenz J, Pizzo PA. Evolving risk factors for invasive fungal infections—all neutropenic patients are not the same. Clin Infect Dis 1994; 18:793–798.

80. Roilides E, Uhlig K, Venzon D, Pizzo PA, Walsh TJ. Prevention of corticosteroid-induced suppression of human polymorphonuclear leukocyte-induced damage of *Aspergillus fumigatus* hyphae by granulocyte colony-stimulating factor and gamma interferon. Infect Immun 1993; 61:4870–4877.

81. Roilides E, Uhlig K, Venzon D, Pizzo PA, Walsh TJ. Enhancement of oxidative response and damage caused by human neutrophils to *Aspergillus fumigatus* hyphae by granulocyte colony-stimulating factor and gamma interferon. Infect Immun 1993; 61:1185–1193.

82. Roilides E, Holmes A, Blake C, Pizzo PA, Walsh TJ. Effects of granulocyte colony-stimulating factor and interferon-γ on antifungal activity of human polymorphonuclear neutrophils against pseudohyphae of different medically important *Candida* species. J Leukoc Biol 1995; 57:651–656.

83. Roilides E, Uhlig K, Venzon D, Pizzo PA, Walsh TJ. Neutrophil oxidative burst in response to blastoconidia and pseudohyphae of *Candida albicans:* augmentation by granulocyte colony-stimulating factor and interferon-γ. J Infect Dis 1992; 166:668–673.

84. Yamamoto Y, Klein TW, Friedman H, Kimura S, Yamaguchi H. Granulocyte colony-stimulating factor potentiates anti-*Candida albicans* growth inhibitory activity of polymorphonuclear cells. FEMS Immunol Med Microbiol 1993; 1:15–22.

85. Yamamoto Y, Uchida K, Klein TW, Friedman H, Yamaguchi H. Immunomodulators and fungal infections: use of antifungal drugs in combinations with G-CSF. Adv Exp Med Biol 1992; 319:231–242.

86. Coffey MJ, Phare SM, George S, Peters-Golden M, Kazanjian PH. Granulocyte colony-stimulating factor administration to HIV-infected subjects augments reduced leukotriene synthesis and anticryptococcal activity in neutrophils. J Clin Invest 1998; 102:4–663.

87. Roilides E, Blake C, Holmes A, Pizzo PA, Walsh TJ. Granulocyte-macrophage colony-stimulating factor and interferon-γ prevent dexamethasone-induced immunosuppression of antifungal monocyte activity against *Aspergillus fumigatus* hyphae. J Med Vet Mycol 1995; 34:63–69.

88. Yamamoto Y, Klein TW, Tomioka M, Friedman H. Differential effects of ganulocyte/macrophage colony-stimulating factor (GM-CSF) in enhancing macrophage resistance to *Legionella pneumophila* vs *Candida albicans*. Cell Immunol 1997; 176:75–81.

89. Wang M, Friedman H, Djeu JY. Enhancement of human monocyte function against *Candida albicans* by the colony-stimulating factors (CSF): IL-3, granulocyte-macrophage-CSF, and macrophage-CSF. J Immunol 1989; 143:671–677.

90. Levitz SM. Activation of human peripheral blood mononuclear cells by interleukin-2 and granulocyte-macrophage colony stimulating factor to inhibit *Cryptococcus neoformans*. Infect Immun 1991; 59:3393–3397.

91. Kowanko IC, Ferrante A, Harvey DP, Carman KL. Granulocyte-macrophage colony-stimulating factor augments neutrophil killing of *Torulopsis glabrata* and stimulates neutrophil respiratory burst and degranulation. Clin Exp Immunol 1998; 83:225–230.

92. Vitt CR, Fidler JM, Ando D, Zimmerman RJ, Aukerman SL. Antifungal activity of recombinant human macrophage colony-stimulating factor in models of acute and chronic candidiasis in the rat. J Infect Dis 1994; 169:369–374.

93. Cenci E, Bartocci A, Puccetti P, Mocci S, Stanley ER, Bistoni F. Macrophage colony-stimulating factor in murine candidiasis: serum and tissue levels during infection and protective effect of exogenous administration. Infect Immun 1991; 59:868–872.

94. Brummer E, Stevens DA. Macrophage colony-stimulating factor induction of enhanced macrophage anticryptococcal activity: synergy with fluconazole for killing. J Infect Dis 1994; 170:173–179.

95. Nassar F, Brummer E, Stevens DA. Macrophage colony-stimulating factor (M-CSF) induction of enhanced anticryptococcal activity in human monocyte-derived macrophages: synergy with fluconazole for killing. Cell Immunol 1995; 164:113–118.

96. Spielberger RT, Falleroni MJ, Coene AJ, Larson RA. Concomitant amphotericin B therapy, granulocyte transfusions, and GM-CSF administration for disseminated infection with *Fusarium* in a granulocytopenic patient. Clin Infect Dis 1993; 16:528–530.

97. Leong KW, Crowley B, Crotty GM, O'Briain DS, Keane C, McCann SR. Cutaneous mucormycosis due to *Absidia corymbifera* occurring after bone marrow transplantation. Bone Marrow Transplant 1997; 19:513–515.

98. Fukushima T, Sumazaki R, Shibasaki M, et al. Successful treatment of invasive thorocopulmonary mucormycosis in a patient with acute lymphoblastic leukemia. Cancer 1995; 76:895–899.

99. Kreisel JD, Adderson EE, Gooch WM III, Pavia AT. Invasive sinonasal disease due to scopulariopsis candida: report and review of scopulariopsosis. Clin Infect Dis 1994; 19:317–319.

100. Williamson PR, Kwon-Chung KJ, Gallin JI. Successful treatment of *Paecilomyces varioti* infection in a patient with chronic granulomatous disease and a review of *Paecilomyces* species infections. Clin Infect Dis 1991; 14:1023–1026.

101. Cohen-Abbo A, Edwards KM. Multifocal osteomyelitis caused by *Paecilomyces varioti* in a patient with chronic granulomatous disease. Infection 1995; 23:55–57.

102. Grauer ME, Bokemeyer C, Bautsch W, Freund M, Link H. Successful treatment of a *Trichosporon beigelii* septicemia in a granulocytopenic patient with amphotericin B and granulocyte colony-stimulating factor. Infection 1999; 22:283–285.

103. Fanci R, Pecile P, Martinez RL, Fabbri A, Nicoletti P. Amphotericin B treatment of fungemia due to unusual pathogens in neuropenic patients: report of two cases. J Chemother 1997; 9:427–430.

104. Gonzalez CE, Couriel DR, Walsh TJ. Disseminated zygomycosis in a neutropenic patient: successful treatment with amphotericin B lipid complex and granulocytic colony-stimulating factor. Clin Infect Dis 1998; 24:192–196.

Index